ADVANCES IN HEALTH ECONOMICS AND HEALTH SERVICES RESEARCH

A Research Annual

Editor: RICHARD M. SCHEFFLER
Department of Economics
George Washington University

VOLUME 2 · 1981

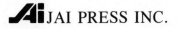 JAI PRESS INC.

Greenwich, Connecticut   *London, England*

Volume 1 published as: RESEARCH IN HEALTH ECONOMICS

CONTENTS

LIST OF CONTRIBUTORS

Martha Blaxall	Department of Commerce, Washington, D.C.
Linda N. Edwards	Department of Economics, Queens College
Jon Gabel	National Center for Health Services Research, Hyattsville, Maryland
Michael Grossman	National Bureau of Economic Research, New York
Teh-wei Hu	Institute for Policy Research and Evaluation, Pennsylvania State University
Laurence A. Miners	Department of Economics, State University of New York—Stony Brook
Joseph P. Newhouse	The Rand Corporation, Santa Monica, California
Michael Redisch	Interstate Commerce Commission, Washington, D.C.
David Whipple	Administrative Sciences Department, Naval Postgraduate School

INTRODUCTION

Volume two contains six extremely important papers which are also quite timely given the ongoing discussions of methods to increase competition in the health sector. Joseph Newhouse's paper on "The Erosion of the Medical Marketplace" helps to set the tone for the papers that follow. His paper looks at three alternative types of competitive models in the health sector: (1) the standard competitive model, (2) the standard model modified to take account of technological changes, (3) the standard model modified to take account of search behavior. Using time series from 1944 to 1974 empirical versions of these three models are estimated. His empirical work supports the conclusion that the competitive model needs to be modified if reimbursement via a third party is present and for the first time, his work takes this fact into account at the market level. The final section of the paper compares the use of regulation and the market-orientated strategy in the health sector.

Linda Edwards and Michael Grossman examine the relationship between family characteristics and the health status of the children in these families, using an economic model of fertility as a framework for their empirical work. Three measures of child health are employed in the empirical work—birth weight, overall health at age one as perceived by the parent, and the physician's impression of the child's health. In my view, some interesting findings are that the independent effect of family income on child health is small in magnitude; however, the years of schooling of the parents is a quite important variable in its relationship to the health of the child. Parents having a positive attitude towards preventive medical care appears to relate to healthier children.

Using Grossman's demand model for health care, Larry Miners constructs a household model of the demand for medical care. His model employs a household utility model which is maximized subject to a time and family income (earned and unearned income) constraint. Specific attention in the theoretical model is given to the impact of prices and wages on the demand schedule of the family for medical care. He develops a test to determine when medical care among different members of the family is substitute or complement. The empirical results are based on micro data set from a rural community and are estimated using a Tobit model. The results suggest that travel time in this rural community is a more important determinant of demand than price. Household size reduces demand and the demand by household members who are not parents is positively related to the wife's wages.

The demand for dental care has received much less attention by researchers. Following the work of Paul Felstein, Teh-wei Hu used the 1970 National Opinion Research Center to study the demand for dental care by different income classes. Following an excellent literature review on dental care, Hu specifies his three equation simultaneous model. Dental insurance, dental visits and expenditures are the endogenous variables in the model. As expected, income has a significant positive effect on dental visits and prices have a negative effect. The overall income elasticity is .20 but is .14 for those above the poverty line as compared to .25 for those below it. Individuals without dental insurance have a higher elasticity of demand with respect to price than those with insurance. As Miners found for medical care, family size has a negative impact on the demand for dental care. Of interest is the finding that whites and females spend more on dental care than blacks and males. Education of the head of the household was positively related to dental expenditures.

Utilizing data from a unique national survey of over a thousand physicians in private practice, Michael Redish, Jon Gabel and Martha Blaxall explore the hypothesis that the price mechanism in the medical care market does not properly perform its allocation function. Hence, increases in the supply of physicians tend to increase prices rather than reduce them. They discuss three interrelated questions about the market for medical care: (1) is the health care market competitive or monopolistic?, (2) do supply parameters enter into the demand function?, (3) are physicians utility or income maximizers? Redish, Gabel and Blaxall emphasize the preliminary nature of their empirical results. Among some of the interesting findings is that increases in supply are related to lower levels of physician productivity as well as an overall reduction in output. As has been suggested by Mark Pauly, they find evidence that physicians use the hospital as a rent-free workshop and that hospital beds are a complementary input in the production of medical care. They also conclude that their empirical evidence is consistent with the notion that physicians maintain their income in the face of increasing supplies by raising fees and offering a more complex service mix.

David Whipple's paper on incentives in HMOs is extremely timely, given the current national debate on Alain Enthoven's consumer choice proposal. The paper discusses the organization, structure and the types of incentives used in HMOs, as well as how these factors relate to productivity and costs. He outlines both the strengths and weaknesses of HMOs with specific attention given to how they might restructure their incentives systems. Whipple uses a case study method to examine three HMOs in order to illustrate how important the role of incentives is. He also discusses the military health care system's use of capital budgeting in place of workload budgeting. He suggests a method for organizing an "integrated, goal-congruent resource allocation methodology and performance measure" for HMOs. His suggestion has the potential for making an important contribution to the delivery of services in HMOs.

I am also pleased to report that volume III of the annual series is completed and is already in press. Also beginning with this volume, Louis Rossiter will be working with me as the associate series editor. His position at the National Center for Health Services Research is consistent with the notion that the series will include papers in health services research as well as those limited to health economics. The contents of volume III of the series are listed below.

A Short History, *William D. White, University of Illinois, Chicago Circle.* Some Indirect Evidence of Economies of Scale in Retail Pharmacy: A Duopoly Model, *Louis F. Rossiter, National Center for Health Services Research.* Distribution of Medical Input Across SMSAS and Implications for Health, *Charles Stewart, George Washington University.* Short Term Illness and Labor Supply: The Impact of Sick Leave, *Lynn Paringer, The Urban Institute.* Permanently Disabling Injuries: A General Model and an Application to Florida Work Injuries, *Wayne Vroman, The Urban Institute.* Health Manpower Credit Subsidies, *Richard C. McKibbin, Wichita State University.* Index.

*Richard M. Scheffler**
Series Editor

*Richard M. Scheffler is currently a visiting associate professor of Health Economics, School of Public Health, University of California, Berkeley.

THE EROSION OF THE MEDICAL MARKETPLACE

Joseph P. Newhouse

I. INTRODUCTION

Many have observed that increases in prices and expenditures for medical care, especially hospital services, show few signs of abating. As a result, concerns have been voiced that too many resources are being allocated to medical care and that factor prices may be above competitive rates. The Carter administration responded to these concerns by introducing hospital cost containment legislation in 1977. The legislation passed the Senate in 1978 but was not brought to a vote in the House. Although currently dormant, one might anticipate the reintroduction of such a proposal at some time in the future.

As part of the case for the cost-containment legislation, the then Secretary of Health, Education, and Welfare termed the hospital industry obese and alleged that it is noncompetitive. To date, however, such

Advances in Health Economics and Health Services Research, Vol. 2, pgs. 1–34.
(Volume 1 published as Research in Health Economics)
Copyright © 1981 by JAI Press Inc.
All rights of reproduction in any form reserved.
ISBN: 0-89232-100-8

allegations have not been embedded in any of the formal models of the medical care marketplace whose predictions have been tested. The objective of this paper is to provide such models and tests.

It is important for the reader not well acquainted with health insurance to understand the nature of the contract between the insurer and the insured. In general, an individual's health insurance policy pays benefits that are a stipulated fraction, often 100 percent, of the individual's medical expenses. The insurer typically does not question the nature of the medical services provided to a patient as long as they fall within a general description of those covered by the patient's policy, such as the services of a hospital or physician. To monitor these services would apparently involve prohibitive costs.

In the case of hospitals—and to a considerable degree other providers of medical services—the insurer places little or no effective limit on the unit price of the service. Blue Cross and government insurance plans (Medicare and Medicaid) reimburse hospitals on the basis of cost, i.e., they reimburse, approximately, the institution's incurred costs times the fraction of the costs attributable to the patients they insure. Commercial insurance companies reimburse hospitals on the basis of charges, i.e., in accordance with a stated price that the hospital quotes for its services to any given patient.

The insured's premium is negligibly affected by his own experience; in particular, it does not reflect his choice of medical provider (i.e., physician or hospital). An individual who uses a physician who tends to hospitalize more frequently, or to admit his patients to more expensive hospitals, pays the same premium as others.

The distortion of the individual consumer's demands caused by these institutional arrangements has long been recognized in the literature (Pauly, 1968; Feldstein, 1973). Much less attention has been given to their effect on providers of medical services and the medical marketplace. In this report I inquire into how such institutional arrangements affect prices and then assess their long-term viability.

I explore three different models of the medical marketplace: (1) the standard competitive model, (2) the competitive model modified to account for technological change, and (3) the competitive model modified to account for search behavior on the part of consumers. I present evidence favoring the third model.

A number of implications for both research and policy can be derived from the third model. The most important is that present institutional arrangements, i.e., the type of contract described above—may well not be viable in the long run and that alternative arrangements will probably evolve. These alternatives could be either increased regulation or contractual forms that would increase price competition. The report concludes with some thoughts on the implications of these alternatives.

II. THE THREE MODELS

A. The Standard Competitive Model in Medical Care

If relative prices for a product change, a natural vehicle for explaining such changes is the standard competitive paradigm. This paradigm, or a model quite close to it, is a standard approach to explaining inflation in medical care.[1] The familiar model is sketched in Figure 1, where SS^1 is an industry supply curve; DD^1 (c_0) and DD^1 (c_1) are two market demand curves that are drawn for two levels of insurance coverage.

Insurance is assumed to pay a fixed proportion of total expenditure. Thus, insurance subsidizes the marginal unit so that at the margin net price to the consumer equals c times gross price, where c is the coinsurance rate (the proportion of total expenditure paid by the patient). In Figure 1, $c_1 < c_0$. As shown by Frech and Ginsburg (1975), a lower coinsurance rate rotates the demand curve so as to make it less elastic.[2] The rotation serves to increase the equilibrium price, save for the special case in which SS^1 is perfectly elastic.[3]

Muth (1964) gives a general expression for the equilibrium price change when demand changes in the case of a two-factor production function, homogeneous of the first degree. The percentage change in equilibrium price dp* equals

$$dp^* = \{\eta(\sigma + k_B e_A + k_A e_B)/[\sigma\eta - \sigma(k_A e_A + k_B e_B) \\ + \eta(k_B e_A + k_A e_B) - e_A e_B]\}\alpha \\ = K\alpha, \tag{1}$$

where α = the percentage increase in price at any given quantity on the new demand schedule,

η = the elasticity of product demand,

σ = the elasticity of substitution,

k_i = the share of receipts of factor i,

e_i = the elasticity of supply of factor i.

Letting $E(p^*,C) = E$ be the elasticity of equilibrium price with respect to coinsurance, we have $E(p^*,C)$ equal to $-K$.[4] We are interested in the behavior of price as C changes. Clearly E is negative, but in general the sign of dE/dC cannot be evaluated. Two special cases can, however, be distinguished. In the first case, η, σ, k_i, and e_i are constants, and hence K is a constant. Clearly, in this case dE/dC is zero; a given percentage change in coinsurance will everywhere result in the same percentage change in price. A second special case is that of linear supply and demand curves. In this case, it can be shown that dE/dC is negative, i.e., the elasticity of price with respect to coinsurance will be larger in absolute value the smaller the coinsurance rate (save for the special case of a perfectly elastic supply curve).

Figure 1.   Insurance and the Price of Medical Care Services in the
Standard Competitive Model.

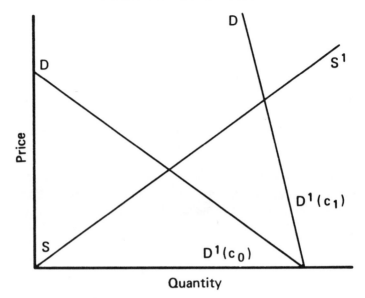

These results pertain to a given medical service and show the consequences of changes in coinsurance for equilibrium price, other factors being constant. In the empirical work below, I compare observed price behavior across four medical services. In addition to changes in demand caused by changes in coinsurance, observed price changes in a competitive world will be influenced by changes in the supply schedule and changes in demand other than those caused by changes in insurance.

In the empirical work, I shall take account of changes in demand caused by changes in income and of changes in the supply schedule caused by changes in factor prices; but I will ignore (consign to the error term) the effect of increases in supply and productivity on medical care prices because I am unable to measure them with any precision.[5] In both cases I see no reason to expect that omission has biased the results in a way that affects the conclusions drawn. However, some discussion of the effects of these two variables may be helpful.

The supply of most medical inputs has steadily increased over the past several years, so shifts in supply cannot explain persistent price *increases*. Although it is difficult to measure supply for a constant-quality product, crude measures of supply have increased the most for hospital services relative to other services. In particular, the bed/population ratio increased 33 percent over the 1950–1974 period, whereas the number of physicians per person increased less than half that amount and the dentist/ population ratio was nearly unchanged.[6]

As will be seen in the following discussion, we must explain differentially large increases in hospital prices and expenditure; it appears that, if anything, changes in supply have worked in the other direction. To be sure, an increase in the supply of beds does not correspond to an equivalent shift in the supply schedule. Nonetheless, there is no evidence of the supply schedule's shifting to the left for hospital services for a given product, holding factor prices constant. Nor is there any reason why the supply curve for hospital services should be markedly less elastic than that for other services; indeed, it might well be more elastic than for physician or dental services. We shall have to look further for an explanation of differentially large hospital price increases.

Changes in productivity would explain some of the price increases in medical care generally. Medical care is a service industry, and it is known that productivity change in service industries is below the economy average (Fuchs, 1968). But the quantitative amount of price change accounted for in this manner is the differential between productivity in medical care and the rest of the economy. Therefore, assuming that productivity in medical care is not decreasing, an upper limit on the amount of (relative) price change that could be attributed to differential productivity change is the increase in productivity in the remainder of the economy. John Kendrick (1973, Table 3-2) estimates this increase to be around 3 percent annually in the 1948–1966 period. Fuchs (1968, Table 15) estimated that the differential increase in productivity between all services and the rest of the economy was around 2 percent per year. We do not have an estimate of productivity change for medical care (as opposed to all services), but an estimate of productivity change for physician services concluded that over the 1955–1965 period it was around 3 percent per year (Reinhardt, 1975, Table 3-5), the same as the economy average. Thus, differential changes in productivity could explain perhaps a 1 to 2 percentage point increase in relative price each year—maybe less. As will be seen, most of the hospital price increase remains to be explained.

An important conclusion from the competitive model is that price changes are related to *changes* in supply or demand schedules. In order to focus on the role of insurance in increasing price, assume for the moment that effects of other factors are either small or tend to reduce price. In this case, continued price increases should not be observed unless insurance continues to increase. Hence, if one observes continuing price changes (for a given product) when insurance and other factors are constant, one must conclude that either (a) the market has not yet adjusted to equilibrium, in which case the standard model is not very helpful in a practical sense because it explains equilibrium behavior while observed variation is taking place out of equilibrium, or (b) the standard model needs modification. One modification frequently mentioned is that the hospital's product has changed and these changes have caused the price increase. Reliance upon an *exogenous* product change to explain price changes, however, robs the competitive model of explanatory power. A modification of the standard model that makes product change endogenous is considered next.

B.   The Standard Model Modified to Take Account of Technological Change

The foregoing discussion assumed a given technology and a given product. As is well known, there has been considerable technological change in the medical area. It is frequently stated that technological change in medical care has led to cost increases. In fact, as Feldstein pointed out several years ago, technological change could reduce cost as well as increase it (Feldstein, 1971a).[7] While this argument is correct in a general market, I shall argue that insurance (as presently structured) introduces a distortion, so that technological change tends to increase the rate of medical care price and expenditure increases relative to a competitive market.[8]

A standard distinction in the literature on technological change is between product and process innovation. Product innovation leads to new products that enable new capabilities to be attained (e.g., computed tomography, coronary care units); process innovations reduce the cost of existing products. In a competitive industry, process innovations will always be adopted; product innovations may or may not be adopted, depending on whether a sufficient market exists for the product.

As the level of insurance increases, the rate of product innovation should rise; even if uninsured consumers were not willing to pay the entire cost of certain products, they (or physicians acting as their agents) may be willing to pay some fraction of the cost (with their insurance paying the rest). Therefore, for a given rate of change in knowledge, there should be a greater rate of observed product innovation, the greater the level of insurance. For empirical purposes, I assume that knowledge increases at a reasonably constant rate from year to year.[9] The rate of adopted technological change in medical care is then a constant that depends on the level of insurance. The higher the *level* of insurance, the higher the constant. It follows that the rate of expenditure growth will be higher with more insurance because some new medical care products will be bought each year that would not otherwise be bought.[10]

Whether the rate of measured price increase (as opposed to expenditure increase) will be higher if the level of insurance is higher depends on accounting conventions for unit price. Conceptually, a price index is for a given market basket, and problems arise when new goods are introduced.[11] In practice, medical care price indices are typically measured per visit, per admission, or per day in the hospital. Because product change will typically add to the products (services) that can be consumed during a visit, day, etc., the usual price indices will increase faster, the faster the product-enhancing technological change. (Drugs are an exception to this statement because the same drug is priced over time.) Because the rate of change is a function of the level of insurance, the measured rate of price change will also be related to the *level* of insurance.

In sum, insurance as it is now structured induces more rapid technological change than would be observed in a competitive market. Assuming that optimality prevails everywhere else, there are too many resources devoted to product-enhancing technological change.

C. *The Standard Model Modified to Take Account of Search Behavior*

A much more drastic modification of the competitive model focuses on the incentives facing the consumer (and/or the physician acting as an agent) to search for the lowest-cost supplier of a given product. A fundamental result of the competitive model is that inefficient firms are driven out of business. This result follows from the assumption that consumers maximize utility for a given level of income, but it is also assumed that the consumer actually receives the monetary difference in price between any two suppliers; indeed, models of optimal search behavior focus upon the trade-off between this saving and the cost of search.

With complete insurance ($C = 0$), the consumer does not receive any benefits from receiving services at an efficient supplier. If he searches at all, it is because the "quality" (i.e., productivity) of services may vary among providers and he is interested in the highest-quality provider. Even though any single consumer is insured, a competitive *market* may continue to exist if completely (or nearly completely) insured consumers constitute a relatively small fraction of the market. In that case, there are a substantial number of uninsured (or nearly uninsured) consumers, and those consumers should be willing to arbitrage among alternative suppliers. It might be thought that some firms could specialize in insured patients and avoid the arbitrage; however, if insurance companies pay only the market rate, there is no advantage to specialization.

It is interesting to consider the phrase found in many health insurance policies—reimbursement at "usual, customary, and reasonable" rates— in this light. When insurance was a small factor in the market, insurers could observe a meaningful market rate and define that rate as usual, customary, and reasonable. Insurance is, however, no longer a small factor in the market. At the present time, 92 percent of hospital expenditures are insured. Of the 8 percent that are not insured, most may be for certain relatively uninsured services, such as maternity, or may be spent on deductibles that are exceeded during the stay and so do not affect choice of supplier.[12]

In this context, a market rate cannot be observed (or has little meaning because firms can ignore the noninsured market in making price decisions). In practice, the phrase *usual, customary, and reasonable* for a given supplier is defined relative to what other suppliers are charging the insurance company. If suppliers move their prices up together, say, 15 percent per year, there is no constraint from usual, customary, and reasonable. Thus, results obtained in the small on the effect of insurance on expenditure do not necessarily obtain in the large; there is a fallacy of composition. If widespread, insurance as presently structured should reduce the amount of price competition in the marketplace. It should convert the medical firm either into a monopolist facing a nearly perfectly inelastic demand curve or into a firm that competes on the basis of quality with nearly no regard for price.[13]

The diminution in the elasticity of the demand curve facing the medical firm causes the equilibrium price to rise. Will consumers then buy less insurance, thereby reducing the amount of the price rise? The answer is theoretically ambiguous, and existing empirical studies of the question are both conflicting and far from definitive (Phelps, 1976; Frech, 1976). However, the high rate of hospital insurance coverage despite persistently large price and premium increases is prima facie evidence that demand for insurance does not markedly decrease when medical care prices rise. Thus, in this model, the usual link between the price that the firm charges and its volume of business is weakened and, in the limit, eliminated.

This model has an important similarity with the standard competitive model, for in both cases the rotation of the demand curve serves to increase the equilibrium price. However, it differs in the important respect that the competitive supply curve ceases to exist, because firms that charge a higher price for a given product continue in business. In the limiting case of full insurance, the equilibrium price charged by a profit-maximizing monopolist is bounded only by the income effect that ultimately serves to make the demand curve less than perfectly inelastic. This is not a completely satisfactory outcome, for such an equilibrium price is presumptively well above present levels. If so, an explanation of why such a price is not observed is necessary.[14]

Many explanations are rather unpalatable theoretically. One may accept the conclusion that equilibrium is much above present levels and argue that what we in fact observe is a steady adjustment to that equilibrium price. The problem is that we lack a theory of how adjustment occurs, so to accept the conclusion that what we observe is behavior out of equilibrium is to argue that we have no theory to explain the rate of price change. Moreover, this argument does not stand up well empirically, as we shall see.

A second explanation abandons the profit-maximizing assumption, arguing that many institutions in medical care are nonprofit (especially many hospitals) and that nonprofit institutions either do not maximize profit or can appropriately be modeled by a satisficing model. However, nonprofit institutions can earn a return in kind (hence, nonprofit status per se is not a reason to abandon maximization), and we have no theory to predict targets in a satisficing model.

A third explanation incorporates into the supplier's maximand an argument in addition to profit that serves to bound equilibrium price (Evans, 1973). The additional argument might be the price charged to the consumer (on the basis of altruism) or the fear that institutional arrangements may change if price changes are "too large." Both devices are, of course, ad hoc; also, the fear of institutional change argument suffers from a free-rider problem, because price changes in any single institution probably do not jeopardize the institutional framework. All in all, the conclusion from the standard theory of the consumer (that search or arbitrage diminishes as insurance increases) serves to make the standard theory of the market rather impotent.[15]

A fourth explanation, which I favor, is that the equilibrium price may not be feasible because insurance contracts may change. The costs of risk sharing using present contracts may simply be too high at the equilibrium price and so it may not be observed. In short, higher prices may induce a change in insurance contracts. I return to this matter at the end of this paper. (Section V).

The third model leaves us with the prediction that the scope for discretionary price behavior on the part of the medical firm is related to the extent of insurance coverage in the market. Because we do not have a well-accepted theory of discretionary behavior, we do not ultimately have a theory of price changes in this model (given current contractual arrangements); however, it would be surprising if there were not an above-average rate of price increase in the industry as insurance approached completeness. Moreover, the rate of price change should be nonlinearly related to the level of insurance coverage, for insurance could cover a certain portion of consumers without impairing price competition (by reimbursing them at market rates). This nonlinearity will be exploited in the empirical work below to distinguish this model from the other two. A second result from this model that will be used below is that as complete insurance is approached the discretion the medical firm enjoys with respect to passing on factor price changes increases.

D.   Implications of the Models for Factor Price Changes

If factors are price-takers, it appears difficult to distinguish the implications of the three aforementioned models for factor price changes. In the competitive model, a shift in the demand for the product leads to an increase in factor prices (unless factor supply is perfectly elastic); similarly, a decrease in the elasticity of demand for the product leads to a decline in the elasticity of demand for the factor (Hicks, 1968, Appendix; Muth, 1964). Thus, increased insurance coverage should lead to increased factor prices; and the increase may well be larger, the higher the level of insurance coverage.

No general statement can be made about the effect on factor prices of a more rapid rate of product innovation except that those particular factors that are used intensively by the new product will face a higher demand than otherwise would be the case. Similarly, a decline in price competition in the product market would not necessarily imply a decline in competition in the factor market. However, if the third model is correct, there are potentially large gains to collective behavior by factors in highly insured industries. Although one could examine whether the extent of collective behavior by factors (e.g., unionization of nurses) varied by the extent of insurance coverage in the local market, I have not pursued this implication here.

E.   Some Tests of the Three Models

Although both modifications of the competitive model described above (Sections II.A and II.B) follow from the theory of the consumer and so have some a priori claim to validity, it is important to construct empirical tests that discriminate among them. The empirical tests I use are based on the following equation, which is a linear functional form in the variables specified above and can be regarded as the first-order Taylor series expansion of a reduced form equation for changes in price:

$$DP_{it} = \alpha_i + \beta_i DC_{it} + \gamma_i C_{it} + \delta_i DGNP_t + \mu_i DGNPDEF_t, \quad (2)$$

where DP_{it} = the percentage change in price of the ith service in year t,

DC_{it} = the percentage change in coinsurance for the ith year t,

C_{it} = the level of coinsurance for the *i*th service in year t,

DGNP$_t$ = the percentage change in the gross national product (GNP) in year t,

DGNPDEF$_t$ = the percentage change in the GNP deflator in year t,

and α_i, β_i, γ_i, δ_i, and μ_i are constants to be estimated. DGNP and DGNPDEF are included to control for changes in demand caused by income and changes in factor prices, respectively.[16]

I have used Eq. (2) to conduct several tests of the standard competitive model. I begin straightforwardly by testing the hypothesis that with coinsurance, GNP, and the GNP deflator unchanging, predicted DP will differ insignificantly from zero. A common form of the standard model, namely, constant elasticities implying a constant K in Eq. (1), would predict this to be the case; the second and third models would predict that the more insured the service, the more likely the price changes will differ from zero, other variables being unchanged. The test, then, computes a predicted rate of price change when DC, DGNP, and DGNPDEF are set to zero; I have set C at both the mean value in the sample and the "current" (1974) value for the purpose of this test.

Unfortunately, this test is not entirely satisfactory. As shown above, in certain forms of the standard model (e.g., linear supply and demand curves), the elasticity E of equilibrium price with respect to coinsurance falls (rises in absolute value) as coinsurance falls. Now note that if both sides of Eq. (2) are divided by DC, E appears on the left-hand side. For empirical purposes, I approximate the elasticity by evaluating the right-hand side of Eq. (2) divided by DC at DC = 1 (C ranges from 0 to 100). Then a term in C on the right-hand side could merely account for a potentially negative interaction between E and C for a given service. Thus, it might be argued that differences among services on the basis of the first test could merely reflect a possible within-service interaction between E and C; in particular, a lower C would appear associated with a higher rate of price increase, although such an interaction appears unlikely by itself to cause predicted DP to differ from zero.

The second and third tests avoid the problem just described; they are based on E (more precisely, the approximation to E when DC = 1). In the standard model, the magnitude of E across services depends on supply and demand elasticities; specifically, the more elastic the demand curve and the more inelastic the supply curve for service i, the more negative E should be.[17] No relationship is implied, however, between E and the level of coinsurance *across services,* in contrast to the third model.

The third model predicts that E will be much higher (in absolute value) for a highly insured service such as hospital services; i.e., the relationship between E and C can be described by a nonlinear relationship of the kind shown in Figure 2. (This is the nonlinearity referred to in the discussion of the third model.) The null hypothesis for the second test, therefore, is that E is the same for hospital services as for the other three services.[18]

The third test examines whether E changes more rapidly as a function of coinsurance for hospital services than for other services. Thus, the second test examines whether the levels of E differ across services; the third test examines whether the slope of a curve such as that shown in Figure 2 is much steeper for hospital services.

One can also examine the relationship between a measure of factor prices (DGNPDEF) and medical care prices (DP). In a competitive model, a positive relationship between these two variables should exist. In the third model, however, insurance coverage gives the medical firm considerable discretion and one may not observe such a relationship holding in the short run.

Finally, a test is possible of the hypothesis that we can observe the results of the competitive model, but adjustment to equilibrium is very slow. All results pertaining to this hypothesis, of course, are conditional upon the correct specification of the lag structure. The common (and

Figure 2.   Elasticity of Equilibrium Price as a Function of
Coinsurance in the Third Model.

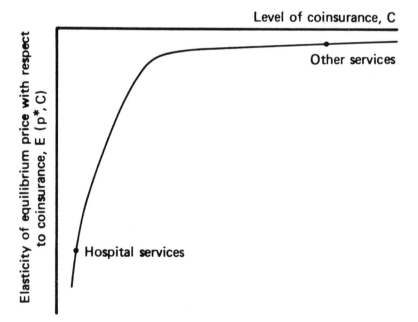

plausible) specification of geometrically declining weights is the maintained hypothesis used below.

Table 1 summarizes the four principal tests employed.

III. DATA AND ESTIMATION METHODS

Data were collected on the changes in price for four medical services: hospital, physician, dental, and drugs. Table 2 shows descriptive statistics for the percentage change in the price of various medical services and the level of third-party payments for these services in the 1949–1974 period. One measure of price change is the Consumer Price Index for the services. However, the Consumer Price Index for a semiprivate hospital room is not entirely satisfactory as a measure of hospital price, and so an additional hospital price variable is shown: the percentage change in expense per adjusted admission.[19] (The adjustment is designed to remove the effect of outpatient services on the costs of the hospital.) Expense per adjusted admission is a more comprehensive measure of unit price than the semiprivate room charge, although the two measures are very similar in their first and second moments, as can be seen in Table 2.

In order to use the second and third tests described in Table 1, the possibility must be ruled out that for these four services the ordering of

Table 1. Tests of Competitive Model vs. Modified Models

Test	Null Hypothesis	Basis for Test
1	Price change for each medical service equals zero when all variables are unchanging (DC = DGNPDEF = DGNP = 0).	Second and third models predict a greater price change for more highly insured services. The first model predicts no change if other variables are unchanging.
2	Elasticity of price change with respect to coinsurance for the most highly insured service is equal to the elasticity for other services.	Third model predicts more negative elasticities for the more highly insured services. The first model predicts no relationship with level of insurance. The second model yields no prediction.
3	Change in the elasticity of price as coinsurance changes is the same for the most highly insured service as for other services.	Third model predicts much greater change in elasticity for very well insured service. The first model predicts no relationship with level of insurance. The second model yields no prediction.
4	No relationship exists between factor price change and product price change.	First and second models predict rejection. The third model does not necessarily predict rejection for highly insured service.

Table 2. Descriptive Statistics

Variable	Mean	Standard Deviation	Minimum	Maximum
Annual percentage change in expense per adjusted hospital admission, 1949–1974	8.66	3.93	3.54	21.18
Annual percentage change in hospital semi-private room charge, 1949–1974	8.10	3.85	3.41	19.76
Annual percentage change in physician fee index, 1949–1974	4.09	1.99	1.47	9.12
Annual percentage change in dental fee index, 1949–1974	3.52	1.77	0.49	7.63
Annual percentage change in drug price index, 1949–1974	0.94	1.36	−1.55	3.53
Annual percentage change in overall Consumer Price Index, 1949–1974	2.83	2.70	−0.97	10.97
Percentage of hospital expenditure reimbursed by third parties, 1949–1974	82.3	6.7	62.7	92.2
Percentage of physician expenditure reimbursed by third parties, 1949–1974	38.7	14.0	13.7	65.1
Percentage of dental expenditure reimbursed by third parties, 1949–1974	3.3	4.9	0	14.7
Percentage of drug expenditure reimbursed by third parties, 1949–1974	4.2	4.5	0.4	14.4

Source: See Appendix A, Sources of Data.

supply and demand elasticities is confounded with the level of insurance. As Table 2 shows, hospital services are nearly completely insured, physician services are partially insured, and there is little insurance for dental services or drugs. Thus, the third model would predict E to be markedly higher (in absolute value) for hospitals than for the other services, with physician services perhaps intermediate (depending on how many consumers can be insured before price competition becomes seriously impaired).

Fortunately, the underlying supply (demand) elasticities do not appear to be smallest (largest) for hospital services and largest (smallest) for dental and drug services. If they were, the first and third models could not be distinguished by using the second and third tests. I have no hard evidence on supply elasticities (indeed, the results below call into question the existence of a competitive supply curve), but I would expect that, if anything, supply elasticities would be smaller for physicians and dentists than for drugs and hospitals, given training and licensure requirements. The relevant demand elasticities are for the range of coinsurance observed in the sample. Phelps and Newhouse (1974) give data on demand elasticities that have been standardized to a range of 0 to 25 percent of coinsurance; hospital, dental, and drug elasticities all appear to cluster around .07 in absolute value in this range, whereas demand elasticities for physician-office visits are somewhat higher (around .14).[20]

Phelps and Newhouse show that, empirically, elasticities fall as coinsurance goes to zero; hence, hospital services should be the most inelastic of the four services when evaluated at the range of coinsurance rates found in the sample. Because $dE/d\eta$ is positive in the first model, and because η for hospital services is closest to zero, the first model would predict that, ceteris paribus, E for hospital services would be closest to zero, exactly the opposite of the third model. Likewise, if the supply curve for hospital services were more elastic than for the other services, the first model would predict E for hospital services to be closest to zero (ceteris paribus). Thus, the second and third tests are not confounded by the ordering of supply-and-demand elasticities; indeed, the ordering means that one should potentially be able to distinguish quite well among the first and third models by using the two tests.

To implement the four tests, an error term e_{it}, with the following properties, has been added to Eq. (2) for the purpose of estimation:

$$e_{it} = r_i e_{it-1} + u_{it}, \tag{3}$$

where r_i is a constant and u_{it} is an independent random variable with mean zero. In addition, nonzero covariances across services are allowed among contemporaneous random components of the error term [$E(u_{it}u_{js})$ $= S_{ij}$ for $t = s$; $= 0$ for $t \neq s$].

The following four-stage procedure was used to estimate the parameters of Eqs. (2) and (3): (1) Each equation (one for each of four services) was estimated using ordinary least squares (OLS), which yielded consistent estimates of the residuals. (2) The estimated residuals were used in a seemingly unrelated regression context to derive new estimates of the residuals of the four equations. These new estimated residuals were used to estimate the r_i values (a least squares estimator was used on the residuals). (3) The estimated r_i values were used to difference each equation; i.e., new variables were defined equal to $y_{it} - \hat{r}_i y_{i,t-1}$ and x_{it}

$- \hat{r}_i x_{i,t-1}$. The error term thus becomes $e_{it} - \hat{r}_i e_{i,t-1} = u_{it}$, which asymptotically satisfies the usual properties (in particular, it is not autocorrelated). OLS was then applied to each equation to yield estimates of the residuals u_{it}. (4) Finally, the estimates of the residuals were used in a seemingly unrelated regression context to obtain final estimates of the coefficients and their standard errors. In effect, seemingly unrelated regressions have been run twice—first to obtain an estimate of the autocorrelation coefficient used to transform the variables, and then on the transformed variables. These estimates are asymptotically efficient and have been shown by Kmenta and Gilbert (1970) to have desirable small-sample properties for the size sample in this study.

IV. RESULTS

Table 3 shows the results obtained from estimating Eq. (2) for the four services, as well as from estimating Eq. (2) with the change in income variable (DGNP$_t$) omitted. The reason for the omission is that the variable enters with an unexpected negative sign, indicating that it may represent not only demand but also unmeasured supply effects. Fortunately, as Table 3 shows, the results for the other variables are scarcely changed if this variable is omitted, and it is the other variables that are important to the tests described earlier. In the tests that follow, we shall report the estimates from the specification with DGNP$_t$ included, although the results are very similar if DGNP$_t$ is excluded.

The results for the first test are shown in Table 4. These results are consistent with the second and third models because of the association between th predicted rates of price change for a service when other variables are not changing and the level of insurance for that service. The price of hospital services, for example, is predicted to increase at a rate of 13 percent per year, other variables being constant, at current levels of coinsurance. We can, with some confidence, reject the hypothesis that the predicted price change is zero for hospital services, the most heavily insured service; for physician services rejection is somewhat more ambiguous; and one would not reject the null hypothesis for dental services or drug services. Rejection is more clearly called for at current levels of coinsurance for hospital and physician services (i.e., more insurance) than at the sample mean levels, consistent with the second and third models. Between-service differences in price behavior not explained by these variables would appear in the intercept. Although differences in the intercept are partially responsible for the difference between hospitals and other services (and not just the term in C), it is important to examine other tests to rule out the possibility that the term in C is merely measuring a within-service interaction between E and C, as might occur in some variants of the first model.

Table 3. Prediction of Percentage Change in Price for Various Medical Services, 1949–1974[a,b]

Dependent Variable	Percentage of Expenditure Paid Out-of-Pocket (C)	Percentage Change in Expenditure Paid Out-of-Pocket (DC)	Percentage Change in GNP Deflator (DGNPDEF)	Percentage Change in GNP (DGNP)	Intercept/ $(1 - r)$	R^2	n	Durbin–Watson Statistic	r
Percentage change in hospital expense per adjusted admission	−.407 (1.79)	−.051 (1.26)	−.176 (.42)	−.060 (.28)	16.25 (3.51)	.27	25	2.13	.39
Percentage change in hospital expense per adjusted admission	−.416 (2.00)	−.056 (1.46)	−.198 (.49)	—	16.21 (3.70)	.27	25	2.14	.38
Percentage change in physician fees	−.032 (1.05)	−.070 (1.12)	.414 (2.62)	−.187 (2.13)	5.26 (2.44)	.61	25	1.92	.28
Percentage change in physician fees	−.049 (1.66)	−.091 (1.49)	.352 (2.10)	—	5.66 (2.65)	.52	25	1.72	.23
Percentage change in dentist fees	−.127 (1.41)	.240 (1.89)	.426 (3.29)	−.197 (3.06)	15.10 (1.70)	.64	25	1.65	.52
Percentage change in dentist fees	−.174 (2.05)	.172 (1.19)	.369 (2.36)	—	19.14 (2.23)	.53	25	1.66	.34
Percentage change in drug fees	+.093 (1.04)	−.169 (1.10)	.447 (4.94)	−.143 (3.10)	−0.12 (1.06)	.64	25	1.35	.67
Percentage change in drug fees	+.066 (.68)	−.216 (1.28)	.431 (4.06)	—	−7.01 (.75)	.47	25	1.46	.63

Notes:

[a] The data used to estimate these equations are given in Appendix B; $t_{.10}$ with 20 degrees of freedom (2-tail) is 1.72; $t_{.05}$ is 2.09; $t_{.01}$ is 2.85. The upper and lower bounds for the Durbin–Watson statistic are 1.04 and 1.77, respectively; r is treated as a constant when estimating the standard error of the intercept.

[b] The explanatory variables, coefficients, and absolute values of t-statistics are given in parentheses.

Table 4. Predicted Annual Percentage Price Change by Service if Coinsurance Were Constant at Mean and Current Levels; All Other Variables Constant[a]

Service	C at Sample Mean Level[b]	Significance Level of 1-Tail t-Test Against Null Hypothesis That Change Is Zero	C at Current Level[b]	Significanct Level of 1-Tail t-Test Against Hypothesis That Change is Zero
Hospital	9.04 (8.30)	.15	13.06 (6.28)	.03
Physician	3.29 (3.99)	.21	4.13 (3.19)	.11
Dentist	2.82 (17.51)	.45	4.27 (16.49)	.40
Drug	−0.21 (17.19)	.50	−1.16 (16.27)	.53

Notes:
[a] Using the specification with DGNP entered. Results omitting DGNP are similar.
[b] Standard errors are given in parentheses.

The results from the second test are shown in Table 5.[21] These results are in the general direction one would anticipate from the third model, but they cannot be called definitive. Using a chi-square test on the combined t-tests representing the three pairwise comparisons (Wallis, 1942), rejection of the null hypothesis that hospital services are like the other three services can be made with 30-percent probability of error by using sample mean coinsurance rates, but rejection can be made with only 10-percent probability of error at current levels of coinsurance rates.

Table 5. Significance Levels for Tests of Whether Elasticities for Hospital Service Differ from the Other Three Services

Comparison of Service	Significance Level at—	
	Sample Mean Coinsurance	Current Coinsurance Rates
Hospital–physician[a]	.26	.09
Hospital–dentist[a]	.36	.30
Hospital–drug[a]	.28	.18
Hospital–other three services[b]	.30	.10

Notes:
[a] Uses 1-tail t-test for difference in means. Test is therefore of null hypothesis that expected values of price changes are similar.
[b] Combines probabilities from the above three t-tests (see Wallis, 1942).

Results from the third test, shown in Table 6, are stronger. The rate of change of the elasticity with respect to the coinsurance rate (with other variables held constant) is much higher for hospital services than for the other three services. The table shows results for the specifications with and without the change in GNP variable; results are very similar. One can, with 2-percent or less chance of error, reject the null hypothesis that hospital services are similar to the other three services (the last row in the table).

Results from the fourth test, shown in Table 3, are also consistent with the third model. The coefficient of the GNP deflator variable is significant and of reasonable magnitudes in the physician, dental, and drug equations, consistent with the hypothesis that those markets are competitive. In the case of hospitals, however, the dependent variable is not price but cost per admission. The logic of the fourth test therefore does not apply to hospitals, because a valid measure of hospital factor costs should by definition correlate with cost per admission irrespective of market organization and performance. The coefficient of DGNPDEF is insignificant and actually negative in the hospital equation, suggesting that the GNP deflator is not a valid measure of factor prices for the hospital sector. Why the GNP deflator performs acceptably for physician, dental, and drug services but not hospitals is not clear.

Some tests of robustness were performed on the estimates in Table 3. In particular, an interaction term, $DC_{it}C_{it}$, was specified in lieu of the C_{it} term to test further whether the C variable only measured a within-service interaction. The fit was not as good as in the results presented, although the qualitative results were unchanged. Additionally, equations that were linear in the logarithms were estimated to test sensitivity to functional form; the results were not changed qualitatively, but the fit was not as good.[22] The equations were also estimated with the insurance variables lagged one year; again, the fit was not as good, but the broad conclusions were unaltered. In sum, the findings presented in Table 3 appear robust.

It was pointed out above that a theoretical model in which price is slowly adjusting to a much higher competitive equilibrium level may be appropriate for highly insured services, especially hospitals. A test of this hypothesis is available, conditional upon the correct specification of the lag structure. As already noted, geometrically declining weights were used in this test. Thus, the specification is as in Eq. (2), with a lagged dependent variable replacing the term C_{it}; the issue is whether the estimated rate of adjustment is slow.[23]

A modified version of Wallis's procedure was used to estimate these equations (Wallis, 1967). The terms $DC_{i,t-1}$, $DGNPDEF_{t-1}$, and $DGNP_{t-1}$ were used as instrumental variables for $DP_{i,t-1}$, and consistent

Table 6. Change in the Elasticity of Price with Respect to Coinsurance as Coinsurance Changes for Four Services and Tests of the Difference Between Hospital and Other Services

Service	Specification with DGNP		Specification without DGNP	
	Change in Elasticity	Significance Level of 2-Tail t-Test Against Null Hypothesis That Change is Zero	Change in Elasticity	Significance Level of 2-Tail t-Test Against Null Hypothesis That Change Is Zero
Hospital	−.407	.09	−.416	.06
Physician	−.032	.31	−.049	.11
Dentist	−.127	.17	−.174	.05
Drug	+.093	.31	+.065	.50

Comparison of Service	Significance Level of 1-Tail t-Test Against Null Hypothesis of Equal Change	Significance Level of 1-Tail t-Test Against Null Hypothesis of Equal Change
Hospital–physician	.06	.04
Hospital–dentist	.11	.13
Hospital–drug	.04	.03
Hospital–other three services[a]	.02	.01

Note:
[a] Uses chi-square test (see Wallis, 1942).

20

estimates of the error term e_{it} were obtained. The estimated e_{it} were used to make estimates of the parameter r in the error term. This parameter was estimated from the corrected first-order serial correlation coefficient.[24] The corrected serial correlation coefficient was then used to transform the equation by differencing, and OLS was used to estimate the transformed equation. Thus, OLS was used to estimate:

$$
\begin{aligned}
DP_{it} - r_i DP_{i,t-1} &= a_i(1 - r_i) + b_i(DC_{it} - r_i DC_{i,t-1}) \\
&+ c_i(DGNPDEF_t - r_i DGNPDEF_{t-1}) \\
&+ d_i(DGNP_t - r_i DGNP_{t-1}) + u_{it}, \\
&i = 1 - 4; t = 1950 - 1974.
\end{aligned}
\tag{4}
$$

The resulting estimates were then used in a seemingly unrelated regression framework to obtain Generalized Least Squares estimates.

The estimates are shown in Table 7. Again, the equations have been estimated with and without the $DGNP_t$ term because of its unexpected negative sign, and again the results are not sensitive to the inclusion of the $DGNP_t$ variable.[25]

The most important result is that the estimated mean length of the lag is very short, usually a year or less, and is not associated with the level of insurance (across services). Thus, conditional upon geometrically declining weights, the hospital sector does *not* appear to be slowly responding to changes in coinsurance, as hypothesized by Feldstein (1971b). In fact, these results are quite similar to those shown in Table 3; the short lag implies that the decision not to allow for a lag in the specification in Table 3 is approximately correct. Moreover, the effect of a change in insurance is of similar magnitude to that in Table 3, and price changes for hospital services are still not related to the GNP deflator, although price changes for other services are. The robustness of the results in Table 3 to a change in specification is encouraging.

V. IMPLICATIONS AND CONCLUSIONS

I have argued that high levels of insurance, given the nature of present insurance contracts, can permit medical care prices and expenditures to increase at above-average rates independent of a change in demand that a change in insurance induces. Present insurance heavily subsidizes the marginal unit, and insurance premiums do not reflect choice of supplier. Therefore, it is likely that the rate of technological change is higher than would be observed in the absence of such insurance and that price competition among medical firms is diminished (in the limit eliminated), thereby potentially giving the firm considerable discretion over its price. Both effects can serve to increase the rate at which prices and expenditures rise above what they would be without such insurance. One

Table 7. Distributed Lag Equations

Dependent Variable	Explanatory Variables[a]			Lagged Dependent Variable	Intercept/ $(1 - r)$	R^{2b}	n	Estimated Mean Lag (years)	r
	Percentage Change in Coinsurance (DC_i)	Percentage Change in GNP Deflator $(DGNPDEF)$	Percentage Change in GNP $(DGNP)$						
Percentage change in hospital price	−.074 (1.70)	.124 (.38)	−.129 (.52)	.504 (3.30)	4.26 (2.46)	.46	24	1.00	−.25
Percentage change in hospital price	−.069 (1.65)	.223 (.73)	—	.509 (3.52)	3.47 (2.63)	.48	24	1.04	−.28
Percentage change in physician price	−.057 (.89)	.496 (3.88)	−.190 (2.01)	.234 (1.60)	2.21 (2.75)	.66	24	.31	.03
Percentage change in physician price	−.070 (1.07)	.501 (3.77)	—	.298 (2.01)	1.21 (1.80)	.61	24	.42	.02
Percentage change in dental price	.136 (.80)	.531 (4.76)	−.178 (2.12)	.320 (2.01)	1.44 (2.15)	.68	24	.47	.09
Percentage change in dental price	−.035 (.18)	.461 (3.92)	—	.449 (2.88)	.50 (.97)	.70	24	.81	−.15
Percentage change in drug price	−.075 (.50)	.392 (4.87)	−.147 (2.72)	.485 (3.45)	−.36 (.80)	.70	24	.94	.41
Percentage change in drug price	−.294 (2.04)	.421 (4.63)	—	.391 (2.36)	−1.06 (1.63)	.57	24	.64	.68

Notes:
[a] Coefficients with absolute values of t-statistics are shown in parentheses.
[b] The apparent anomalies in R^2 as percentage change in GNP (DGNP) is added—i.e., the fall in the hospital and dental equations—occur because $DGNP_{t-1}$ is used as an instrumental variable to predict the lagged dependent variable in those equations that use DGNP as an explanatory variable.

would expect that current institutional arrangements are not viable in the long run; the price of risk aversion accomplished in this manner will become too high.

In addition to these a priori arguments about the effect of insurance, I have presented a number of tests suggesting that the standard competitive model needs modification if reimbursement insurance is present. Most prior literature (e.g., Feldstein, 1973) has recognized the implications of reimbursement at the individual level; much less attention has been paid to its effects at the market level.

If these arguments are valid, there are implications for both research and policy. For research, these include:

1. Estimated or theoretical models of the medical care sector frequently assume a competitive supply curve. Especially in the case of the hospital sector, this assumption is dubious. Thus, theories that seek to explain price rises from reimbursement insurance as simply an increase in demand that presses against an inelastic supply curve may be missing an important part of the story.

2. Estimates of welfare loss from reimbursement insurance based on the assumption of a competitive supply curve may be greatly understated (see, for example, the estimates of Feldstein, 1973; and Keeler et al., 1977).

3. Work is needed on theories of the medical firm (especially the hospital). In particular, the nature of the constraints facing the firm needs attention.

4. The debate over demand-pull vs. cost-push as an explanation of hospital cost inflation does not seem fruitful. Cost-push theories have been tested by including in regressions of hospital cost a measure of the percentage of revenues derived from insurance that reimbursed cost (Pauly and Drake, 1970; Davis, 1973). This variable has not been found to be associated with cost, and so cost-push theories have been rejected.[26] However, there is no reason to expect that the extent of cost reimbursement would be significantly related to cost; whether the hospital obtains reimbursement by quoting the insurance company a "price," which the insurance company pays, or by having its "costs" reimbursed should not be expected to affect costs in any of the models specified earlier. Thus, the existing tests do not really distinguish the two theories. However, the introduction of widespread insurance may serve both to raise demand (demand-pull) and to grant to the medical firm some element of discretion (cost-push). One may argue that the discretion is arbitraged away by consumers and/or their physicians seeking the highest "quality" care (demand-pull). Either way, however, there is a substantial market failure. If the firm has discretion, it can produce goods that provide it

with utility but may provide little or no utility to consumers; if discretion is arbitraged away in the name of quality, resources that have little or no value to the consumer may be devoted to producing "quality." Moreover, it does not appear that the answer to the cost-push or demand-pull question has differential policy implications. Hence, resolution of the demand-pull vs. cost-push issue would not seem to be of pressing importance.

5. The models developed herein could potentially explain the rate of price change across physician specialties. In particular, services of hospital-related specialists, such as surgeons, have traditionally been more heavily insured than services of primarily office-based specialists, such as pediatricians. One would predict that the price of hospital-related specialty services would therefore have shown a more rapid rate of increase than that of other specialties. For lack of data I have not attempted to test this implication.

For policy, the results are consistent with the view that hospital prices and expenditures could continue to increase at above-average rates for a very long time if present institutions are not changed. They are also consistent with the contention that additional insurance for other services could cause an increase in the rate that prices and expenditures for those services change. If these arguments are correct, three broad strategies may be pursued:

Do nothing. Proponents of doing nothing could argue that not enough evidence has yet been marshaled to reject the first model. They might also argue that the proposed cures are worse than the disease.

Regulate. This is the strategy that was pursued in the 1970's; it argues that public sector agencies (or quasi-public sector entities such as Health Systems Agencies) should set budgets, at least for hospitals. More incremental interventions, such as control of the entry of capital through certificate-of-need legislation, are also consistent with this strategy. Proponents of this strategy either argue that a market solution is inappropriate in medical care (on equity grounds) or that it is infeasible (on political grounds).

Use a market-oriented strategy. A market-related strategy must reject public-utility type regulation because its goal is to foster price competition. Methods for ensuring price competition can differ between hospital and nonhospital services. For nonhospital services (although the above results do not reject the standard model for nonhospital services), insurance policies would be structured so that most individuals, most of the time, paid for their medical care services by including substantial deductibles in health insurance policies (which could be income-related and need not apply to the poor). For hospital services, however, something else is needed. Individual demand for risk aversion implies that the marginal unit of care is likely to be subsidized for most individuals who are hospitalized, potentially creating the problems discussed earlier. These problems would *not* arise, however, if the premium for the health insurance policy was related to the choice of supplier and was higher for suppliers that imposed higher costs on their users. In that case, inefficient suppliers (including suppliers who introduced technological change at a rate consumers were unwilling to support) would lose business, just as in a standard market.

A health maintenance organization (HMO) is a device for relating choice of supplier to the magnitude of the insurance premium; and if HMOs were more widespread, the amount of price competition could markedly increase.[27] HMOs are difficult to organize, however, and do not command a large market share. Fortunately, there may be other ways to increase the amount of price competition. Several years ago, Vincent Taylor and I proposed rating hospital premiums, and possibly physician premiums, on the basis of the unit price of the hospital (and physician) (Newhouse and Taylor, 1971); more recently, Paul Ellwood (1978) has proposed rating physicians on the expenses they engender. Both proposals could serve to strengthen price competition in medical care. There are questions of feasibility about both proposals; in addition, the Ellwood proposal (or expansion of HMOs) could introduce access difficulties for poor health risks.[28] In my view, both proposals deserve a trial.[29] Widespread indemnity insurance could also potentially bring about price competition, although in practice it appears to make information more costly to the consumer than do the foregoing proposals.

Thus, market-oriented solutions for hospital services may well be feasible. In the absence of regulatory efforts that hinder them, one would predict their growth. And growth is occurring. Although their market share is still only 3 percent, from 1977 to 1978 the number of HMOs grew 21 percent, and the number of enrollees grew 14 percent (Interstudy, 1978). One would therefore predict continuing institutional change in the medical care marketplace; present contractual arrangements do not appear to represent a long-run equilibrium.

APPENDIX A
SOURCES OF DATA

Consumer Price Index: U.S. Department of Labor, Bureau of Labor Statistics, *Handbook of Labor Statistics, 1973* (U.S. Government Printing Office, Washington, D.C., 1973, Bulletin 1790) gives values through 1972; U.S. Department of Health and Human Services, Social Security Administration, *Medical Care Expenditures, Prices, and*

Costs: Background Book [U.S. Government Printing Office, Washington, D.C., 1975, Publ. No. (SSA) 75-11909, p. 27] gives values for 1973 and 1974.

Expense per Adjusted Admission: U.S. Department of Health and Human Services, Social Security Administration, op. cit., page 37, gives values for the adjusted measure from 1963 to 1973, and for the unadjusted measure from 1960 forward. *Hospitals, Guide Issue,* August 1, 1964, gives values of the unadjusted measure from 1960 and before. An adjusted measure was calculated from the unadjusted measure by multiplying the latter by 0.9, approximately the ratio of the two measures in the 1963–1966 period. The 1974 value is estimated from data in American Hospital Association, *Guide Issue to the Hospital Field,* 1975; the value of 878.95 equals the expense per unadjusted admission times the ratio of adjusted expense per day/unadjusted expense per day.

Third Party Payments: Calculated at 100 [1-(Direct Payments/Total Expenditure)]. Data on hospital and physician service coverage through 1973 are from U.S. Department of Health and Human Services, Social Security Administration, *Compendium of National Health Expenditures Data* [U.S. Government Printing Office, Washington, D.C., 1976, Publ. No. (SSA) 76-11927, Table 12]; 1974 data (91.31 percent for hospital, 65.075 percent for physician services) are unpublished estimates from the Social Security Administration. Data on dental and drug coverage are not available separately before 1970. For 1970 and forward, data on these services are unpublished estimates made available by the Social Security Administration. Prior to 1970, two estimates were used that will bracket the true value. The first estimate is the total of direct payment and private insurance payment; these values are again unpublished data provided by the Social Security Administration. This measure is probably quite accurate, but the resulting percentage of third-party payment is somewhat understated. The second estimate uses the percentage of third-party payment observed in 1970 (9.96 percent for dental and 10.72 percent for drugs) for all previous years. This percentage almost surely overstates the true coverage in these years. The first estimate is used to derive the results presented, but the conclusions are not changed if the second estimate is used.

Gross National Product and Gross National Product Deflator: *Economic Report of the President,* 1977 (U.S. Government Printing Office, Washington, D.C., 1977, Tables B-2 and B-3).

APPENDIX B
DATA USED IN ESTIMATION

Year	Service[a]	Percentage Change in Price	Percentage of Total Expenditure Reimbursed by Third Parties (100-C)	Percentage Change in GNP Deflator
1949	HOSP	4.381	62.693	−1.016
1949	PHYS	1.873	13.673	−1.016
1949	DENT	4.000	0.0	−1.016
1949	DRUG	1.510	0.385	−1.016
1950	HOSP	6.570	70.086	1.997
1950	PHYS	1.471	16.818	1.997
1950	DENT	2.404	0.0	1.997
1950	DRUG	1.259	0.637	1.997
1951	HOSP	9.056	77.221	6.767
1951	PHYS	3.804	21.862	6.767

APPENDIX B DATA USED IN ESTIMATION (*cont.*)

Year	Service[a]	Percentage Change in Price	Percentage of Total Expenditure Reimbursed by Third Parties (100-C)	Percentage Change in GNP Deflator
1951	DENT	3.912	0.0	6.767
1951	DRUG	2.825	0.754	6.767
1952	HOSP	6.654	78.143	1.275
1952	PHYS	4.363	23.702	1.275
1952	DENT	2.108	0.0	1.275
1952	DRUG	0.879	0.869	1.275
1953	HOSP	7.080	77.345	1.517
1953	PHYS	2.676	25.839	1.517
1953	DENT	3.245	0.0	1.517
1953	DRUG	0.871	0.976	1.517
1954	HOSP	7.082	75.827	1.376
1954	PHYS	2.932	27.280	1.376
1954	DENT	3.286	0.0	1.376
1954	DRUG	1.188	1.100	1.376
1955	HOSP	5.952	77.661	2.161
1955	PHYS	3.481	30.171	2.161
1955	DENT	0.968	0.0	2.161
1955	DRUG	1.067	1.174	2.161
1956	HOSP	3.541	81.755	3.149
1956	PHYS	3.058	31.301	3.149
1956	DENT	1.918	0.0	3.149
1956	DRUG	2.112	1.191	3.149
1957	HOSP	6.428	83.198	3.370
1957	PHYS	4.303	33.673	3.370
1957	DENT	2.419	0.0	3.370
1957	DRUG	2.689	1.196	3.370
1958	HOSP	8.351	82.737	1.600
1958	PHYS	3.414	33.462	1.600
1958	DENT	3.150	0.0	1.600
1958	DRUG	3.525	1.696	1.600
1959	HOSP	9.772	83.074	2.210
1959	PHYS	3.301	33.461	2.210
1959	DENT	2.417	0.0	2.210
1959	DRUG	1.556	2.014	2.210
1960	HOSP	3.777	80.158	1.703
1960	PHYS	2.530	34.624	1.703
1960	DENT	1.988	0.152	1.703
1960	DRUG	0.096	1.613	1.703
1961	HOSP	9.337	81.635	0.888
1961	PHYS	2.597	37.523	0.888
1961	DENT	0.487	0.194	0.888
1961	DRUG	− 1.148	1.935	0.888
1962	HOSP	5.261	82.652	1.833
1962	PHYS	2.911	37.673	1.833

APPENDIX B   DATA USED IN ESTIMATION (*cont.*)

Year	Service[a]	Percentage Change in Price	Percentage of Total Expenditure Reimbursed by Third Parties (100-C)	Percentage Change in GNP Deflator
1962	DENT	2.667	1.074	1.833
1962	DRUG	− 1.549	2.271	1.833
1963	HOSP	6.257	81.476	1.474
1963	PHYS	2.214	38.282	1.474
1963	DENT	2.834	1.186	1.474
1963	DRUG	− 0.885	2.574	1.474
1964	HOSP	6.249	81.602	1.564
1964	PHYS	2.527	36.565	1.564
1964	DENT	2.641	1.246	1.564
1964	DRUG	− 0.298	2.834	1.564
1965	HOSP	8.679	82.756	2.214
1965	PHYS	3.638	37.118	2.214
1965	DENT	3.132	1.282	2.214
1965	DRUG	− 0.299	2.928	2.214
1966	HOSP	8.607	82.725	3.283
1966	PHYS	5.776	39.635	3.283
1966	DENT	3.254	1.923	3.283
1966	DRUG	0.299	3.579	3.283
1967	HOSP	21.183	87.677	2.944
1967	PHYS	7.066	48.634	2.944
1967	DENT	5.042	3.750	2.944
1967	DRUG	− 0.498	4.140	2.944
1968	HOSP	15.221	89.472	4.493
1968	PHYS	5.600	54.329	4.493
1968	DENT	5.500	6.725	4.493
1968	DRUG	0.200	5.028	4.493
1969	HOSP	14.418	87.986	5.026
1969	PHYS	6.913	54.327	5.026
1969	DENT	7.014	5.218	5.026
1969	DRUG	1.098	5.915	5.026
1970	HOSP	13.139	89.681	5.351
1970	PHYS	7.529	56.011	5.351
1970	DENT	5.757	9.958	5.351
1970	DRUG	2.270	10.717	5.351
1971	HOSP	10.639	92.161	5.101
1971	PHYS	6.919	56.230	5.101
1971	DENT	6.365	11.010	5.101
1971	DRUG	1.737	12.287	5.101
1972	HOSP	10.351	89.748	4.145
1972	PHYS	3.082	58.601	4.145
1972	DENT	4.173	12.328	4.145
1972	DRUG	0.190	12.633	4.145
1973	HOSP	6.900	88.560	5.920
1973	PHYS	3.288	60.423	5.920
1973	DENT	3.099	14.255	5.920
1973	DRUG	0.284	13.591	5.920

APPENDIX B DATA USED IN ESTIMATION (*cont.*)

Year	Service[a]	Percentage Change in Price	Percentage of Total Expenditure Reimbursed by Third Parties (100-C)	Percentage Change in GNP Deflator
1974	HOSP	10.382	91.310	9.705
1974	PHYS	9.117	65.075	9.705
1974	DENT	7.625	14.730	9.705
1974	DRUG	3.494	14.427	9.705

[a] HOSP, hospital; PHYS, physician; DENT, Dentist; DRUG, prescription drug.

Year	Percentage Change in GNP
1949	0.615
1950	8.722
1951	8.060
1952	3.816
1953	3.893
1954	− 1.303
1955	6.697
1956	2.138
1957	1.809
1958	− 0.206
1959	6.019
1960	2.276
1961	2.511
1962	5.799
1963	3.954
1964	5.261
1965	5.890
1966	5.951
1967	2.722
1968	4.376
1969	2.567
1970	− 0.324
1971	2.995
1972	5.743
1973	5.456
1974	− 1.700

ACKNOWLEDGMENTS

The author owes a considerable debt to Lindy Friedlander and Sally Carson for careful data collection and computation. Rodney Smith, Charles Phelps, Michael Grossman, Willard Manning, Bridger Mitchell, David Salkever, and participants in the University of Chicago's Industrial Organization Workshop all gave me helpful comments. Because the advice of these individuals was not always heeded, they cannot be held responsible for the content. I am grateful to the Social Security Administration for providing me with unpublished data on dental and drug insurance coverage.

The research reported herein was performed pursuant to Health Insurance Study Grant No. 016B-7501/2-P2021 from the U.S. Department of Health and Human Services, Washington, D.C. The opinions and conclusions expressed are solely those of the author and should not be construed as representing the opinions or policy of any agency of the United States government.

NOTES

1. See Feldstein, 1971a,b, 1973, 1977; Feldstein and Friedman, 1976; Intriligator, 1976; Leffler and Lindsay, 1976; Newhouse and Taylor, 1971; Yett et al., 1975.

2. Indemnity insurance that only paid a fixed dollar amount per unit of service would only shift the demand curve upward and would not rotate it. I have not taken account of existing indemnity insurance in this report, but to do so would not alter my conclusions because the estimates implicitly include whatever indemnity insurance exists.

3. The long-run supply curve for hospital care may be (approximately) perfectly elastic, because there are no obvious limitations on factor supplies. If so, the empirical results presented in this chapter are strengthened.

4. More precisely, E equals the negative of the limit of K as dC tends toward zero. To see this, note that $E = KE(\alpha,C)$ but $E(\alpha,C) = -1$, because a change in coinsurance causes an equiproportionate rotation of the demand curve about its intersection with the x axis (see Figure 1).

5. This is especially true of productivity (see Reder, 1969).

6. Data on hospital beds relate to private short-term general hospital beds from the American Hospital Association, deflated by the civilian population; active physician data (M.D. and D.O.) are from the American Medical Association; dentist data are from *Health Resources Statistics*, 1975, DHEW Publ. No. HRA 76-1509, p. 80.

7. In the health services research literature, cost-enhancing technological change is often referred to as *halfway technology*.

8. Feldstein also reaches this conclusion, although his meaning is different from mine. His argument applies to a given state of knowledge and would not predict that the rate of price and expenditure increase would be related to the level of insurance. Put another way, if insurance were unchanging (but at a high level), Feldstein's model does not imply price increases whereas mine does.

9. There is no evidence for medical care, but this appears to be the case in the aircraft industry (see Alexander and Nelson, 1972; see also Evenson and Kislev, 1976).

10. This argument is a dynamic version of the standard argument that a subsidy will serve to shift productive resources along a production possibility frontier in the direction of a subsidized product (Friedman, 1953). Although the argument in the text is heuristic, it can be made rigorous by assuming a utility function in health and other goods and by assuming that health is produced by medical care of a given technology. Health and other goods are superior goods subject to diminishing marginal utility; medical technology can be made everywhere more productive by greater investment in research and development, units of which (it is assumed) can be "bought" by consumers at a constant price but with diminishing marginal returns. The constant price of medical care and technological research and development are subject to a common coinsurance rate. Reductions in the coinsurance rate lead to a greater demand for both medical care and medical technology; in effect, the subsidy represented by the coinsurance rate induces more allocation on both the intensive and extensive margins.

It might be thought that there is no welfare loss because the consumer purchases insurance in a competitive market. This is not so, however, when insurance distinguishes states of the world only on the basis of total expenditure. Confronted with a choice of this type of insurance or no insurance, the consumer may well purchase the insurance to diminish risk.

11. Fisher and Shell (1972) propose the following treatment of new goods in price indices: The utility function is defined to include the new good, and in the base period its quantity is constrained to equal zero. Under the usual conditions, the Laspeyres index still bounds the true index from above, but for a Paasche index to bound from below the new good needs to be assigned the demand reservation price (i.e., the shadow price on the constraint that quantity be zero). Although this conceptually integrates new goods into index theory, we are concerned here with analyzing variation in the conventional indices.

12. The most common type of policy is "service" benefits, which reimburses the hospital stay in full. There are also "indemnity" benefits; this is something of a misnomer, however, because the policy will usually pay in full, provided a rate less than $X per day is charged. Available evidence suggests that most consumers with such policies use providers whose rates are less than $X. (Note that the overall reimbursement rate is 92 percent; see also Phelps and Newhouse, 1974, p. 30.) Indemnity benefits could provide some check on unit price, but do not appear sufficiently widespread to do so (see Section IV).

The deductible in the Medicare program alone can account for about two percentage points of the out-of-pocket expenditure; deductibles in private policies account for an unknown additional amount.

13. The caveat "nearly" appears to take account of income effects that may become important in ranges of price above those now observed.

14. One must also explain why a voluntary community hospital would engage in a labor dispute over wages and why some voluntary hospitals go bankrupt, phenomena that are not consistent with the theory. I do not have a good explanation, but the events appear sufficiently rarely that an explanation may not be necessary.

15. One may ask what governs entry. The third model per se puts no restrictions on entry (although nonprofit status, licensure, etc., are barriers). However, price competition is unavailable to the entrant because fully insured consumers, by assumption, are indifferent to the cost of the supplier. Hence, entry will not preserve price competition. Insofar as entrants compete on the basis of quality, price and expenditure increases may be exacerbated. Entry need not, therefore, compete away rents.

16. It can be argued that the gross national product (GNP) deflator measures the price of other goods and that this would induce a positive effect on demand. Although this effect is incorporated in the coefficient, it is thought to be swamped empirically by changes in the general price level and resulting changes in factor prices. A question can also be raised about the exogeneity of DC and C. I interpret the existing empirical literature (Frech, 1976; Phelps, 1976) as consistent with no change in demand for insurance as medical prices rise. Under this assumption, C is exogenous.

17. That E is greater (in absolute value) as demand is more elastic follows from differentiating K in Eq. (1) with respect to η. That the price change is larger the more inelastic the supply curve is obvious graphically, but a formal demonstration is as follows: Let $p(q)$ be the demand function and $s(q)$ be the supply function. Then the new equilibrium is $p(q) + \alpha - s(q) = 0$. Taking the total differential, we obtain $dq/d\alpha = -1/(p' - s')$. But $dp/d\alpha = p'dq/d\alpha = -p'/(p' - s')$. Since p' is negative and s' is positive, as s' rises (supply becomes more inelastic), $dp/d\alpha$ rises $[d^2p/(d\alpha ds') = (-p')/(p' - s')^2$, which is positive].

18. Note that the coefficient of C in the estimated equation is picking up the effect of the within-service variation in C. The second and third tests are based on between-service comparisons.

19. The Consumer Price Index measure for hospital services was for many years based on the semiprivate room charge. Room charges account for only about half of all hospital revenue, the remainder coming from charges for ancillary services, such as laboratory, X-ray, and operating room, and these prices may have moved somewhat differently from room charges.

20. Although there are no data on demand elasticities for physician procedures in the hospital, it is possible, by taking account of such procedures, to lower the elasticity for physician services below .14 (though probably not to .07), because such services are a smaller part of the total bill (which includes hospital charges) than they are for outpatient services.

21. These results are approximate because I have ignored the term in DC to simplify the computations. This term is very small relative to the total value (only 1 percent of the elasticity for hospital services, for example), and so the approximation should be quite good.

22. There were several observations with negative values prior to taking logarithms. Arbitrarily, unity was added to each variable prior to taking its logarithm, and any observation remaining with a negative value was deleted.

23. It was felt that allowing for an interaction term between DC_{it} and C_{it} would place too large a demand on the data; hence, C_{it} was omitted.

24. The correlation was Wallis's correction 3, which required adding 3/25 to the estimated serial correlation coefficient.

25. $DGNP_{t-1}$ was not used as an instrumental variable in the equations in which $DGNP_t$ was omitted.

26. Davis finds the variable related to cost when data from across 3 years are pooled; but it is not related when each year's data are analyzed separately, and not when year dummies are included in the pooled regression. She infers that the extensiveness of cost reimbursement is not the "true explanator."

27. Edwards (1977) has recently tested the hypothesis that the more competitive the environment for commercial banks, the less the ability of a single bank to engage in expense-preference behavior. Edwards's test of expense-preference behavior is whether banks in more sheltered markets spend more on wages and salaries (add staff); he finds that they do. There is an obvious opportunity to test the same hypothesis for HMOs relative to the fee-for-service system, given that HMOs must compete on the basis of price, whereas firms within the fee-for-service system (especially hospitals) may not.

28. In particular, a provider who engenders expenses because he treats (on average) patients with expensive diseases must be distinguished from one who is simply inefficient or providers will not wish to treat patients with expensive diseases. How well this can be done is an open issue.

29. One may reasonably ask why such schemes have not emerged. The answer may be that the fallacy of aggregation, described above, was not realized, that medicine has colluded against them, that legislation somehow precludes them, that administrative costs render them impractical, or that there are unforeseen problems with them. A trial would settle most, if not all, of these issues.

REFERENCES

Alexander, Arthur J., and Nelson, J. R. (1972), *Measuring Technological Change: Aircraft Turbine Engines*. The Rand Corporation, R-1017-ARPA/PR (June).

Davis, Karen (1973), "Theories of Hospital Inflation: Some Empirical Evidence," *Journal of Human Resources 8*(2), 181–201.

Edwards, Franklin R. (1977), "Managerial Objectives in Regulated Industries: Expense-Preference Behavior in Banking," *Journal of Political Economy 85*(1), 147–162.

Ellwood, Paul M., Jr. (1978), "The Health Care Alliance," in *National Commission on the Cost of Medical Care, 1976–1977,* Vol. 2: *Collected Papers.* Chicago: American Medical Association.

Evans, Robert G. (1973), *Price Formation in the Market for Physician Services.* Ottawa: Information Canada.

Evenson, Robert E., and Kislev, Yoav (1976), "A Stochastic Model of Applied Research," *Journal of Political Economy 84*(2), 265–281.

Feldstein, Martin S. (1971a), *The Rising Cost of Hospital Care.* Washington, D.C.: Information Resources Press.

—— (1971b), "Hospital Cost Inflation: A Study in Nonprofit Price Dynamics," *American Economic Review 61*(5), 853–872.

—— (1973), "The Welfare Loss from Excess Health Insurance," *Journal of Political Economy 81*(2), 251–280.

—— (1977), "Quality Change and the Demand for Hospital Care," *Econometrica 45*(7), 1681–1702.

Feldstein, Martin S., and Friedman, Bernard (1976), "The Effect of National Health Insurance on the Price and Quantity of Medical Care," in R. Rosett (ed.), *The Role of Health Insurance in the Health Services Sector.* New York: National Bureau of Economic Research.

Fisher, Franklin M., and Shell, Karl (1972), *The Economic Theory of Price Indices.* New York: Academic Press.

Frech, H. E. (1976), "Comment on Paper by Charles E. Phelps," in *The Role of Health Insurance in the Health Services Sector* (R. Rosett, ed.). New York: National Bureau of Economic Research.

Frech, H. E., and Ginsburg, Paul B. (1975), "Imposed Health Insurance in Monopolistic Markets: A Theoretical Analysis," *Economic Inquiry 13*(1), 55–70.

Friedman, Milton (1953), "The Welfare Effects of an Income Tax and an Excise Tax," in *Essays in Positive Economics.* Chicago: Univ. of Chicago Press.

Fuchs, Victor R. (1968), *The Service Economy.* New York: National Bureau of Economic Research.

Hicks, J. R. (1968), *The Theory of Wages,* 2nd ed. New York: St. Martin's Press.

Interstudy (1978), "HMO Growth: 1977 to 1978," Excelsior, Minn.: Interstudy.

Intriligator, Michael D. (1976), "Comment on Feldstein-Friedman Paper," in *The Role of Health Insurance in the Health Services Sector* (R. Rosett, ed.). New York: National Bureau of Economic Research.

Keeler, Emmett B., Newhouse, Joseph P., and Phelps, Charles E. (1977), "Deductibles and Demand: A Theory of the Consumer Facing a Variable Price Schedule Under Uncertainty," *Econometrica 45*(3), 641–655.

Kendrick, John W. (1973), *Postwar Productivity Trends in the United States,* New York: Columbia Univ. Press.

Kmenta, Jan, and Gilbert, Roy F. (1970), "Estimation of Seemingly Unrelated Regressions with Autoregressive Disturbances," *Journal of the American Statistical Association 65*(329), 186–197.

Leffler, Keith B., and Lindsay, Cotton M. (1976), "The Long-Run Effects of National Health Insurance on Medical Care Prices and Output," in *New Directions in Public Health Care* (Cotton M. Lindsay, ed.). San Francisco: Inst. for Contemporary Studies.

Muth, Richard F. (1964), "The Derived Demand Curve for a Productive Factor and the Industry Supply Curve," *Oxford Economic Papers 16,* 221–234.

Newhouse, Joseph P., and Taylor, Vincent (1971), "How Shall We Pay for Hospital Care?" *The Public Interest 23,* 78–92.

Pauly, Mark V. (1968), "The Economics of Moral Hazard: Comment," *American Economic Review 58*(3), 531–536.

Pauly, Mark V., and Drake, David (1970), "The Effect of Third-Party Methods of Reim-
    bursement on Hospital Performance," in *Empirical Studies in Health Economics*
    (Herbert Klarman, ed.). Baltimore: Johns Hopkins Press.
Phelps, Charles E. (1976), "Demand for Reimbursement Insurance," in *The Role of Health
    Insurance in the Health Services Sector* (R. Rosett, ed.). New York: National Bureau
    of Economic Research.
Phelps, Charles E., and Newhouse, Joseph P. (1974), *Coinsurance and the Demand for
    Medical Services,* The Rand Corporation, R-964-1-OEO/NC, October.
Reder, Melvin W. (1969), "Some Problems in the Measurement of Productivity in the
    Medical Care Industry," in *Production and Productivity in the Service Industries*
    (Victor Fuchs, ed.). New York: Columbia Univ. Press.
Reinhardt, Uwe E. (1975), *Physician Productivity and the Demand for Health Manpower.*
    Cambridge, Mass.: Ballinger.
Wallis, Kenneth F. (1967), "Lagged Dependent Variables and Serially Correlated Errors:
    A Reappraisal of Three-Pass Least Squares," *Review of Economics and Statistics*
    49(4), 555–567.
Wallis, W. Allen (1942), "Compounding Probabilities from Independence Significance
    Tests," *Econometrica 10,* 229–248.
Yett, Donald E., Drabek, Leonard, Intiligator, Michael D., and Kimbell, Larry (1975),
    "A Microeconomic Model of the Health Care System in the United States," *Annals
    of Economic and Social Measurement 4*(3), 407–433.

CHILDREN'S HEALTH AND THE FAMILY

Linda N. Edwards and Michael Grossman

I. INTRODUCTION

Children's health care has been and continues to be provided primarily within the family. This is in marked contrast to the provision of children's education, which for the past 100 years has been among the responsibilities of government.[1] State governments determine how many years children must attend school, how many days per year they must attend, and to a large extent the content of that schooling. Further, recent rulings of the Supreme Court stipulate that all children are entitled to schooling of equal quality. Only recently has the focus returned to the role of the preschool years and, consequently, the family, in determining the intellectual development of children.[2]

In the case of children's health, it has been widely recognized that it is the family rather than the public or medical care sectors that plays

Advances in Health Economics and Health Services Research, Vol. 2, pgs. 35–84.
(Volume 1 published as Research in Health Economics)
Copyright © 1981 by JAI Press Inc.
All rights of reproduction in any form reserved.
ISBN: 0-89232-100-8

the fundamental role. For example, a recent Carnegie Council on Children report says "Doctors do not provide the bulk of health care for children; families do" (Keniston, 1977, p. 179). With the exception of immunization, which clearly has important externalities, there has been no form of compulsory health care for children,[3] and with the advent of relatively simple and effective treatments for important childhood diseases of the past (influenza, pneumonia, and tuberculosis), one might even imagine that the doctor's role is declining. Indeed, the expanding interest of pediatricians into the area of the "new morbidity"—"learning difficulties and school problems, behavioral disturbances, allergies, speech difficulties, visual problems, and the problems of adolescents in coping and adjusting"—is a response to the decline in importance of the traditional health problems of children.[4]

While the overall importance of the family in providing health care for children is widely acknowledged, information about the nature of the association between various family characteristics and the health status of children is relatively scarce.[5] Only family income and race have been related to various children's health characteristics. It is well known that infant mortality is higher for blacks than for whites and that the incidence of low birth weight (a good indicator of risk or damage to surviving infants) is greater among poor and black families.[6] There is also evidence that both black families and low-income families evaluate their children's health as poorer than do white or high-income families. Similar differences are reported in the proportion of children for whom "significant abnormalities" are found on a physical exam.[7] Less uniform findings are evident when various specific conditions and illnesses are examined. For example, chronic conditions are more prevalent among high-income families.[8] The extent to which the aforementioned differences are the result of income and/or race alone, as opposed to correlated factors like parental education, family size, mother's work status, and place of residence, has hardly been studied. In order to formulate sensible and effective programs to improve the health of children, we need a much more complete understanding of how these and other family characteristics work in producing healthy children.[9]

The objective of this paper is to examine the relationship between a number of family characteristics and some measures of the health of children in those families. This multivariate analysis is carried out within the framework of an economic model of the family. Such a framework explicitly recognizes not only the family's function as health care provider but also that it is faced with resource constraints and that some of its objectives for its children may conflict with maximizing their health level. Although our primary focus is on analyzing the health of the child as recorded at the time the data were collected, we also look at some measures of the child's health status at birth and during early infancy.

These early health status variables are then related, in combination with the family characteristics, to the current health of the child.

The data set used, Cycle II of the Health Examination Survey, is an exceptional source of information about a national sample of 7,119 non-institutionalized children aged 6–11 years in the 1963–1965 period.[10] The data comprise complete medical and developmental histories of each child provided by the parent, information on family socioeconomic characteristics, birth certificate information, and a school report with information on school performance and classroom behavior provided by teachers or other school officials. Most important, there are objective measures of health from detailed physical examinations. The physical examinations (as well as associated psychological and achievement tests) were administered by the U.S. Public Health Service (PHS). There is little direct information about the medical care received by these children, but some attempt will be made to control for variations in the availability of local medical care.

The amount of health information for the children in the Cycle II sample is prodigious. To illustrate the exact nature of this information, as well as to provide a description of the overall health of the children in the sample, selected summary data are presented in Table 1. Almost

Table 1. Summary of Selected Health Information From Cycle II of the Health Examination Survey

Panel A. Parent's Assessment of Children's Current Health

	Percent of Children Whose Parent Rates Present Health as:				Percent of Children Whose Parent Considers Present Health a Problem
	Very Good	*Good*	*Fair*	*Poor*	
Both sexes	51.8	42.9	4.9	0.4	19.0
Boys	51.6	43.2	4.8	0.4	19.0
Girls	51.8	42.7	5.1	0.4	19.0

Panel B. Physician's Findings on Survey Examination

	Percent of Children with Finding of		Distribution of Those with Significant Abnormality by Type of Abnormality (Percent)				
	Otitis Medina	*Significant Abnormality*	*Cardiovascular*	*Injury Residual*	*Neuromuscular Joint*	*Other Congenital*	*Other Major Diseases*
Both sexes	1.6	11.2	22.9	13.7	31.8	23.6	28.6
Boys	1.8	12.2	21.8	13.5	32.9	22.6	28.9
Girls	1.4	10.2	24.4	14.1	30.4	24.7	28.1

Table 1. (cont.)

Panel C. Medical History as Reported by Parent

Medical History Item	Percent of Children with History of Indicated Condition		
	Both Sexes	Boys	Girls
Infective diseases			
Chickenpox	—	—	—
Measles	85.8	85.5	86.2
Mumps	48.8	50.1	47.3
Scarlet fever	3.8	3.8	3.9
Whooping Cough	9.4	8.9	9.8
Accidents			
Broken bones	7.8	8.5	7.0
Knocked unconscious	3.4	4.0	2.8
Scars from burns	4.5	4.4	4.7
Other accidents	4.2	4.7	3.7
Allergies and related conditions			
Asthma	5.3	6.5	4.0
Hay fever	4.6	5.5	3.6
Other allergies	11.4	12.2	10.7
Kidney condition	3.9	2.6	5.1
Heart condition	3.7	4.2	3.1
Respiratory conditions			
Sore throat	11.7	10.2	13.2
Colds	21.0	19.9	22.1
Coughs	10.7	11.0	10.4
Bronchitis	15.7	16.9	14.4
Chest colds	6.2	6.5	5.9
Pneumonia	—	—	—
Sensorineurological conditions			
Convulsions or fits	3.3	3.5	3.1
Eye trouble	14.0	12.7	15.3
Trouble hearing	4.3	4.8	3.7
Earaches	26.8	24.8	28.8
Running ears	11.9	12.2	11.6
Problem talking	8.4	10.0	6.8
Trouble walking	2.3	2.5	2.1
Arm or leg limitation	1.3	1.3	1.2
Operations	30.8	35.3	26.1
Hospitalized more than 1 day	26.8	30.0	23.6
Exercise restricted			
Ever	5.4	5.6	5.2
Now	1.5	1.4	1.6
Taking medicine regularly	4.1	4.0	4.2

Source: National Center for Health Statistics (1973b): Panel A—Table 1; Panel B—Tables 1 and 3; Panel C—Table 4.

95 percent of parents rate their child's health as good or very good. At the same time, 19 percent of these parents also consider their child's present health to be a problem (see Panel A). The PHS physicians affirm this assessment in the sense that they find that 11.2 percent of the children had at least one "significant abnormality" (see Panel B). An indication of the types of problems that may be bothering parents is given by the incidence of various items in the medical history (Panel C). The total picture, then, is of a cohort whose overall health is good but who are nevertheless disturbed by particular health problems.

The present paper proceeds as follows. Section II briefly describes the economic model of the family used to generate the relationships to be estimated. Section III discusses the nature of the estimated relationships and defines the variable measures. The estimates are presented and discussed in Section IV. The final sections highlight and interpret the statistical findings of the study.

II. THE ECONOMISTS' VIEW OF CHILDREN AND CHILDREN'S HEALTH

An important focal point of recent economic models of fertility (Becker and Lewis 1973; Willis 1973; Ben Porath and Welch 1976) is that children are not homogeneous. In particular, these models distinguish between two aspects of children that enter the parents' consumption (or investment) portfolio—the number of children and the "quality" of each child. By quality of the child is meant those characteristics of the child which generate utility (or disutility) for the parents: his health, sex, wealth, social adjustment, intellectual development, sense of humor, etc. Therefore, when parents choose their optimal family composition, they choose not only how many children they will have but also what portion of the family's resources will be devoted to each child.[11] This choice is made in the usual way: parents choose the number and quality of children, as well as of other consumption goods, so as to maximize their utility subject to the constraints imposed by their wealth (their potential earned income and their nonearned income) and the various prices they face. In the case of children, there is a further constraint in the form of children's genetic endowments, which in part determine their quality. Genetic endowments act as a constraint because they are, for the most part, outside of the family's control.[12]

The prices of children and of the various components of their quality are determined by recognizing that children are produced within the home using goods bought in the market and the time of family members. The cost of producing a child of a given quality depends on the prices of the purchased inputs—parents' time, medical care, food, toys, lodging, etc.—and on the efficiency with which these inputs are used. The marginal cost of a child, then, depends on the quality chosen and on the cost of one unit of that amount of quality. Similarly, the cost of an increment in quality depends on how many children will receive this increment (i.e., family size) and on the cost of an incremental unit of quality.[13] To take the case of that aspect of child quality of interest in this paper, children's health, the cost (price) of increasing the average health level of all children in the family depends on the number of children there are in the family and on the costs of medical care, nutrition, the parents' or other caretakers' time, and any other purchased inputs used to improve children's health. In addition, to the extent that there are systematic differences in the ability of families to produce children's health with given inputs, these differences in efficiency are also relevant. For example, more educated parents are more likely to be able to follow doctors' instructions, to have general information about nutrition, and to be willing and able to acquire medical information from published materials. Consequently, one would expect more educated parents to be more efficient at producing healthy children.[14]

A final consideration in the determination of the cost of children's health is introduced by the nature of the relationship between the marginal cost of investment in children's health and the level of investment. In particular, given rising marginal costs, parents have an incentive to spread out investments over many periods. Thus, even if parents care only about the ultimate health of their children (say, at age 18 years), prices of health inputs such as medical care and parents' time at different stages of a child's life cycle (infancy, early childhood, adolescence) will influence the cost of health.

Given these considerations, the following factors are expected to influence children's health levels: the child's exogenous (genetic) health endowment, family wealth, parents' wage rates, family size, parents' educational attainment and other measures of their efficiency in household production, costs and availability of medical care and of other market health inputs (vitamins, sanitation, etc.), the prices of inputs used to produce other aspects of child quality, and the prices of other forms of parents' consumption. The relationship between the child's ultimate health and these factors may be termed a demand function for the output health. Associated with this output demand function are input demand functions for parents' time, medical care, and other market health inputs at various stages of the child's life cycle. Moreover, there are also demand functions for infant, early childhood, and adolescent health, which may be regarded as intermediate health outputs. The input and intermediate output demand functions depend on the same set of variables as the final output demand function. Since our main concern in this paper is with the last function, we focus on its properties.

Given that children's quality and, in particular, their health, is a normal good, one would expect to observe a positive association between children's ultimate health and family wealth. Similarly, a positive association is expected between both parents' education and children's endowed health status and children's ultimate health status.[15] Negative associations would be anticipated between all of the prices of health inputs and children's health and between family size and children's health. Parents' wage rates may have negative or positive effects on children's health levels, depending on whether the household production of children's health is more or less time intensive than the production of other aspects of child quality and/or other types of parents' consumption commodities. Finally, to the extent that there is substitutability between the various aspects of child quality, the prices of inputs into the nonhealth aspects of child quality (say, music lessons) might be positively associated with children's health.

These predictions concerning the effects of various family characteristics and market prices do not necessarily apply when some realistic twists are incorporated into the model. An important instance is the introduction of joint production between various aspects of child quality and/or between child quality and other consumption commodities. Such joint production can make both wealth effects and input price effects ambiguous. To take a simple example, both athletic development and health may be regarded as aspects of children's quality. If athletic development has a high income elasticity and also has some negative health effects, a negative relationship between income or wealth and certain health measures may be observed. Indeed, the incidence of broken bones is greater in high-income families than it is in low-income families.[16] Alternatively, suppose that parents' time in child care yields direct utility rather than generating utility only through its effect on children's quality. In this case, parents may appear to choose inefficient modes of producing child quality, modes that use "too much" time relative to its cost.

The basic model outlined here is also modified when one takes account of the fact that the human capital dimensions of child quality are by necessity embodied in the child. Because of this embodiment, for some types of human capital there are natural minimum and maximum states that cannot be reduced or exceeded. In the case of children's health, increased expenditures on health inputs or increased production efficiency cannot continually increase the child's health. For this reason, one would not predict constant absolute effects of the various determinants of children's health but rather that these effects attenuate in the region of the minimum and maximum health levels.

Recent models of intergenerational transfers utilize this embodiment insight in a somewhat different way. In these models investments in children's human capital are assumed to be subject to decreasing returns in terms of the future earnings of the child. This assumption, along with the assumption that parents measure a child's quality by his expected lifetime wealth, generates additional predictions concerning the effects of the set of variables discussed earlier on various components of children's quality.[17] In particular, this type of model yields a distinction between two types of families: (1) those for whom the optimal quantity–quality calculation involves making a financial transfer to their children and (2) those for whom a financial transfer is not optimal. These two types of families differ systematically with respect to the effects of the various explanatory variables on the human capital dimensions of child quality. The strongest prediction is that the wealth effect on the child's human capital (health, in our case) will be zero in families which plan to make financial transfers to the children but positive in families who do not plan such a transfer.[18]

The various models outlined here so far generate somewhat different types of predictions, but the point of reviewing them is not to demonstrate that one gets from an economic model what one puts into it. Rather, our objective is bifold. First, the foregoing discussion illustrates that, even though the exact nature of the predictions of these models may differ, the list of relevant factors to consider in understanding the determination of children's health—parents' wealth, wage rates, and education, family size, other input prices, etc.—does not. Second, these models provide ready structures within which to interpret empirical findings. Thus, the greater incidence of broken bones among children from high-income families is seen not as an anomalous finding but rather as a result of conflicting family objectives concerning various aspects of child quality. Or, a finding that for high-income families increases in wealth are not associated with increased children's health is not viewed as evidence that wealthy parents do not care about their children but rather as being a result of the fact that wealthy parents have already made the optimal health investment for their children. In the sections to follow, both the choice of variables to be investigated and the interpretation of the results of that investigation are guided by the general framework outlined here.

III.   VARIABLES AND RELATIONSHIPS
TO BE ESTIMATED

As is typical with economic modeling in the field of human resources (and, although somewhat less obviously, in other fields as well), the fundamental and inescapable problem associated with empirical estimation is that of finding measures of the variables described by the model. This difficulty is intensified here because the object of our study, children's health, is not itself well defined even in the public health literature. In this section we first discuss alternative ways of measuring children's health and define the current and early health measures to be used. Second, we describe the available measures of the explanatory variables and how the use of these measures affects the estimation and interpretation of the child health–family characteristics relationship. Finally, the endogeneity of family size is pointed out and the implications of this endogeneity for estimation and interpretation are explored.

A. Measurement of Child Health

The issue of defining and measuring children's health is very much an unresolved one, even among professionals in the area of public health.[19] Definitions of health range from all-encompassing positive conceptualizations like that of the World Health Organization (WHO), "Health is a state of complete physical, mental and social well-being and not merely the absence of disease and illness,"[20] to more restricted notions that involve simply measuring mortality and morbidity.[21] Undoubtedly, no single definition or measure is appropriate for all purposes, so that the use to which a measure is to be put will partly govern one's choice.

The economist's approach to defining health is somewhere between these two extremes. Economists view health as a form of human capital which determines the amount of time available for consumption and for work in the home and labor market.[22] (Individuals may also derive disutility, or even utility, from the state of being ill.) With this type of definition, an appropriate measure of health status over some time period would be the proportion of potential available time that is actually available for the usual consumption, maintenance, and work activities. Similarly, the complementary measure of ill-health would be the proportion of potential available time lost due to inability to function or to imperfect functioning. While such disability may seem to be relatively easy to measure when dealing with adults who are members of the labor force (a good approximation would be days lost from work because of illness), it is not easy to measure for other adults. Moreover, even a measure of days lost from work might not capture losses in consumption time. Therefore, in economists' studies of adults' health, both the incidence of particular physical conditions and the individual's own assessment of his health status have been used as supplementary health status variables in addition to measures of time lost from work (Grossman, 1972).

We use the same type of restricted, morbidity-oriented definition of children's health—focusing on the child's physical health rather than his overall well being—and similar types of measures, i.e., disability, physical conditions, and parental assessment of health status. The use of disability measures (time lost from usual activities), however, and of the incidence of certain physical conditions is somewhat less appropriate for children than for adults.[23] This is because there is a natural sequence of childhood diseases and acute conditions which prevent children from carrying out their normal activities but which do not reflect on the child's health capital or on the child's future prospects for life preservation and normal functioning. A useful distinction to make here is between "permanent" health, which is what we mean by health capital, and "transitory" health, those short-run deviations from one's normal state of health caused by the acute conditions of childhood.[24] It is the child's permanent health status that we wish to study, and we attempt to use those factors which will be good predictors of that permanent health status.[25]

In some situations a single overall index of permanent health might be desired—say, to parsimoniously describe the health status of a population or to allocate public funds. Health, however, clearly is a multidimensional concept. Hence, a single index is not feasible and might not even be desirable from a medical point of view. In particular, even if it were clear what the components of such an index should be, there would be no agreement about the weights assigned to each component. Deriving such weights is especially complicated in the case of children's health because some of the components would be development related: a condition that might be an indication of low capital at one stage of development may not be at another stage of development. Finally, although a single health status index would be conceptually neat, it is possible that the various components of health will be differentially affected by family characteristics. Analysis of a set of components rather than a single index will allow us to detect such differential effects.[26]

The actual choice of components of children's current (measured at the time of the Cycle II survey) physical health status to be examined is controlled by the Cycle II data set and guided by the child health literature,[27] as well as by discussions with public health pediatricians.[28] They are listed and described below.

1. *The parent's assessment of the child's overall current health, represented by* PFGHEALTH. PFGHEALTH is a dichotomous variable indicating whether the parent views the child's health as poor, fair, or good (as opposed to very good).

2. *Current height and weight, represented by* IHEIGHT *and* IWEIGHT. These are standard indicators of children's nutritional status (for example, see National Center for Health Statistics, 1970b, 1975; Seone and Latham, 1971), and good nutrition is an obvious and natural

vehicle for maintaining children's health. Height is a better summary measure of the lifetime nutritional status of the child, whereas weight conveys information primarily about his or her current nutritional status. Since it is well known that physical growth rates differ by age and sex, our height variable is computed as the difference between the child's actual height and the mean height for his or her age-sex group divided by the standard deviation of height for that age-sex group. Current weight is computed in a similar manner.[29]

3. *The child's hearing acuity, represented by* IHEAR.   IHEAR is a dichotomous variable indicating that the child has abnormal hearing. A child is defined to have abnormal hearing if his average threshold decibel reading in his best ear over the range of 500, 1,000, and 2,000 Hz (hertz, or cycles per second) is greater than 15; 500, 1,000, and 2,000 Hz are the frequencies that occur most frequently in normal speech. A threshold of 15 or more decibels above audiometric zero at these frequencies is classified as corresponding to "significant difficulty with faint speech" by the Committee on Conservation of Hearing of the American Academy of Ophthalmology and Otolaryngology (National Center for Health Statistics, 1970a).

4. *The child's visual acuity, represented by the dichotomous variable* ABVIS.   ABVIS indicates whether the child has abnormal distance vision. All children were examined *without* their eyeglasses; their uncorrected binocular distance vision is defined as abnormal if it is worse than 20/30 (National Center for Health Statistics, 1972).[30]

5. *The child's blood pressure, represented by* HDBP.   HDBP is a dummy variable which indicates whether the child's diastolic blood pressure exceeds the 95th percentile for his or her age and sex.

6. *Whether or not the child has hayfever or other allergies, represented by the dummy variable* ALLEG.

7. *An assessment of the child's level of tension, represented by the dummy variable* TENS.   TENS characterizes children who are rated by their parents as "high-strung" or "moderately tense." Both the tension and allergy variables may be regarded as measures of the "new morbidity."

8. *The presence of one or more "significant acquired abnormality" on physical examination of the child, represented by the dummy variable* ACABN.   These abnormalities include heart disease; neurological, muscular, or joint conditions; and other major diseases.[31]

9. *The child's peridontal index, represented by* APERI.   APERI is a good overall indicator of oral health as well as a positive correlate of nutrition (Russell 1956). Due to the significant age and sex trends in this variable, it is standardized by age and sex in the same manner as height and weight. Higher values of APERI denote poorer values of oral health.[32]

10. *Excessive absence from school for health reasons during the past 6 months, represented by the dichotomous variable* SCHABS.   This variable is taken from information provided by the child's school.[33]

In addition to these current health variables, we also analyze a set of measures relating to the child's early health status—his birth weight, his overall health level at the end of his first year, and whether or not he has any congenital abnormalities. These early health measures are analyzed in addition to the set of current health measures for several reasons. First, as indicated in Section II, the assumption of rising marginal cost of investments in health generates demand functions for intermediate health outputs. The child's early health status can be regarded, in part, as an intermediate health output in the sense that it will determine the child's current health. Second, an understanding of how the various family characteristics relate to these early health measures is of intrinsic interest because early health is itself frequently the object of government policy.[34] This is because the child's early health status has been found to have far-reaching impacts not only on his future health but also on other aspects of his future development.[35] Finally, these variables will also appear as explanatory variables in estimating the determinants of the child's current health status as proxies for exogenous health endowments and input prices in infancy and early childhood. Estimates of how various family characteristics relate to early health measures will help unravel the mechanism by which these family characteristics work to effect children's current health.

The exact definitions of the early health variables follow:

1. The child's birth weight is represented by two dummy variables LIGHT$_1$ and LIGHT$_2$. LIGHT$_1$ indicates whether the child was under 2,000 grams (4.4 pounds) at birth, and LIGHT$_2$ indicates whether the child was between 2,000 and 2,500 grams (between 4.4 and 5.5 pounds) at birth. Infants of low birth weight are generally considered to be "at risk" with respect to their health.[36] When LIGHT$_2$ is the dependent variable, observations for which LIGHT$_1$ equals 1 are deleted. Similarly, when LIGHT$_1$ is the dependent variable, observations for which LIGHT$_2$ equals 1 are deleted. Restricting these dependent variables to take on only two values (low birth weight vs. normal birth weight, or very low birth weight vs. normal birth weight) permits clearer interpretation of the coefficients of the explanatory variables.

2. The child's overall health at age 1 year is represented by the dummy variable FYPH, indicating whether the parents' assessment of the child's health at 1 year is poor or fair (as opposed to good).

3. The overall diagnostic impression of the physician concerning whether or not the child had any "significant" abnormalities of a congenital nature is represented by the dummy variable CABN, indicating when the child has such an abnormality.

Precise definitions of the above current and early health measures appear in Table 2, along with a notation concerning the source of each variable (medical history, physician's exam, birth certificate, or school form). Their means and standard deviations are contained in Table A1 in the Appendix.

B. Measurement of Explanatory Variables

The theoretical variables needed for investigating children's health were listed earlier: family wealth, parents' wage rates, parents' educational attainment (or other measures of their efficiency in household production), the child's health endowment, the costs and availability of medical care and other market health inputs, the prices of other inputs used to produce child quality, and family size. Aside from family size, these are the variables that would enter the reduced form demand function for children's health.[37]

Not surprisingly, the actual measures available in the Cycle II survey correspond only very roughly to the aforementioned theoretical variables. We shall discuss these measures and indicate how they relate to the theoretical variables. A complete list of the measures and their precise definitions appear in Table 3. Their means and standard deviations are in Table A1 in the Appendix.

Family wealth and the father's wage rate are both represented by the family income measure. Two income variables are used (FINC, HFINC) in order to allow for the possibility that the relationship between family wealth and children's health differs for high and low-income families.[38] Low-income families are defined as families with an annual income of under $7,000. High-income families are defined as families with an annual income of $7,000 or more. A $7,000 cutoff point is used because it is approximately equal to the median family income in the sample.

The mother's wage rate cannot be measured in any direct way in this survey. We attempt to control for variations in her wage rate by using three variables: (1) her educational attainment (MEDUCAT); (2) her current work status (MWORKFT, MWORKPT); and (3) whether or not she breast-fed her child (BFED). More educated women are likely to have higher market opportunity costs. Similarly, women who are currently in the labor force and who did not breast-feed their children are likely to have higher

Table 2. Definition of Health Measures

Variable Name	Definition	Source[a]
Current health measures		
1. PFGHEALTH	Dummy variable that equals 1 if parental assessment of child's health is poor, fair, or good and 0 if assessment is very good	1
2. IHEIGHT	Height, standardized by the mean and standard deviation of 1-year age-sex cohorts	3
3. IWEIGHT	Weight, standardized by the mean and standard deviation of 1-year age-sex cohorts	3
4. IHEAR	Dummy variable that equals 1 if hearing is abnormal	3
5. ABVIS	Dummy variable that equals 1 if uncorrected binocular distance vision is abnormal and child does not wear glasses	3,1
6. HDBP	Dummy variable that equals 1 if the child's diastolic blood pressure is above the 95th percentile for his age and sex	3
7. ALLEG	Dummy variable that equals 1 if the child has had hayfever or any other kind of allergy	1
8. TENS	Dummy variable that equals 1 if the parent rates the child as high-strung or moderately tense	1
9. ACABN	Dummy variable that equals 1 if the physician finds a "significant" acquired abnormality in examining the child (other than an abnormality resulting from an accident or injury)	3
10. APERI	Peridontal index, standardized by the mean and standard deviation of 1-year age-sex cohorts	3
11. SCHABS	Dummy variable that equals 1 if child has been excessively absent from school for health reasons during the past six months	4
Early health measures		
1. LIGHT$_1$	Dummy variable that equals 1 if child's birth weight was under 2,000 grams (under 4.4 pounds)	2
2. LIGHT$_2$	Dummy variable that equals 1 if child's birth weight was equal to or greater than 2,000 grams but under 2,500 grams (under 5.5 pounds)	2
3. FYPH	Dummy variable that equals 1 if parental assessment of child's health at one year was poor or fair, and zero if it was good	1
4. CABN	Dummy variable that equals 1 if the physician finds a "significant" congenital abnormality in examining the child	3

Notes: [a] The sources are 1 = medical history form completed by parent; 2 = birth certificate; 3 = physical examination; 4 = school form completed by teacher or other school official.

Table 3. Explanatory Variables[a]

Variable Name	Definition

FINC   Continuous family income computed by assigning midpoints to the following closed income intervals, $250 to the lowest interval, and $20,000 to the highest interval. The closed income classes are

$500– $999
$1,000– $1,999
$2,000– $2,999
$3,000– $3,999
$4,000– $4,999
$5,000– $6,999
$7,000–$9,999
$10,000–$14,999

HFINC   Same as FINC for incomes of $7,000 and over; equals 0 for incomes below $7,000

MWORKPT

MWORKFT   Dummy variables that equal 1 if the mother works part-time or full-time, respectively

BFED   Dummy variable that equals 1 if the child was breast-fed

MEDUCAT   Years of formal schooling completed by mother

FEDUCAT   Years of formal schooling completed by father

FLANG   Dummy variable that equals 1 when a foreign language is spoken in the home

MALE   Dummy variable that equals 1 if child is male

LMAG   Dummy variable that equals 1 if the mother was less than 20 years old at birth of child

HMAG   Dummy variable that equals 1 if the mother was more than 35 years old at birth of child

FIRST   Dummy variable that equals 1 if child is the first born in the family

TWIN   Dummy variable that equals 1 if child is a twin

NEAST

MWEST

SOUTH   Dummy variables that equal 1 if child lives in the Northeast, Midwest, or South, respectively; omitted class is residence in West

URB_1

URB_2

URB_3

NURB   Dummy variables that equal 1 if child lives in an urban area with a population of 3 million or more (URB_1); in an area with a population between 1 million and 3 million (URB_2); in an urban area with a population less than 1 million (URB_3); or in a nonrural and nonurbanized area (NURB); omitted class is residence in a rural area

$DENT_{12}$ Dummy variable that equals 1 if child has been to a dentist sometime in his life but not within the last 12 months

$DENTIST_3$ Dummy variable that equals 1 if child has never been to a dentist

LESS 20   Number of persons in the household 20 years of age or less

NOFATH   Dummy variable that equals one if child lives with mother only

Note: [a] All of these variables are taken from the medical history form.

49

opportunity costs both currently and when the child was an infant. (The labor force status measure in Cycle II pertains only to the time of the survey; information about breast-feeding is used as a crude proxy for the mother's opportunity cost at an earlier period in the child's life because mothers who breast-feed are less likely to have been in the labor force during the child's infancy.)

Of course, interpretation of the coefficient of both of the labor force status and breast-feeding variables is very much affected by their endogenous nature. That is, women in families with a stronger preference for high-quality children will be less likely to be in the labor force during their children's youth and more likely to breast-feed, no matter what their opportunity cost is. Thus, a negative relationship between mother's work status and her child's health or a positive relationship between breast-feeding and the child's health may be interpreted either as a taste effect or a price (wage) effect, or both.[39] Put differently, these variables can be regarded as endogenous inputs in a child health production function as well as measures of the mother's wage rate.[40]

Mother's and father's educational attainment (MEDUCAT, FEDUCAT) represent the parents' efficiency in producing healthy children. A supplementary efficiency (or taste) measure is a variable indicating whether a foreign language is spoken in the home (FLANG). Foreign-born and native families are likely to exhibit differences in tastes and/or household production efficiency.

The child's endowed health status is represented by a set of variables relating to his early health. Four of these, mentioned earlier, are clearly endogenous to some extent: birth weight (LIGHT$_1$, LIGHT$_2$), the child's health at age one (FYPH), and the presence of congenital abnormalities (CABN). Two additional measures are the child's sex (MALE) and the age of the mother at the time of the child's birth (LMAG, HMAG). Two mother's age variables are used—one identifying very young mothers (LMAG), and one identifying those over age 35 at the time of the child's birth (HMAG). Mother's age is included among the health endowment measures because older mothers are more likely to bear children with health defects whereas young mothers are more likely to have unwanted births and consequently receive poorer prenatal care.[41] The child's sex is included because of the well-documented higher incidence rates of certain health problems among males at young ages (for example, see National Council for Health Statistics, 1973b). Note that if genetic factors are not fully captured by the endowed and early health measures, the observed effects of variables such as parents' education may contain a genetic component.

In addition to these early health endowment measures, we also control for several exogenously determined characteristics of the child which may cause him to receive better or worse treatment within the family simply by virtue of his luck in possessing these characteristics. They are his sex (MALE), his birth order (FIRST), and whether or not he is a twin (TWIN). For example, first-born children (or nontwins) will have greater access to individual parental attention because they arrived in the family first (or they arrived alone). Similarly, male children may receive larger investments than female children if males are preferred to females (see Ben Porath and Welch, 1976).

Direct information about the prices of inputs in the health production function and in the other household production functions is not available in the Cycle II data. Moreover, since the precise locality of each observation cannot be identified at the present time,[42] it is not possible to estimate these prices with local market data. Therefore, to partially control for these prices we use a set of three *region* and four *size of place of residence* variables. (These variables will also control for other regional differences that are not otherwise accounted for.) In addition, information about the last time the child visited a dentist (DENT$_{12}$ and DENTIST$_3$) is used to provide a somewhat more specific index of the price and availability of medical care. The latter variables not only are proxies for the price and availability of medical care in the area but also for the family's preferences and attitudes concerning preventive care.[43]

Finally, family size is represented by the number of people in the family who are under 20 years of age (LESS 20).[44]

C. A Note on the Role of Family Size

Earlier, in discussing the various economic models of child quality, we pointed out that family size acts as one determinant of the marginal cost of various aspects of child quality, including children's health. We also pointed out that both the number of children in a family and the quality of each child are jointly determined by the family (subject to chance events). This endogeneity of family size poses the usual problem of bias in its coefficient estimate unless appropriate simultaneous estimation techniques are used.[45] Such techniques cannot be used in this case, however, because the same set of exogenous explanatory variables determine both the number and the quality of children.

As an alternative procedure, we estimate children's health equations in two ways, both with and without the family size variable included. When family size is included, the other variable coefficients will reflect effects in children's health with family size held constant. The coefficient of the family size variable will indicate (with bias) the substitutability in family demand between the quantity and quality dimensions of children. When the family size variable is excluded from the children's health equations, the other explanatory variables will reflect both direct effects on child health and those indirect effects that operate via family size.[46]

We conclude this section with a recapitulation of the type of equations to be estimated. The dependent variables are the health measures listed in Table 2, and the explanatory variables are those listed in Table 3. In addition, when current health measures are the dependent variables, the four endogenous early health measures in Table 2 (LIGHT$_1$, LIGHT$_2$, FYPH, and CABN) are also used as explanatory variables. These equations are not pure reduced form demand equations for the various aspects of children's health for two reasons. First, some of the relevant input prices are missing, and proxy measures are used that in many cases also represent endogenous input quantities. For example, mother's work status not only reflects her potential wage but also (and even more directly) the amount of time she spends with her children. A similar comment can be made with respect to the breast-feeding and dentist visit variables as well as some of the early health measures. Thus, when family size is excluded, a hybrid of a reduced form demand equation for children's health and a production function of children's health is estimated. Second, when family size is included, we are including an endogenous variable from a structural demand equation. The estimated relationship is then a mixture of a structural demand equation, a reduced form demand equation, and a production function. Interpretation of our results will allow for the hybrid nature of the estimating equations.

IV. EMPIRICAL RESULTS

The equations described in the previous section are estimated using white children who live with either both of their parents or with their mothers only. There were 5,768 such children in the Cycle II sample. The exclusion of children for whom there were missing data brings the final sample to 4,196.[47] Data for both types of family composition are pooled for analysis because preliminary estimates indicated that there were no significant differences in the sets of slope coefficients for all dependent variables except SCHABS. A dummy variable identifying children who live with their mothers only (NOFATH) is included to allow for differences in children's health that may be uniquely associated with the absence of a father.

We do not use data for black children in estimating the equations because preliminary analysis revealed significant race differences in slope coefficients for more than half of our measures of health.[48] It was felt that including these children would lead to misleading results in the sense that a race dummy variable would not reflect true differences in health associated with race. Nor would the pooled coefficient estimates of the family characteristics variables be appropriate for interpreting health variations within the black sample. While we do not present separate estimates for black children in this paper (the black sample is too small to allow for reliable coefficient estimates), we do comment briefly on black–white differences in children's health in Section V.

The method of estimation is ordinary least squares. Although this is not the optimal econometric procedure to use when the dependent variable is dichotomous, use of LOGIT[49] or another appropriate nonlinear estimation procedure is not feasible given the sample size and number of variables in our empirical work. To determine whether this misspecification is likely to greatly affect our results when the dependent variables are dichotomous, we experimented with alternative estimation procedures on a subsample of one-third of our basic sample. Using two dependent variables with a low incidence (LIGHT$_1$ and LIGHT$_2$) and one with an incidence near .5 (PFGHEALTH), we obtained both ordinary least squares (OLS) and LOGIT estimates of our equations for this subsample. In all cases the differences between alternate estimators are small: OLS coefficients and the analogous marginal effects in LOGIT are of similar magnitudes and signs, and the patterns of statistical significance do not alter. Indeed, the differences between these OLS and LOGIT estimates for the one-third subsample are much less than are the differences between OLS estimates for the full sample and for the one-third subsample. On the basis of these experiments we believe that OLS estimation applied to the full sample provides the most reliable picture of the relationship between measures of health and the various explanatory variables. Of course, the usual statistical tests on a single coefficient or on sets of coefficients can only be interpreted as suggestive when the dependent variable is dichotomous because the assumptions underlying these tests are not satisfied.

We organize our discussion of the results around groups of explanatory variables. Therefore, rather than presenting estimates of the equations in a single massive table, we have chosen to partition the results into several tables, each showing the coefficients of a subset of explanatory variables. It should be emphasized, however, that the coefficients in each of these tables are taken from multiple regression estimates that contain the complete set of explanatory variables listed in Table 3 (plus the four endogenous early health variables, when relevant). These coefficients, therefore, reflect the partial effects of the associated explanatory variables. Results based on the inclusion of both family size and the endogenous early health measures are the focus of our discussion because it was found that the results were, on the whole, insensitive to the inclusion or exclusion of these variables. Exceptions will be noted in the discussions below.

A. Overview

The first and most obvious question to ask is are these health measures amenable to statistical explanation with the set of variables considered here? To answer this question we present adjusted R^2 values and F statistics for the entire equations (Table 4). In all cases except for hearing acuity, excessive school absence, and poor vision, the equations are statistically significant at the 1 percent level of significance.[50] Thus, we can conclude that for most of the health measures we study, observed variations in our sample are not caused solely by chance but rather are systematically related to the set of family, endowment, and region and city size characteristics considered here.

B. Exogenous Family Characteristics

Since the prime focus of this paper is the relationship between family characteristics and children's health, we begin by looking at the measures of exogenous family characteristics—income, parents' education, whether

Table 4.   Adjusted R Squares for the Basic Equations[a]

Dependent Variable	Adjusted R^2	F Statistic
Early health		
LIGHT$_1$	.027	(5.76*)
LIGHT$_2$	.041	(8.23*)
FYPH	.011	(2.86*)
CABN	.005	(1.94*)
Current health[b]		
PFGHEALTH	.102	(17.95*)
IHEAR	− .002	(0.76)
ABVIS	− .001	(0.86)
HDBP	.010	(2.62*)
ALLEG	.049	(8.65*)
TENS	.024	(4.68*)
ACABN	.009	(2.42*)
SCHABS	.004	(1.49)
IHEIGHT	.072	(13.00*)
IWEIGHT	.060	(10.88*)
APERI	.111	(20.39*)

Notes:
* Statistically significant at the 1 percent level of significance; F statistics are for the entire equations.
[a] These statistics are based on estimates which include all variables in Table 3 as explanatory variables.
[b] These statistics are based on estimates which also include the four early health variables as explanatory variables.

or not a father lives with the family, and whether or not a foreign language is spoken in the home. The coefficients of these variables appear in Table 5.

The partial effects of income on the various current and early health measures are surprisingly small and are statistically significant only for the variables PFGHEALTH, SCHABS, IWEIGHT, and APERI. In some cases, the sign of FINC reflects a perverse relationship in the sense that higher income is associated with poorer rather than better health (IHEAR, HDBP, FYPH, ALLEG, ACABN, TENS, SCHABS). Among the health measures for which income is statistically significant, such a perverse relationship is reported for SCHABS, and this effect disappears in the higher income class (the coefficient of HFINC is opposite in sign and similar in magnitude to the coefficient of FINC). In two of the other cases where there are statistically significant income effects (i.e., PFGHEALTH, APERI), the relationship between income and health is positive and is virtually constant over both income classes (the coefficient of HFINC is small and nonsignificant). The relationship between income and weight reflects positive health effects for low weight levels and negative health effects for high weight levels. To summarize, while income does have a significant relationship with four of the fifteen health measures, the weight of the evidence leads one to conclude that, overall, income is not an important factor for explaining health variations among children.

Unlike family income, the parents' educational attainment measures have positive and significant effects on many of the current health measures. In fact, for every current health measure but IHEAR, ABVIS, IWEIGHT, and SCHABS, at least one of the parents' education measures is statistically significant. This result is consistent with the notion that children's health is produced in the home and that higher parental education leads to greater efficiency in health production.

One might predict that mother's education is more important in explaining variations in children's health than is father's education since most child care is done by the mother. We do not consistently observe this in our results. One reason might be the high correlation between mother's and father's education ($r = .67$ in mother–father families). Contrary to expectations, however, significant *inverse* relationships between health and parents' education are reported for ALLEG, TENS, and ACABN. For the first two, this may be a result of a reporting bias in that more educated parents may be more sensitive to subtle aspects of ill health in their children. An alternative explanation is that more educated parents may be more demanding regarding their children's behavior and achievement, creating greater tension and accompanying allergies. For the third variable, ACABN, we have no explanation for the inverse relationship.

Table 5. Coefficients of Exogenous Family Characteristics[a] (F statistics in parentheses)

Explanatory Variables	Early Health Dependent Variables[b]				Current Health Dependent Variables		
	LIGHT$_1$	LIGHT$_2$	FYPH	CABN	PFGHEALTH	IHEAR	ABVIS
FINC	.0002	.003	.0003	−.0003	−.012	.0001	−.003
	(0.02)	(1.66)	(0.01)	(0.20)	(5.81)	(0.005)	(1.15)
HFINC	−.0002	−.003	.0006	.0005	.0001	−.0001	.002
	(0.05)	(3.25)	(0.09)	(0.11)	(0.003)	(0.04)	(1.58)
FEDUCAT	·.000	−.002	−.006	−.001	−.010	−.0005	.002
	(0.00)	(0.03)	(12.31)	(0.69)	(10.56)	(0.92)	(1.73)
MEDUCAT	−.0009	−.003	−.004	−.002	−.007	−.0003	−.003
	(0.92)	(2.66)	(2.87)	(0.83)	(3.42)	(0.35)	(2.56)
FLANG	.007	−.011	−.025	.008	−.002	−.004	.004
	(1.18)	(0.92)	(2.75)	(0.42)	(0.00)	(0.82)	(0.10)
NOFATH	−.013	.002	−.070	.010	−.132	−.008	.018
	(1.56)	(0.01)	(7.97)	(0.27)	(10.01)	(1.47)	(0.70)

Notes: [a] Coefficients are statistically significant at the 5 percent level if the F is greater than 3.84 for a two-tailed test, or 2.69 for a one-tailed test.

[b] These coefficients are taken from equation estimates which include all variables in Table 3 as explanatory variables.

[c] These coefficients are taken from equation estimates which include all variables in Table 3 plus LIGHT$_1$, LIGHT$_2$, FYPH, and CABN as explanatory variables.

With respect to the early health measures, parents' education has significant positive health effects only on FYPH, the parents' retrospective assessment of the child's health at age 1 year. It is not related to the other three early health measures.

Children from families where a foreign language is spoken in the home do not have significantly different current or early health levels from other children with the exception of the two measures ACABN and TENS. Children from such families are more likely to exhibit an acquired abnormality, but they are less likely to be considered tense by their parents.

Differences in children's health associated with the presence or absence of a father in the household at the time of the survey are not clear-cut. The coefficient of the dummy variable NOFATH indicates significant positive associations with better health when FYPH, PFGHEALTH, HDBP, and APERI are the health measures, and significant negative associations with better health when health is measured by school absenteeism. The Coefficient of NOFATH, however, does not tell the whole story; in fact, it tells only a biased version of the story. This is because for the children with absent fathers there are no data on the educational attainment of their fathers. Given alternative assumptions about the relationship be-

Table 5.   (cont.)

				Current Health Dependent Variables[c]			
HDBP	ALLEG	TENS	ACABN	SCHABS	IHEIGHT	IWEIGHT	APERI
.002	.001	.001	.002	.004	.001	.019	− .017
(0.97)	(0.08)	(0.04)	(0.93)	(3.72)	(0.02)	(3.62)	(4.83)
− .002	.0002	− .002	− .002	− .004	.007	− .008	.004
(1.09)	(0.004)	(0.45)	(1.79)	(5.43)	(0.93)	(1.23)	(0.75)
− .003	.006	− .003	.002	.002	.010	.006	− .020
(3.71)	(6.86)	(0.68)	(3.52)	(1.15)	(2.81)	(0.81)	(18.13)
− .003	.007	.007	− .0002	− .002	.013	.003	− .017
(2.56)	(7.09)	(3.58)	(0.02)	(0.78)	(2.96)	(0.16)	(9.74)
− .013	− .014	− .069	.025	− .012	− .066	.025	− .013
(1.67)	(0.51)	(6.79)	(6.12)	(1.14)	(1.70)	(0.24)	(0.12)
− .057	.052	− .051	− .001	.046	.091	.015	− .185
(8.29)	(2.73)	(1.38)	(0.00)	(5.54)	(1.20)	(0.03)	(8.52)

tween father's education and children's health within families where the father is absent, minimum and maximum estimates of the pure effect of an absent father can be obtained. Both types of estimates are presented in Table 6. "Minimum" estimates (which are the same as those in Table 5) are shown in the second column; they are minimum in the sense that their derivation is based on the assumption that father's education has no effect on child health if the father is absent. "Maximum" estimates are shown in the fourth column; they are based on the assumption that father's education has the same effect on child health whether or not the father is actually present.[51] Obviously, reality lies somewhere in between: while there is every reason to believe that the effect of father's education on child health will be smaller for children in families where the father is no longer present, it is hard to believe that his education had no impact, even if his tenure in the family was very short.[52] Without data on the education of missing fathers, however, we must settle for the range of estimates in Table 6.

Even when we look at this range of estimates, however, the impact on children's health of having an absent father cannot be readily summarized. Both negative and positive effects are still observed, sometimes for the same health measure. The only two health measures for which both the minimum and maximum estimates are of the same sign and are significant are SCHABS (children with absent fathers are more likely to be absent from school for health reasons) and HDBP (children with absent fathers are less likely to have very high diastolic blood pressure readings).

Table 6.   Minimum and Maximum Effects of Not Having a Father
Living with the Family[a]

Dependent Variables	Mininum Effect[b]	F Statistic	Maximum Effect[c]	F Statistic
Early Health				
LIGHT$_1$	− .013	(1.56)	− .013	(3.04)
LIGHT$_2$	.002	(0.01)	.004	(0.11)
FYPH	− .070	(7.97)	.003	(0.02)
CABN	.010	(0.27)	.023	(2.71)
Current Health				
PFGHEALTH	− .132	(10.01)	− .019	(0.38)
IHEAR	− .008	(1.47)	− .003	(0.32)
ABVIS	.018	(0.70)	− .006	(0.13)
HDBP	− .057	(8.29)	− .025	(3.00)
ALLEG	.052	(2.73)	− .017	(0.53)
TENS	− .051	(1.38)	− .021	(0.44)
ACABN	− .001	(0.001)	− .026	(4.77)
SCHABS	.046	(5.54)	.027	(3.71)
IHEIGHT	.091	(1.20)	− .025	(0.17)
IWEIGHT	.015	(0.03)	− .049	(0.61)
APERI	− .185	(8.52)	.040	(0.75)

Notes:[a] All results are taken from regressions that include LESS 20 and, where applicable, the four
  endogenous early health measures. Coefficients are statistically significant at the 5 percent
  level if the F is greater than 3.84 for a two-tailed test or 2.69 for a one-tailed test.
  [b] See note 51 for a definition of the minimum effect.
  [c] See note 51 for a definition of the maximum effect.

For the other measures, either one of the two estimates is not significant
or they change signs, or both.[53] The only conclusion that can be drawn
from these ambiguous results is that having an absent father is neither
a clear health disadvantage nor health advantage to a child.

C.   Endogenous Family Characteristics

Table 7 contains coefficients of the mother's current work status
(MWORKFT, MWORKPT) and whether or not she breast-fed her child (BFED).
In general, breast-feeding is an important correlate of favorable early
health outcomes and is statistically significant for three of these four
measures. Special caution, however, must be used when interpreting the
strong negative relationship between BFED and the two low birth weight
measures. The most likely explanation for this relationship is drawn from
the nature of hospital procedures: low-birth-weight babies require special
care and medical procedures that may not be altogether compatible with
breast-feeding. Thus, the reported coefficients of BFED in the LIGHT$_1$ and
LIGHT$_2$ equations may simply mean that hospital personnel discourage

Table 7.   Coefficients of Endogenous Family Characteristics[a]

Dependent Variables	BFED Coefficient	F	MWORKPT Coefficient	F	MWORKFT Coefficient	F
Early health[b]						
LIGHT₁	− .015	(14.51)	− .001	(0.35)	.009	(2.93)
LIGHT₂	− .017	(5.74)	− .006	(0.38)	.013	(2.13)
FYPH	− .008	(0.69)	.009	(0.47)	.015	(1.48)
CABN	− .016	(4.59)	− .014	(1.92)	− .011	(1.27)
Current Health[c]						
PFGHEALTH	− .047	(8.22)	.030	(1.89)	.028	(1.79)
IHEAR	− .001	(0.26)	− .004	(1.51)	− .001	(0.09)
ABVIS	− .004	(0.20)	− .017	(2.16)	.008	(0.49)
HDBP	.004	(0.26)	− .001	(0.01)	.003	(0.11)
ALLEG	.023	(3.61)	− .004	(0.05)	.010	(0.40)
TENS	− .019	(1.18)	− .013	(0.31)	− .035	(2.50)
ACABN	− .005	(0.61)	− .006	(0.51)	.011	(1.86)
SCHABS	− .005	(0.46)	− .0004	(0.00)	.001	(0.02)
IHEIGHT	.053	(2.59)	− .126	(8.21)	− .057	(1.87)
IWEIGHT	.027	(0.63)	− .017	(0.15)	.019	(0.19)
APERI	.008	(0.11)	.006	(0.04)	.084	(6.88)

Notes:[a] Coefficients are statistically significant at the 5 percent level if the F is greater than 3.84 for
a two-tailed test, or 2.69 for a one-tailed test.
[b] These coefficients are taken from equation estimates which include all variables in Table 3
as explanatory variables.
[c] These coefficients are taken from equation estimates which include all variables in Table 3
plus LIGHT₁, LIGHT₂, and CABN as explanatory variables.

mothers from breast-feeding low-birth-weight babies. The relationships between breast-feeding and the various current health measures are not statistically significant except when PFGHEALTH or ALLEG is the dependent variable. Breast-feeding lowers the probability that a child is rated as having poor, fair, or good current health (raises the probability that he is rated as having very good health) and raises the probability that he has an allergy.

The dichotomous variable that compares the health of children whose mothers currently work part-time to the health of children whose mothers do not currently work (MWORKPT) has a statistically significant negative coefficient in the height equation alone. The estimate indicates that children are shorter if their mothers work part-time. The analogous variable comparing the health of children whose mothers currently work full-time to that of children whose mothers do not work at all (MWORKFT) is statistically significant in two instances—when very low birth weight (LIGHT₁) or the peridontal index (APERI) is the dependent variable. In each instance health is lower if the mother works full-time. In general the results reveal that participation by mothers in the labor market is not particularly detrimental to the health of their children, subject to the qualification that birth weight, current height, and oral health are worse when the mother works.[54]

Interpretations of the roles of mother's labor force status and breast-feeding in the health equations must take into account the hybrid nature of these equations. As was indicated in Section III, the estimated health equation is a mixture of a demand curve for health and a production function of health. In a demand setting, mother's labor force status reflects the value of her time and her preferences for children. In a production setting, it is an indicator of the amount of time she spends with her children. Similarly, breast-feeding is an indicator of preferences, the amount and value of time mothers spent with their children, as well as being a direct physical input into good health. In addition, the breast-feeding variable may serve as proxy for the amount and quality of pre-natal care received by the mother.

D. Exogenous Endowments

Regression coefficients of the child's exogenous health endowment measures are given in Table 8. Significant male–female health differentials are present in the case of very low birth weight, parental rating of health at one year, abnormal vision, allergies, and tension. Except for the vision and birth weight effects, the differentials indicate more health problems for male children. These sex effects replicate, in general, the results of other studies and do not merit additional discussion.

Not surprisingly, twins weigh less at birth than most other children do. The only other significant twin-status coefficient is for allergies. We offer no explanation of the lower reported incidence of allergies among twins.

First-born children are in better health than other children according to some of our health measures, but they are in worse health according to others. First-borns are taller and heavier than their peers, although they weigh somewhat less at birth. They also are more likely to have an allergy and to be tense. These current health effects are consistent with the notion that first-born children receive relatively more time and attention from their parents than do other children: their rate of physical development is more rapid, despite their lower weight at birth; and they exhibit a greater incidence of allergies and tension. The latter finding is similar to the positive effects of mother's schooling on these two variables.

There is no evidence in Table 8 that a mother's age at the birth of her child has a significant impact on her child's early health status, but there are significant impacts on the current height and weight measures. The

Table 8. Coefficients of Exogenous Endowments[a]
(F statistics in parentheses)

	MALE	TWIN	FIRST	LMAG	HMAG
Early Health[b]					
LIGHT$_1$	−.008	.164	.007	−.009	.002
	(5.15)	(154.91)	(2.80)	(1.77)	(0.07)
LIGHT$_2$	−.006	.022	.011	.014	.008
	(0.97)	(94.00)	(1.87)	(1.28)	(0.53)
FYPH	.020	.016	−.017	.018	−.003
	(5.26)	(0.30)	(2.62)	(1.05)	(0.04)
CABN	.009	−.004	−.004	−.020	.007
	(1.77)	(0.03)	(0.28)	(2.08)	(0.42)
Current Health[c]					
PFGHEALTH	−.009	−.023	−.024	−.060	.058
	(0.35)	(0.20)	(1.69)	(4.07)	(5.77)
IHEAR	.002	−.005	.000	−.005	−.001
	(0.75)	(0.42)	(0.03)	(0.95)	(0.13)
ABVIS	−.023	.017	.004	−.015	−.003
	(9.41)	(0.44)	(0.15)	(1.00)	(0.07)
HDBP[d]	—	−.025	.009	−.012	.022
	—	(1.05)	(1.08)	(0.74)	(3.65)
ALLEG	.031	−.080	.025	−.005	−.011
	(8.02)	(4.48)	(3.26)	(0.05)	(0.38)
TENS	.054	−.004	.131	−.018	.033
	(12.62)	(0.01)	(47.49)	(0.32)	(1.65)
ACABN	−.004	−.020	.007	−.010	.0002
	(0.44)	(0.96)	(1.07)	(0.68)	(0.01)
SCHABS	−.007	.011	−.001	−.013	.009
	(1.14)	(0.24)	(0.02)	(0.88)	(0.73)
IHEIGHT[d]	—	.133	.132	−.176	.127
	—	(1.75)	(13.35)	(8.80)	(6.87)
IWEIGHT[d]	—	.121	.140	−.185	.169
	—	(1.37)	(14.20)	(9.25)	(11.67)
APERI[d]	—	−.037	.018	.120	.017
	—	(0.24)	(0.42)	(7.12)	(0.21)

Notes: [a] Coefficients are statistically significant at the 5 percent level if the "F" is greater than 3.84 for a two-tailed test or 2.69 for a one-tailed test.
[b] These coefficients are taken from equation estimates which include all variables in Table 3 as explanatory variables.
[c] These coefficients are taken from equation estimates which include all variables in Table 3 plus LIGHT$_1$, LIGHT$_2$, FYPH, and CABN as explanatory variables.
[d] Variable is sex adjusted.

coefficient of LMAG indicates that children whose mothers were less than 20 years old when they gave birth are lighter and shorter than children whose mothers were between the ages of 20 and 35 when they gave birth. In contrast, children whose mothers were over the age of 35 when they gave birth are heavier and taller than children whose mothers were between the ages of 20 and 35. The only other significant effects of mother's age are in the PFGHEALTH equation. Young mothers are more likely, and older mothers less likely, to rate their children's current health status as very good.

The observed relationships between mother's age at birth and children's health reflect two forces that go in opposite directions. As suggested in Section III, relatively young mothers are probably in better physical health when they give birth but are more likely to have unwanted births and consequently receive poorer prenatal care and spend less time with their children. Births at relatively old ages pose health risks both to mothers and children, but older mothers might spend more time with their children. Our results imply that the time and prenatal care effects outweigh the purely physical health factor associated with mother's age at birth. In the case of parental assessment of the child's current health, the observed effects might also be partially a result of a reporting bias in that older mothers apply higher standards than do younger mothers in evaluating their children's health.

E. Endogenous Early Health Measures

The regression coefficients of the endogenous early health measures—LIGHT$_1$, LIGHT$_2$, FYPH, and CABN—capture exogenous health endowment effects as well as early input and input price effects. These estimates, in Table 9, show that favorable early health is an important predictor of favorable current health. In ten of the eleven current health equations, at least one of the four early health variables has a statistically significant regression coefficient (the exception is when ABVIS is the dependent variable). Both LIGHT$_1$ and LIGHT$_2$ are significant in the current height and current weight equations, and one of these two variables is a significant correlate of parental rating of current health, presence of acquired abnormalities, and excessive school absence. The presence of congenital abnormalities (CABN) increases the probabilities of the presence of poor hearing and acquired abnormalities and lowers height and weight. FYPH has significant effects on all current health measures except weight and abnormal vision. This last result is noteworthy because it indicates a close association between a subjective health measure reported by parents and objective health measures based on physical examinations.

Table 9. Coefficients of Endogenous Early Health Measures[a] (F statistics in parentheses)

Explanatory Variable	PFGHEALTH	IHEAR	ABVIS	HDBP	ALLEG	TENS	ACABN	SCHABS	IHEIGHT	IWEIGHT	APERI
$LIGHT_1$	−.052	−.007	−.002	.037	−.021	.081	.049	.052	−.481	−.380	.070
	(0.60)	(0.43)	(0.00)	(1.34)	(0.17)	(1.34)	(3.41)	(2.84)	(13.09)	(7.75)	(0.49)
$LIGHT_2$	.070	−.001	−.011	−.007	−.020	.030	−.008	.009	−.431	−.380	−.040
	(3.64)	(0.01)	(0.35)	(0.17)	(0.52)	(0.60)	(0.29)	(0.26)	(34.69)	(24.91)	(0.51)
CABN	.034	.003	.011	.003	−.002	.042	.035	−.020	−.140	−.151	.081
	(1.03)	(3.69)	(0.38)	(0.03)	(0.00)	(1.39)	(6.83)	(1.62)	(4.36)	(4.86)	(2.54)
FYPH	.236	.008	.012	.047	.141	.112	.044	.038	−.108	−.030	.130
	(79.84)	(3.99)	(0.80)	(14.14)	(50.27)	(16.25)	(17.78)	(9.61)	(4.20)	(0.31)	(10.59)

Note: [a] Coefficients are statistically significant at the 5 percent level if the F is greater than 3.84 for a two-tailed test or 2.69 for a one-tailed test. Coefficients are taken from equation estimates which include all variables in Table 3 plus $LIGHT_1$, $LIGHT_2$, FYPH, and CABN as explanatory variables.

63

Despite the importance of the early health variables in the current health functions, the parameter estimates of the other independent variables are hardly altered when the early health variables are excluded. For this reason we show results only for the full equations. The parameter estimates of family characteristics are not sensitive to the exclusion of early health because the relationships between these characteristics and early health are weak, as has already been indicated. In those instances in which family characteristics and early health are significantly related, the magnitudes of the effects are small. This implies that early health measures are important independent determinants of current health.

F.   Medical Care Measures

Table 10 shows regression coefficients of the dichotomous variables that identify children who last saw a dentist more than one year ago (DENT_{12}) and children who have never seen a dentist (DENTIST_3). Except in the peridontal index equation, these variables serve as negative proxies of the amount of preventive medical care and positive proxies of the

Table 10.   Coefficients of Proxy Variables for Medical Care[a]

Dependent Variables	DENT_{12}		DENTIST_3	
	Coefficient	F Statistic	Coefficient	F Statistic
Early health[b]				
LIGHT_1	− .001	(0.03)	− .003	(0.29)
LIGHT_2	− .010	(1.26)	− .010	(1.16)
FYPH	.014	(1.36)	− .003	(0.07)
CABN	− .007	(0.49)	− .010	(1.05)
Current health[c]				
PFGHEALTH	.096	(21.60)	.088	(15.91)
IHEAR	.003	(0.76)	.002	(0.21)
ABVIS	.007	(0.44)	.009	(0.69)
HDBP	− .022	(4.95)	− .011	(1.07)
ALLEG	− .045	(8.39)	− .045	(7.29)
TENS	− .028	(1.63)	.001	(0.00)
ACABN	.015	(3.55)	.015	(3.05)
SCHABS	.002	(0.07)	.015	(2.27)
IHEIGHT	− .104	(6.39)	− .209	(22.50)
IWEIGHT	− .016	(0.15)	− .106	(5.53)
APERI	.070	(5.00)	.090	(7.21)

Notes: [a] Coefficients are statistically significant at the 5 percent level if the F is greater than 3.84 for a two-tailed test or 2.69 for a one-tailed test.
   [b] These coefficients are taken from equation estimates which include all variables in Table 3 as explanatory variables.
   [c] These coefficients are taken from equation estimates which include all variables in Table 3 plus LIGHT_1, LIGHT_2, FYPH, and CABN as explanatory variables.

price of preventive care. Put differently, parents of children who saw a dentist within the past year are more likely to obtain preventive medical care services for their children and to face a lower price of care. These parents may also have preferences for high-quality children.

The dental variables never have significant impacts on the early health functions. The picture is somewhat different, however, in the current health function. Both dental variables are statistically significant in the peridontal index, height, acquired abnormality, allergy, and parental assessment of health equations. In addition, the coefficient of DENTIST$_3$ is significant in the weight equation, and the coefficient of DENT$_{12}$ is significant in the diastolic blood pressure equation. Except for the allergy and blood pressure relationships, children who saw a dentist within the past year have higher levels of health than children who saw a dentist more than 1 year ago or children who never saw a dentist. The dentist visit–allergy relationship probably reflects a greater awareness of allergy problems among parents who took their children to a dentist within the past year. The dentist visit–blood pressure relationship is puzzling, and we offer no explanation of it.

In the height, weight, and peridontal index equations, the coefficient of DENTIST$_3$ is large relative to the coefficients of other independent variables. In the height regression its coefficient equals 21 percent of the standard deviation in height. The corresponding figures in the weight and peridontal index regressions are 11 percent and 12 percent, respectively. The importance of DENTIST$_3$ is underscored by noting that 18 percent of the children in the sample never saw a dentist. Thus, our proxies for preventive medical care appear to have important impacts on those health measures that reflect basic nutritional status. The statistically significant effects of the two dental variables on the peridontal index are particularly noteworthy. In this case our estimates directly measure the effect of oral health input on oral health output. Therefore, the beneficial input effects that we report are likely to be understated due to reverse causality that runs from a reduction in oral health to an increase in the probability of contacting a dentist.

G. Region and City Size Effects

Table 11 contains estimates of the effects of region and city size on early and current health. The significant relationships in Table 11 can be traced to a number of factors. There are differences in the availability and price of medical care by region and city size that are not captured by the other independent variables in the regressions. Moreover, there are differences in climate, air pollution levels, fluoridation levels, and ethnic composition of the population. Finally, there are factors associated

Table 11.   Coefficients of Region and City Size[a] (F statistics in parentheses)

Explanatory Variables	Early Health Dependent Variables[b]				Current Health Dependent Variables[c]		
	LIGHT$_1$	LIGHT$_2$	FYPH	CABN	PFGHEALTH	IHEAR	ABVIS
NEAST	.015	.007	.0001	.014	−.077	.0001	.005
	(8.04)	(0.60)	(0.00)	(1.74)	(11.80)	(0.000)	(0.19)
MWEST	−.011	.006	−.004	.036	−.034	−.001	.005
	(5.22)	(0.47)	(0.09)	(15.56)	(2.89)	(0.12)	(0.23)
SOUTH	−.010	.026	.010	.019	.066	−.005	.006
	(3.16)	(6.76)	(0.54)	(3.14)	(8.02)	(1.91)	(0.29)
URB$_1$	−.002	.016	−.018	−.022	.019	−.004	.013
	(0.09)	(2.77)	(1.84)	(4.44)	(0.69)	(1.08)	(1.31)
URB$_2$	−.003	−.0003	−.025	−.007	−.068	−.001	.003
	(0.21)	(0.001)	(2.88)	(0.37)	(7.21)	(0.08)	(0.07)
URB$_3$	−.005	.013	−.007	−.017	.007	.001	.003
	(0.98)	(2.07)	(0.29)	(2.83)	(0.10)	(0.04)	(0.07)
NURB	−.002	.014	.006	−.003	−.046	.0005	.008
	(0.10)	(1.97)	(0.18)	(0.08)	(3.94)	(0.02)	(0.52)

Notes: [a] Coefficients are statistically significant at the 5 percent level if the F is greater than 3.84 for a two-tailed test or 2.69 for a one-tailed test.
     [b] These coefficients are taken from equation estimates which include all variables in Table 3 as explanatory variables.
     [c] These coefficients are taken from equation estimates which include all variables in Table 3 plus LIGHT$_1$, LIGHT$_2$, FYPH, and CABN as explanatory variables.

with the stress and tension of residence in large metropolitan areas. This list of factors is not meant to be exhaustive; we leave a complete explanation of the differences in Table 11 as an area for future research.

H. Family Size

Family size (LESS 20) had a special role in our theoretical discussion because of its clearly endogenous nature. Consequently, estimates of our basic equations were promised (and were in fact calculated) with family size excluded as well as included. Yet all of the results discussed so far are taken from estimates with family size included. The reason we have discussed only these results is that family size turned out to be a statistically significant variable for only four of the health measures—PFGHEALTH, IHEIGHT, IWEIGHT, and ALLEG (see Table 12). In all other cases, it was not significant and its inclusion did not appreciably alter the coefficients of other explanatory variables.

When health is measured by the four variables PFGHEALTH, IHEIGHT, IWEIGHT, and ALLEG, children coming from larger families have significantly poorer health. Whether this relationship reflects quality–quantity

Table 11. (Cont.)

			Current Health Dependent Variables[c]				
HDBP	ALLEG	TENS	ACABN	SCHABS	IHEIGHT	IWEIGHT	APERI
.009	− .071	− .004	.022	.013	.045	.028	.491
(0.78)	(17.38)	(0.03)	(6.30)	(1.58)	(1.00)	(0.38)	(207.53)
.004	− .060	− .006	.025	.007	.101	.143	.124
(0.16)	(16.14)	(0.10)	(10.04)	(0.63)	(6.64)	(12.53)	(17.16)
.014	− .053	.015	.016	− .006	− .003	.008	.364
(1.57)	(9.22)	(0.36)	(2.81)	(0.27)	(0.003)	(0.03)	(105.32)
.011	− .004	.056	− .013	− .008	.006	.096	− .015
(0.99)	(0.05)	(5.67)	(2.08)	(0.53)	(0.02)	(4.29)	(0.19)
− .001	− .047	.088	− .033	− .001	.049	.100	.015
(0.002)	(6.12)	(10.96)	(0.10)	(0.01)	(0.95)	(3.74)	(0.15)
.012	.019	.057	− .005	− .007	− .013	− .098	.042
(1.27)	(1.41)	(6.32)	(0.37)	(0.49)	(0.10)	(4.86)	(1.59)
− .032	.005	.039	− .001	.008	− .036	− .005	− .044
(8.35)	(0.10)	(2.66)	(0.01)	(0.59)	(0.61)	(0.01)	(7.12)

Table 12. Coefficients of Family Size[a]

Dependent Variable	Coefficient of LESS 20	F Statistic
Early health[b]		
LIGHT$_1$	.0004	(0.09)
LIGHT$_2$	− .0002	(0.01)
FYPH	− .001	(0.21)
CABN	.002	(0.05)
Current health[c]		
PFGHEALTH	.009	(3.06)
IHEAR	.001	(0.90)
ABVIS	− .001	(0.12)
HDBP	− .003	(1.16)
ALLEG	− .014	(15.56)
TENS	− .0001	(0.00)
ACABN	− .001	(0.12)
SCHABS	.002	(0.94)
IHEIGHT	− .056	(30.54)
IWEIGHT	− .079	(62.18)
APERI	.011	(2.18)

Notes: [a] Coefficients are statistically significant at the 5 percent level if the F is greater than 3.84 for a two-tailed test or 2.69 for a one-tailed test.
[b] These coefficients are taken from equation estimates which include all variables in Table 3 as explanatory variables.
[c] These coefficients are taken from equation estimates which include all variables in Table 3 plus LIGHT$_1$, LIGHT$_2$, FYPH, and CABN as explanatory variables.

substitution on the part of the parents or some alternative mechanism (such as the effects of an exogenous constraint on the amount of parents' time available to each child) cannot be determined. What our empirical work does show, however, is that the strong effects of family size on these four health measures are not primarily the result of other family characteristics operating through family size (a possibility that was suggested in an earlier section).[55] In particular, we find that when family size is *excluded* from the equations for these four health measures, the coefficients of the family characteristics listed in Tables 5 and 7 hardly change:[56] there are no changes in sign, no changes in patterns of significance, and minimal changes in magnitudes (though the coefficients diminish in some cases).[57] Our overall conclusion, then, regarding the effect of family size is that it has a significant negative relationship with only four of the measures of current or early child health—PFGHEALTH, IHEIGHT, IWEIGHT, and ALLEG. In addition, we find that the inclusion of a family size measure does not appreciably alter the coefficients of measures of other family characteristics, suggesting that family size is not an important mechanism by which these other family characteristics operate on children's health.

V.   INCOME AND RACE DIFFERENCES IN CHILDREN'S HEALTH

Much of the attention policy makers and health professionals direct at children's health focuses on differences related to family income levels and differences related to race. In this section, we discuss how our results can be used to provide additional insight into the nature and causes of these differences.

A.   Income Differences

Our findings of small and, in most cases, nonsignificant income effects on children's health may appear to be at variance with accepted opinion. Indeed, in our introduction we refer to large reported differences in health associated with differences in family income. One explanation of these divergent conclusions is that the "conventional wisdom" is based to some extent on income differentials in infant mortality and low birth weight. In our estimates we have not dealt with infant mortality, and we have examined the incidence of low birth weight only in a cohort of children who survived beyond the first year of life. It is well known that low birth weight has a strong positive effect on subsequent infant mortality (for example, see Lewit, 1977).

To the extent that the conventional wisdom deals with children more than 1 year old, our results diverge from it because our estimates control for many family characteristics that are highly correlated with income while simple income comparisons do not. To demonstrate how large a portion of the apparent (or gross) income differences would be attributed to associated family characteristics, in Table 13 we provide illustrative calculations for the measures PFGHEALTH, IHEIGHT, IWEIGHT, ALLEG, and APERI. These are the only health measures for which statistically significant gross income differences are observed in our sample. The third column of Table 13 shows the gross differences in these measures between children in families with annual income under $7,000 and those in families with annual income of $7,000 or more. These gross differences are to be compared to health differences that are allocated to income when all other explanatory variables in our basic equations are held constant (column 5). The "true" income effects are less than one-half (and in some cases, one-quarter) of the observed gross income differences for the five current health measures. The conclusion to be drawn is clear: gross income differences in health greatly overstate the true relationship between family income and health.

If the reported gross income differences are not primarily a result of differences in income, what does account for them? To answer this question we calculate how much of the gross high- vs. low-income differences in the above five health variables—PFGHEALTH, IHEIGHT, IWEIGHT, APERI, and ALLEG—can be attributed to specific explanatory variables or sets of these variables. The procedure is simply to multiply the coefficients of these variables by the differences in their mean values in the high- and low-family-income samples of children. The resulting estimates (in Table 14) illustrate how much of the gross difference would disappear if the low-income class is given the same mean values of the independent variables as the high-income class and if the relationship between health

Table 13.   Income Differences in Selected Current Health Measures

Variable	Mean for Families with Income < $7,000	Mean for Families with Income ≥ $7,000	Gross Difference[a]	Net Difference[b]
PFGHEALTH	.351	.532	− .181	− .080
IHEIGHT	.165	− .103	.268	.083
IWEIGHT	.143	− .041	.184	.045
APERI	.061	− .152	− .212	− .063
ALLEG	.131	.187	.056	.009

Notes: [a] Gross difference equals the second column minus the third. As shown in Table 14, the gross differences vary little from differences that are predicted on the basis of a regression of the health variables on all the independent variables.

[b] Net difference is the difference in mean health levels between the two income classes predicted on the basis of the income coefficients in Table 5 (when all explanatory variables are included in the equations).

and the explanatory variables is the same in both income classes. The estimates also identify which explanatory variables are responsible for the sizable gap between the gross and the net income effect in Table 13.

Several results in Table 14 are noteworthy. It is clear that almost all of the differences in the five health measures between the high- and low-income subsamples can be accounted for by differences in the independent variables that we have included in our empirical work. This suggests similar behavior of high-and-low income parents with respect to their children's health. The two most important components other than family income are parents' schooling and dental care. The parents' schooling component, which includes mother's schooling, father's schooling, and absence of father, is the dominant factor in the determination of the peridontal index and allergies, ranks second in importance in the determination of parental rating of health and height, and ranks third in importance in the determination of weight. The dental care component, which includes both dental variables ($DENT_{12}$ and $DENTIST_3$) ranks second in the allergy equation, third in the peridontal index, height, and parental rating of health equations, and fifth in the weight equation. If both the dental and schooling components are combined, their joint magnitude exceeds the income component in all the equations except the one for PFGHEALTH. Thus, it is these two income-related factors—education and attitudes toward medical care (and its availability)—that account for a major portion of observed gross income differences in four of our five health measures.

Table 14. Components of the Difference in PFGHEALTH, APERI, IHEIGHT, IWEIGHT and ALLEG Between Children from High- and Low-Income Families

Component	PFGHEALTH	APERI	IHEIGHT	IWEIGHT	ALLEG
Family income	−.080	−.063	.083	.045	.009
Parents' schooling	−.044	−.102	.062	.031	.036
Family size	−.004	−.005	.023	.033	.006
Dental care	−.026	−.023	.046	.019	.013
Foreign language	.0001	.001	.003	−.001	.001
Endogenous family inputs	.001	.001	−.001	−.0001	−.0002
Exogenous endowments	.003	−.007	.012	.012	.001
Early health	−.008	−.004	.010	.007	−.004
Region	−.017	.005	.008	.006	−.002
City size	−.002	.003	.008	.020	−.005
Total = Predicted Gross Difference	−.176	−.194	.254	.174	.054
Actual Gross Difference	−.181	−.212	.268	.184	.056

Table 15. Decomposition of Gross Race Differences in Health Measures

Variable	Mean for Whites	Mean for Blacks	Gross[a] Difference	Net Difference	Explained Difference[d]
Early health					
LIGHT$_1$[c]	.013	.034	.021 (13.96)	−.138	.159
LIGHT$_1$[c]	.043	.046	.003 (0.11)	−.030	.033
FYPH[b]	.086	.107	.021 (2.77)	.007	.014
CABN[b]	.050	.076	.026 (6.55)	.035	−.009
Current health					
APERI[c]	−.034	−.073	−.039 (1.42)	−.123	−.084
IHEIGHT[c]	.017	.090	.073 (2.82)	.109	−.036
IWEIGHT[c]	.042	−.127	−.169 (14.98)	.037	−.206
HDBP[b]	.054	.067	.013 (1.65)	.004	.009
PFGHEALTH[c]	.451	.613	.162 (54.23)	−.156	.318
IHEAR[b]	.006	.007	.001 (0.18)	.002	−.001
ABVIS[c]	.055	.096	.041 (14.06)	.004	.037
ALLEG[b]	.156	.088	−.068 (18.98)	−.077	−.061
TENS[b]	.476	.337	−.139 (39.92)	−.138	−.001
ACABN[b]	.037	.043	.007 (0.61)	.014	−.007
SCHABS[b]	.045	.042	−.003 (0.08)	−.007	.004

Notes: [a] Gross difference equals regression coefficient of a race dummy variable (1 = black) from a pooled regression of black and white children that holds no other variables constant; F ratios in parentheses.
  [b] Net difference equals regression coefficient of a race dummy variable (1 = black) from a pooled regression of black and white children that holds constant all other independent variables.
  [c] Net difference equals difference in intercepts between black and white regressions with all independent variables held constant.
  [d] Explained difference equals gross difference minus net difference.

71

B. Race Differences

According to conventional wisdom, black children have lower health levels than white children. As in the case of income differentials, this conclusion is based on differences in infant mortality and low birth weight or on gross differences in health measures between black and white children who survive the first year of life. Column 1 of Table 15 contains gross differences between black and white mean values of the fifteen health measures examined in Section IV.[58] With respect to early health measures, black children are more likely to have had a low birth weight, to have been in poor or fair health at one year of age, and to have a congenital abnormality. With regard to current health measures, blacks have lower health levels when health is measured by weight, parental rating of health, vision, high blood pressure, acquired abnormalities, and hearing (although race differences in the last three variables are not statistically significant). Blacks have *higher* health levels, however, when health is measured by height, presence of allergies, presence of tension, the peridontal index, and excessive school absence due to illness (although race differences for the last two variables are not statistically significant).

The last two columns of Table 15 decompose gross race differences into "net" differences and "explained" differences. We compute the net and explained race differences in two alternative ways. If there are no significant differences in the slope coefficients by race (as is the case for the dependent variables FYPH, CABN, HDBP, IHEAR, ALLEG, TENS, ACABN, and SCHABS), the net race difference is represented by the regression coefficient of a race dummy variable (black = 1) from a pooled regression of black and white children that holds constant all other independent variables. In this case, the explained difference is that portion of the gross difference that can be attributed to differences in mean values of independent variables between black and white families. When there are significant race differences in the slope coefficients (as in the case of the dependent variables LIGHT$_1$, LIGHT$_2$, APERI, IHEIGHT, IWEIGHT, PFGHEALTH, and ABVIS), the net difference is computed as the difference in intercepts from race-specific regressions, with all other variables held constant. In this case, the explained difference reflects differences in means *and* differences in coefficients between black and white families.

Among the nine health measures for which statistically significant gross race differences are reported in Table 15 (these are essentially the same measures for which the gross race differences are largest relative to their respective means in the white sample), blacks have worse health as measured by LIGHT$_1$, FYPH, CABN, IWEIGHT, PFGHEALTH, and ABVIS and they have better health as measured by IHEIGHT, ALLEG, and TENS. When net as opposed to gross race differences are examined, black health deficits diminish substantially. Health as measured by FYPH, CABN, and ABVIS is still worse for blacks, but the difference is greatly reduced for both FYPH and ABVIS (it increases for CABN). On the other hand, health as measured by LIGHT$_1$, IWEIGHT, and PFGHEALTH appears better for blacks on the basis of the computed net differences. For the variables IHEIGHT, ALLEG, and TENS for which the gross race differences indicated that blacks are in better health, the net difference diminished only in the case of ALLEG.

What conclusions do we draw from these results? First, black children have significantly worse current health in a gross sense for only 3 of the 11 current health measures, but for a much larger proportion (3 of 4) of the early health measures. This latter finding is consistent with commonly reported racial differences in infant mortality and birth weight. Second, the gross deficits in the health of black children are greatly diminished when we control for racial differences in the values and impacts of the explanatory variables. In fact, when net rather than gross differences in health are examined, in many cases black children appear in *better* health than white children do. Only in the case of congenital abnormalities do black children appear to be substantially worse off even after all "explained" effects are controlled for. Taken together, these results imply that the pure effect of race on the current health of children aged 6–11 years is smaller than is popularly believed.

VI. SUMMARY AND IMPLICATIONS

In this study multivariate techniques have been employed to examine the determinants of 11 current health measures and 4 early health measures in a national sample of white children between the ages of 6 and 11 years. The most important empirical results and their policy implications are indicated below.

The partial effects of family income on the current health measures are small and seldom statistically significant. In some cases higher income is associated with a greater prevalence of health problems such as high blood pressure, allergies, tension, and obesity. These relationships might be early forerunners of the positive relationships between income and morbidity and mortality rates of adults in the United States (for example, see Auster et al. 1969; Grossman 1972, 1975).

The findings that income- and race-related differences in health are small imply that policies that aim to improve the well-being of children via income transfers, such as those advocated by the recent Carnegie Council on Children (Keniston 1977) would have, at best, very small effects on health. A related implication pertains to proposals by Newberger et al. (1976), Keniston (1977), and Marmor (1977) to restrict national health insurance to rather complete prenatal and pediatric care coverage to offset variations in health associated with race and income. Again, our results indicate that there is not much to offset, even though pediatric care utilization is very sensitive to family income (Colle and Grossman 1978). To be sure, this conclusion would have to be modified if income transfer and national health insurance policies were tailored specifically to deal with unfavorable birth outcomes in high-risk groups. Our results do suggest, however, relatively small payoffs to programs that cover children who survive the first year of life.

As opposed to family income, parents' schooling is an important determinant of children's health. In most instances children of well-educated parents are in better health than those of less educated parents. In fact, for four of the five current health measures that have a significant gross correlation with income, most of this observed income difference is accounted for by associated differences in parents' schooling and preventive medical care. Therefore, if our estimates are taken at face value, policies to raise parents' schooling would not only benefit their children's health but would also reduce differences in health between children from low-income families and those from high-income families.

Caution and more research are required, however, in applying our results to schooling policies. First, the differences in years of parents' schooling between the high- and low-income samples are very large (2 years for mothers; 3 years for fathers), and these would probably be extremely costly to eliminate. Moreover, the mechanisms by which parents' schooling affects children's health still are not well known. Consider, for example, the finding that parents' schooling is an important determinant of children's height. This result has a very definite policy implication if the mechanism at work is a positive correlation between schooling and nutritional intakes or between schooling and the knowledge of what constitutes an appropriate diet. The policy implication is much less clear-cut if the mechanism at work is a positive relationship between parents' schooling and genetic inheritance that is not fully captured by the exogenous endowment and early health variables in the regressions.

Our results are relevant to three striking trends in family characteristics in the United States: (1) the increase in the proportion of families headed by women; (2) the increase in the labor force participation rate of married women with children; and (3) the reduction in family size. We find that the absence of a father in the household has little impact on children's health. Therefore, while the recent rise in the divorce rate might affect certain dimensions of children's well-being, health does not appear to be one of these dimensions. The same comment applies to the increase in labor force participation rates of married women with the exception that our two best measures of long-run nutritional status—height and the peridontal index—are worse if the mother works. Since, however, height is negatively related to family size, the detrimental impacts of increases in labor force participation rates are offset to some extent by the beneficial impacts of reductions in family size.

The measure of attitudes toward preventive medical care and its availability has rather large, positive effects on height, weight, and oral health. Thus returns to preventive care are indicated with regard to three health measures that reflect in part nutritional status. Since the preventive care variable is a proxy, research with a more direct measure of such care is in order. By obtaining medical care inputs in counties in which the children in the Health Examination Survey reside, we will pursue this issue in future work.

The diverse findings in this paper underscore the multidimensional nature of children's health. Use of a single index is misleading because a given family characteristic can have positive impacts on some components of good health and negative impacts on other components. For instance, parents' schooling is positively related to good nutrition (measured by height and oral health) but is also positively related to the "new morbidity" as measured by the presence of allergies and tension. In general, improvements in schooling and income will increase the incidence of the new morbidity; to cite one illustration, black children would have more allergies if their parents had the same socioeconomic characteristics as whites. One can speculate that an upward trend in the new morbidity will lead to more utilization of physicians' services for problems that are in many cases not amenable to treatment by physicians. This suggests that some modification in the training received by pediatricians and in the delivery of pediatric care services would be desirable.

Finally, although we do not altogether resist speculating about the implications of our empirical findings, we fully understand that this paper falls squarely within the sphere of traditional epidemiological research. We document the statistical relationships between family characteristics and measures of children's health in detail, but even though we outline the possible role of economic factors we cannot determine the exact nature of the mechanisms that generate these relationships. Nor was it possible to establish the causal nature of these relationships in a definitive sense. As epidemiological data, however, our findings do highlight two promising areas for future research. The first is an investigation of health and family characteristics at later stages in the child's life cycle. In particular, one could determine if some of the strong relationships reported in this paper taper off as the child grows. The second is a longitudinal study of the change in health for the same child between two different ages as it relates to the initial level of health and to family background variables.

APPENDIX

Table A1. Means and Standard Deviations of Dependent and Independent Variables: Whites[a]

Variable	Mean	Standard Deviation
PFGHEATH	.451	.498
IHEIGHT[b]	.017	.975
IWEIGHT[b]	.042	.994
IHEAR	.006	.074
ABVIS[c]	.055	.227
HDBP	.054	.226
ALLEG	.156	.363
TENS	.476	.500
ACABN	.037	.188
SCHABS[d]	.045	.207
APERI[b]	−.034	.757
LIGHT$_1$	.013	.112
LIGHT$_1$[e]	.013	.114
LIGHT$_2$	.043	.202
LIGHT$_2$[f]	.043	.203
FYPH	.086	.280
CABN	.050	.219
FINC	7.502	4.405
HFINC	5.038	6.138
MWORKPT	.132	.339
MWORKFT	.158	.365
BFED	.305	.460
MEDUCAT	11.095	2.808
FEDUCAT[g]	11.220	3.461
FLANG	.105	.307
MALE	.513	.500
LMAG	.073	.261
HMAG	.105	.307
FIRST	.288	.453
TWIN	.023	.149
NEAST	.236	.425
MWEST	.322	.467
SOUTH	.181	.385
URB$_1$	.199	.400
URB$_2$	.120	.325
URB$_3$	.181	.385
NURB	.148	.355
DENT$_{12}$	.169	.375

Table A1. (*Cont.*)

Variable	Mean	Standard Deviation
DENTIST$_3$	.179	.383
LESS 20	3.635	1.676
NOFATH	.071	.257

Notes:

[a] These means and standard deviations are computed for the "basic" sample of 4,196 children. Excluded are children who did not live either with both parents or with their mother only (418 children), 12-year-olds (72 children), and children for whom there were missing data for the variables we study. The absence of birth certificate information was the main reason for excluding such observations.

[b] The means and standard deviations of these variables are not 0 and 1, respectively, because the standardization was done using the entire Cycle II sample rather than the subsample of 4,196 reported on in this paper.

[c] The mean and standard deviation for this variable are computed for a subsample of 3,729 who do not wear eyeglasses.

[d] The mean and standard deviation for this variable are computed for a subsample of 3,812 for whom the school report is not missing.

[e] The mean and standard deviation for this variable are computed for a subsample of 4,017 for whom LIGHT$_2$ is not equal to 1.

[f] The mean and standard deviation for this variable are computed for a subsample of 4,143 for whom LIGHT$_1$ is not equal to 1.

[g] The mean and standard deviation for this variable are computed for a subsample of 3,899 whose fathers are present.

ACKNOWLEDGMENTS

Research for this paper was supported by PHS Grant No. 1 R01 HS 02917 from the National Center for Health Services Research to the National Bureau of Economic Research (NBER) and by a grant from the Robert Wood Johnson Foundation to the NBER. We would like to thank Ann Colle, Jacob Gesthalter, and Steven Jacobowitz for research assistance. This report has not yet undergone the review accorded official NBER publications; in particular, it has not yet been submitted for approval by the Board of Directors.

NOTES

1. Early compulsory schooling laws are discussed in Landes and Solmon (1972).

2. This change in emphasis is partially the result of the Coleman Report and subsequent research, which showed that the effects of school quality on children's achievement may be small relative to the effects of family characteristics. Averch et al. (1972) provide an excellent review of this literature.

3. Some states require children to receive certain immunizations before they may begin attending school. An analysis of immunization as a public good can be found in Buchanan and Tullock (1964). An exception to the text statement is Connecticut, which requires school children to have physical examinations every 3 years (Foltz and Brown, 1975).

4. This definition of the new morbidity is quoted from Haggerty et al. (1975, p. 316).

5. Starfield (1977) emphasizes that, although many persons have studied the effects of medical care and socioeconomic characteristics on infant mortality, relatively few have examined the effects of these variables on the health of children who survive the first year of life. For a few recent exceptions, see Kaplan et al. (1972), Hu (1973), Kessner (1974); Haggerty et al. (1975), and Inman (1976).

6. See Keniston (1977, p. 156).

7. These data come from Cycles II and III of the Health Examination Survey and are reported in National Center for Health Statistics (1973b, pp. 22–26).

8. *Ibid.*

9. A better understanding of the effects of medical care is also needed, but the data used in this paper do not permit explicit analysis of the effects of medical care.

10. A full description of the sample, the sampling technique, and the data collection is presented in National Center for Health Statistics (1967). The one deficiency of this sample from the point of view of studying children's health is the exclusion of children in institutions. To the extent that these children are more likely to have serious and disabling physical conditions, the reported incidence of certain conditions will be lower in our sample than in the entire population of children. In addition, if the probability of the institutionalization of a child with a given condition depends on the various family characteristics studied here, our results will incorporate unknown biases. The number of institutionalized children is small, however, at about four-tenths of a percent of all children aged 5 through 13 years. [This is the proportion of 5- through 13-year-olds living in "group quarters" in 1970 according to the U.S. Bureau of the Census (1973, Tables 52 and 205). The corresponding percentages by race are 0.38 percent for whites and 0.7 percent for blacks.]

11. Introducing uncertainty about the number and quality of children complicates the model, but many of the basic insights provided by the notion of both a quantity and quality dimension of children remain valid. Ben Porath and Welch (1976) illustrate how uncertainty regarding one aspect of quality—the child's sex—affects fertility.

12. Recent medical advances allow some types of poor genetic endowments to be detected intra utero and defective fetuses aborted, so that parents can now partially control their children's genetic endowments. Genetic or early health endowments also have endogenous components that depend on prenatal medical care and parental characteristics.

13. See Willis (1973) and Becker and Lewis (1973) for a full development of these points.

14. The proposition that higher levels of parents' education lead to more efficient household production is tested in Michael (1972).

15. Presumably, parents' education raises efficiency in the production of many household commodities. Therefore, there is an "own price effect" due to an improvement in the efficiency of producing children's health and a "cross price effect" due to an improvement in the efficiency of producing other commodities. The statement in the text with respect to the impact of parents' education on children's health assumes that the own price effect outweighs the cross price effect if the two effects go in opposite directions.

16. National Center for Health Statistics (1973b), Table 14.

17. Edwards and Grossman (1977a,b) use this model to study children's health and intellectual development; Leibowitz and Friedman (1979) use it to study health inputs; Tomes (1978) uses it to examine years of schooling attained; and Ishikawa (1975) uses it to explain intergenerational transfers of education and financial wealth. Both Ishikawa (1975) and Leibowitz and Friedman (1979) treat family size as exogenous.

18. See Edwards and Grossman (1977a).

19. See, for example, Sullivan (1966), Berg (1973), and, more recently, Ware (1976).

20. World Health Organization (1958).

21. For example, in concluding "Conceptual Problems in Developing an Index of Health," Daniel Sullivan says "a definition of health levels in terms of mortality and morbidity would be realistic and useful in view of today's health problems" (op. cit., p. 15).

22. See Grossman (1972, p. 58). This definition is also very similar to that proposed in Torrance (1976).

23. A good discussion of the subsidiary issue of how one measures disability in children can be found in Schack and Starfield (1973).

24. Of course, there is a positive relationship between the two in the sense that a child with low health capital is more likely to contract some acute conditions and to have them for a more extended time period. For example, Birch and Gussow (1970) discuss how nutrition (which is clearly a determinant of "permanent" health status) and disease are intimately related.

25. The earlier theoretical discussion pertains to children's health status measured at the end of their childhood, while health measures in the Cycle II data are for 6- to 11-year-old children. Our analysis implicitly assumes that health in midchildhood is a good proxy for the health stocks at the end of childhood.

26. In earlier work some attempts were made to condense the health information using principal component analysis. The analysis yielded almost as many equally weighted components as there were initial health measures.

27. The studies we consulted are Wallace (1962), Mechanic (1964), Mindlin and Lobach (1971), Talbot et al. (1971), Kaplan et al. (1972), Hu (1973), Schack and Starfield (1973), Kessner (1974), Haggerty et al. (1975), and Inman (1976).

28. The following physicians gave us extremely helpful advice: John McNamara, M.D., then Assistant Professor of Public Health and Pediatrics at Columbia University School of Public Health and Associate Commissioner in the New York City Department of Health; Roy Brown, M.D., Associate Professor of Community Medicine and Pediatrics at the Mount Sinai School of Medicine of the City University of New York; Thomas Travers, D.D.S., Director of Ambulatory Care in the New York City Department of Health; and Ruth T. Gross, Professor of Pediatrics and Director of Ambulatory Pediatrics, Stanford University Medical Center, Stanford, California.

29. If the actual height or weight of each age-sex group is normally distributed, IHEIGHT and IWEIGHT could be translated directly into the child's height and weight percentile. In addition to these continuous height and weight measures, we also experimented with discrete measures identifying children who are more than two standard deviations from the mean height or weight for their age-sex cohort. These measures were used to allow for noncontinuous relationships between height (or weight) and family characteristics. For example, beyond some weight level, problems with obesity start to develop, so that "more" weight is no longer better than "less" weight. Results using these discrete measures did not differ greatly from those based on using IHEIGHT and IWEIGHT, so we do not report them here.

30. Children who wear glasses are excluded from the vision analysis because it cannot be assumed that the glasses they wear are appropriate for their vision defect. Kessner (1974), for example, finds that 40 percent of children in a low-income sample who were tested with their glasses failed a visual acuity test.

31. In defining ACABN, we exclude abnormalities resulting from accidents or injuries because these are likely to reflect transitory rather than permanent health variations.

32. The peridontal index suffers from the defect that it is subject to intra-rater and inter-rater variability. We have experimented with a somewhat more objective measure of oral health, the number of decayed permanent and primary teeth adjusted for age and sex, and have obtained results similar to those for the peridontal index. Compared to the number of decayed teeth, the peridontal index reflects more serious oral health problems.

33. There is no school form for approximately 500 children in the Cycle II data set. Since excessive absence due to illness is the only variable taken from the school form, children without the school form are eliminated from the empirical analysis *only* when school absence is the dependent variable.

34. For example, there are government programs directed at providing prenatal care to pregnant women. An analysis of such a program appears in Lewit (1977).

35. See Edwards and Grossman (1977b) and the references cited therein.

36. See, for example, Birch and Gussow (1970). Note that Cycle II does not distinguish children who are born prematurely, so we cannot determine to what extent low birth weight is a result of prematurity or of other factors.

37. Family size is an endogenous variable. When it is included in what otherwise would be a reduced form demand equation, the result is a "mixture" of the structural demand equation and the health production function. This issue is discussed in more detail in Section III.C.

38. See Edwards and Grossman (1977a) for a rationale for such a difference. Since this family income measure does not hold constant the mother's labor force status and the father's experience, we experimented with an income measure that held these two factors constant. The adjusted income variable was very highly correlated with FINC (the correlation coefficient was greater than .99) and the regression results were not altered when adjusted income was used in place of FINC. Therefore, we report results based on the use of FINC in this paper.

39. Breast-feeding is not only a measure of the mother's time input; it has also been found to contribute to the nutritional status of infants and to help protect them from acute illnesses (see, for example, Mata, 1978, and the associated references).

40. A subtle point to keep in mind is that given rising marginal costs of investment in health, input prices at various stages of a child's life cycle are arguments of output demand functions. Therefore, to the extent that early health is an intermediate output, a mother's current price of time is a relevant predictor variable of early health. An absolute increase in the current price of time generates a substitution in production toward early health and a substitution in consumption away from ultimate health (and therefore early health) if the production of health is relatively time-intensive. Since the two effects go in opposite directions, the current price of time should have a smaller absolute effect on early health than the past price of time.

41. Mother's age may also be regarded as an endogenous variable, although here we treat it as exogenous.

42. In the future the National Center for Health Statistics might provide us with area-specific input availability and price measures. This will enable us to examine the effects of medical care quantities and prices on health outputs.

43. Information about the time of the child's last visit to a doctor is also available in the data but would be greatly contaminated by the child's health level. We refer to the well-known reverse causality between health and medical care.

44. Since LESS 20 does not actually measure completed family size but rather the number of persons in the household younger than 20 years at the time of the Cycle II interview, it may overstate or understate completed family size.

45. This bias could be positive or negative, and may even be nonexistent. In empirical work in a somewhat different context (looking at years of school completed rather than children's health), Tomes (1978) finds that the magnitudes of this bias is small.

46. A subsidiary point, not directly relevant to the work in this paper, is that when the equation is estimated with family size excluded, the predicted effects of the various other theoretical variables are much more ambiguous than when family size is held constant (see, for example, Becker and Lewis, 1973).

47. Missing information for birth weight (for 818 observations), and to a lesser extent FLANG (for 324 observations) and income (for 290 observations) account for most of the missing observations. In addition, children who turned 12 years old between the time the sample was chosen and the time of the interview were also excluded. (There were 72 such children in the entire Cycle II sample.)

48. Significant race differences were found for the variables LIGHT$_1$, LIGHT$_2$, IHEIGHT, IWEIGHT, PFGHEALTH, ABVIS, and APERI. For the other variables the results for the white sample would be applicable to the black sample.

49. See Nerlove and Press (1973) for a description of this technique.

50. The lack of statistical significance for these three variables may be partially accounted for by their low incidence (see Appendix Table A1). This is not the total explanation, however, because other dependent variables with an even lower incidence (LIGHT$_1$ and LIGHT$_2$, for example) have significant F statistics.

51. Let the true health function be

$$H = a + b_1 \text{ NOFATH} + b_2 [\text{FEDUCAT} \times (1 - \text{NOFATH})]$$
$$+ b_3 (\text{FEDUCAT} \times \text{NOFATH}) + b_4 Y,$$

where Y is a vector of additional independent variables. If b_3 equals zero, an unbiased estimate of b_1 is obtained by fitting the above health function with the variable (FEDUCAT $\times$ NOFATH) omitted. This estimate is termed the minimum estimate. If b_2 equals b_3 and the mean level of father's education is the same whether or not he is present, an unbiased estimate of b_1 is obtained by fitting the health function with father's education represented as a single variable for both samples (no interaction between FEDUCAT and NOFATH) and father's education in the father-absent families coded at the mean of the father-present families. This estimate is termed the *maximum estimate*.

52. If the father left the family before the birth of the child, his educational attainment might still be expected to have an effect on child health if it reflects genetically determined health characteristics.

53. Both estimates imply positive health effects for LIGHT$_1$, FYPH, PFGHEALTH, IHEAR, HDBP, TENS, ACABN; and both imply negative health effects for CABN and SCHABS. The minimum estimate implies a positive health effect and the maximum a negative health effect for APERI, IWEIGHT, and IHEIGHT; and the opposite pattern is reported for LIGHT$_2$, ABVIS, and ALLEG.

54. The weak relationship between mother's current labor force status and early health can be attributed in part to an imperfect correlation between current and past labor force status or to a larger effect of past labor force status on early health than current labor force status on past health.

55. For example, it can be argued that families with more educated mothers choose to have fewer children but of a higher quality, so that the coefficient of LESS 20 will reflect, in part, the effects of mother's education.

56. In the interest of brevity we do not present these estimates in this paper. They are available from the authors on request.

57. The only variables whose coefficients do alter when LESS 20 is excluded are FIRST, HMAG, and BFED. All three of these (although to a lesser extent, BFED) might be regarded as having a mechanical or definitional relationship with LESS 20 so that they act as proxies for LESS 20 when it is excluded. First-born children are more likely to come from smaller families than are later-born children (the simple correlation between LESS 20 and FIRST is $-.34$); older mothers are likely to have smaller families (the simple correlation between HMAG and LESS 20 is $-.07$); and breast-fed children are more likely to be first born (the simple correlation between BFED and FIRST is .08) and therefore to come from smaller families. Thus, when LESS 20 is excluded from the equations for the current health measures discussed in the text, the coefficient of FIRST increases, the coefficient of HMAG increases (for IHEIGHT and IWEIGHT), and the coefficient of BFED decreases (for IHEIGHT and ALLEG).

58. The black sample contains 581 children who live either with both parents or with their mother only.

REFERENCES

Auster, Richard D., Leveson, Irving, and Sarachek, Deborah (1969), "The Production of Health: An Exploratory Study," *Journal of Human Resources 4*, Fall.

Averch, Harvey A., Caroll, Stephen J., Donaldson, Theodore S., Kiesling, Herbert J., Pincus, John (1972), *How Effective is Schooling? A Critical Review and Synthesis of Research Findings*. Santa Monica, Calif.: The Rand Corp.

Becker, Gary S., and Lewis, H. Gregg (1973), "On the Interaction between the Quantity and Quality of Children," in *New Economic Approaches to Fertility* (T. W. Schultz, ed.). Proceedings of a conference sponsored by the National Bureau of Economic Research and the Population Council. *Journal of Political Economy 81*(2), Pt. II, March/April.

Ben-Porath, Yoram, and Welch, Finis (1976), "Do Sex Preferences Really Matter?" *The Quarterly Journal of Economics 90*(2), May.

Berg, Robert L. (1973), *Health Status Indexes: Proceedings of a conference conducted by Health Services Research, Tucson, Arizona, October 1972*. Chicago: Hospital Research and Educational Trust.

Birch, Herbert G., and Gussow, Joan Dye (1970), *Disadvantaged Children: Health, Nutrition, and School Failure*. New York: Harcourt Brace Jovanovich.

Buchanan, Jane, and Tullock, Gordon (1964), "Public and Private Interaction Under Reciprocal Externality," in *Conference on Urban Public Expenditures* (J. Margolis, ed.). Baltimore: Johns Hopkins Press.

Colle, Ann, and Grossman, Michael (1978), "Determinants of Pediatric Care Utilization," National Bureau of Economic Research Working Paper No. 240, April.

Edwards, Linda N., and Grossman, Michael (1977a), "An Economic Analysis of Children's Health and Intellectual Development," National Bureau of Economic Research Working Paper No. 180 (May).

——— (1977b), "The Relationship between Children's Health and Intellectual Development," National Bureau of Economic Research Working Paper No. 213 (Nov.).

Foltz, Anne-Marie, and Brown, Donna (1975), "State Response to Federal Policy: Children, EPSDT, and the Medicaid Muddle," *Medical Care 13*(8).

Grossman, Michael (1972), *The Demand for Health: A Theoretical and Empirical Investigation*. New York: Columbia Univ. Press for the National Bureau of Economic Research.

——— (1975), "The Correlation Between Health and Schooling," in *Household Production and Consumption,* (Nestor E. Terleckyj (ed.). New York: Columbia University Press for the National Bureau of Economic Research.

Haggerty, Robert J., Roghmann, Klaus J., and Pless, Ivan B. (1975), *Child Health and the Community*. New York: Wiley.

Hu, Teh-Wei (1973), "Effectiveness of Child Health and Welfare Programs: A Simultaneous Equations Approach," *Socio-Economic Planning Sciences 7*.

Inman, Robert P. (1976), "The Family Provision of Childrens Health: An Economic Analysis," in *The Role of Health Insurance in the Health Services Sector* (Richard Rosett (ed.). New York: Columbia University Press for the National Bureau of Economic Research.

Ishikawa, Tsuneo (1975), "Family Structures and Family Values in the Theory of Income Distribution," *Journal of Political Economy 83*(5).

Kaplan, Robert S., Lave, Lester B., and Leinhardt, Samuel (1972), "The Efficacy of a Comprehensive Health Care Project: An Empirical Analysis," *American Journal of Public Health 62*(7).

Keniston, Kenneth, and the Carnegie Council on Children (1977), *All Our Children: The American Family Under Pressure*. New York: Harcourt Brace Jovanovich.

Kessner, David M. (1974), *Assessment of Medical Care for Children*. Contrasts in Health Status, Vol. 3 Washington, D.C.: Institute of Medicine.

Landes, William M., and Solmon, Lewis C. (1972), "Compulsory Schooling Legislation: An Economic Analysis of Law and Social Change in the Nineteenth Century." *Journal of Economic History 32*(1).

Leibowitz, Arleen, and Friedman, Bernard (1979), "Family Bequests and the Derived Demand for Health Inputs," *Economic Inquiry 17*(3).

Lewit, Eugene M. (1977), "Experience with Pregnancy, The Demand for Prenatal Care and the Production of Surviving Infants," Ph.D. dissertation, City University of New York.

Mata, Leonardo (1978), "Breast-Feeding: Main Promoter of Infant Health," *American Journal of Clinical Nutrition 31*, May.

Marmor, Theodore R. (1977), "Rethinking National Health Insurance," *The Public Interest 46*, Winter.

Mechanic, David (1964), "The Influence of Mothers on Their Children's Health, Attitudes and Behavior," *Pediatrics 33*, March.

Michael, Robert T. (1972), *The Effect of Education on Efficiency in Consumption*. New York: Columbia University Press for the National Bureau of Economic Research.

Mindlin, Rowland L., and Lobach, Katherin S. (1971), "Consistency and Change in Choice of Medical Care for Preschool Children," *Pediatrics 48*, September.

National Center for Health Statistics (1975), *Anthropometric and Clinical Findings*. U.S. Public Health Service, Vital and Health Statistics, Publ. No. (HRA) 75-1229, April.

—— (1972), *Binocular Visual Acuity of Children: Demographic and Socioeconomic Characteristics*. U.S. Public Health Service, Vital and Health Statistics, Ser. 11, No. 112, February.

—— (1973a), *Body Weight, Stature, and Sitting Height: White and Negro Youths 12–17 Years, United States*. U.S. Public Health Service, Vital and Health Statistics, Ser. 11, No. 126, August.

—— (1973b), *Examination and Health History Findings Among Children and Youths, 6–17 Years*. U.S. Public Health Service, Vital and Health Statistics, Ser. 11, No. 129, November.

—— (1970a), *Hearing Levels of Children by Age and Sex: United States*. U.S. Public Health Service, Vital and Health Statistics, Ser. 11, No. 102, February.

—— (1970b), *Height and Weight of Children: United States*. U.S. Public Health Service, Vital and Health Statistics, Ser. 11, No. 104, September.

—— (1967), *Plan, Operation, and Response Results of a Program of Children's Examinations*. U.S. Public Health Service, Vital and Health Statistics, Ser. 1, No. 5.

Nerlove, Marc, and Press, S. James (1973), "Notes on the Log-Linear or Logistic Model for the Analysis of Qualitative Socioeconomic Data." Santa Monica, Calif.: The Rand Corp.

Newberger, Eli H., Newberger, Carolyn Moore, and Richmond, Julius B. (1976), "Child Health in America: Toward a Rational Public Policy," *Milbank Memorial Fund Quarterly 54*(3), Summer.

Schack, Elisabeth, and Starfield, Barbara. "Acute Disability in Childhood: Examination of Agreement between Various Measures," *Medical Care 11*(4).

Seoane, Nicole, and Latham, Michael C. (1971), "National Anthropometry in the Identification of Malnutrition in Childhood," *Journal of Tropical Pediatric and Environmental Child Health* (Sept.).

Starfield, Barbara (1977), "Health Needs of Children," in *Children's Medical Care Needs and Treatment*. Harvard Child Health Project Report, Vol. II. Cambridge, Mass.: Ballinger.

Sullivan, Daniel F. (1966), "Conceptual Problems in Developing an Index of Health," U.S. Public Health Service Publ. No. 1000, Vital and Health Statistics, Ser. 2, No. 17. Rockville, Md.: National Center for Health Statistics.

Talbot, Nathan B., Kagan, Jerome, and Eisenberg, Leon, eds. (1971), *Behavioral Science in Pediatric Medicine*. Philadelphia: Saunders.

Tomes, Nigel (1978), "Intergenerational Transfers of Human and Non-Human Capital in a Model of Quality–Quantity Interaction," Ph.D. dissertation, University of Chicago.

Torrance, George W. (1976), "Health Status Index Models: A Unified Mathematical View," *Management Science 22*(9).

U.S. Bureau of the Census (1973), *1970 Census of Population,* Vol. I: *Characteristics of the Population,* Pt. 1, U.S. Summary, Secs. 1 and 2. Washington, D.C.: U.S. Government Printing Office.

Wallace, Helen M. (1962), *Health Services for Mothers and Children.* Philadelphia: Saunders.

Ware, Jr., John E. (1976), "The Conceptualization and Measurement of Health for Policy Relevant Research in Medical Care Delivery." Paper presented at the annual meeting of the American Association for the Advancement of Science, Boston, Massachusetts, February.

Willis, Robert (1973), "A New Approach to the Economic Theory of Fertility Behavior," in *New Economic Approaches to Fertility* (T. W. Schultz, ed.). Proceedings of a conference sponsored by the National Bureau of Economic Research and the Population Council. *Journal of Political Economy 81*(2), Pt. II.

World Health Organization (1958), "Constitution of the World Health Organization, Annex I." in *The First Ten Years of the World Health Organization.* Geneva: WHO.

THE FAMILY'S DEMAND FOR HEALTH:

EVIDENCE FROM A RURAL COMMUNITY

Laurence A. Miners

I. INTRODUCTION

The continued escalation of medical care costs as well as the growth of
the egalitarian concept that all members of society deserve adequate
medical care has spurred economists and other social scientists to study
the health care sector of the economy extensively. Newhouse (1978)
indicates that between 1960 and 1970 medical care prices increased (on
average) by 4.3 percent per annum; between 1970 and 1976 the annual
percentage increase averaged 7.4 percent. The annual rates of increase
for all other goods and services over the same time periods were 2.7
and 6.6 percent, respectively. According to Fuchs and Newhouse (1978),
total health care expenditures have been growing at a high rate as well—
an average increase of 10.5 percent a year from 1960 to 1977.

Advances in Health Economics and Health Services Research, Vol. 2, pgs. 85–142.
(Volume 1 published as Research in Health Economics)
Copyright © 1981 by JAI Press Inc.
All rights of reproduction in any form reserved.
ISBN: 0-89232-100-8

It is not surprising, then, that the demand for and utilization of medical care has become a topic of widespread interest and research among economists. The determinants of the demand for health care are important for a number of reasons. In the first place, the quantification of these factors is necessary to properly assess the health status and medical care needs of the community and to provide programs to increase consumer awareness and knowledge of the health care sector. Secondly, data pertaining to consumer demand can be used by both policy makers and physicians to more accurately meet the needs of the patient and to provide health care in a setting more conducive to the patient's requirements.

The purpose of this study is to construct a household model of the demand for medical care and to test the theoretical results of the model with data from a rural southern community. The theoretical model differs from earlier health demand studies in that the household unit, rather than the individual, is the basic unit of analysis. My concern with the household as a unit of analysis stems from the (maintained) existence of a central decision-making unit within the family, the public nature of many medical goods and services, and the communicability and hereditary aspects associated with many diseases. Individual demand curves are developed from the model and emphasis is placed on the effects of cross-price changes on demand.[1]

Along with the effects of cross-price changes, the indirect costs of receiving medical care are also accentuated. Medical care, like most other goods and services, is a scarce good and hence subject to rationing. The rationing of a good can be accomplished in many ways, although the price of the good is the most common rationing device. However, in the case of medical care, the fee paid for service may not be the most important price. This is due, in part, to the widespread increase in health insurance coverage and the possibility of national health insurance. An alternative explanation for the reduced (relative) importance of money price lies in the investigation of indirect (or nonmonetary) prices. Economists have long been aware of the opportunity costs associated with choices among scarce commodities; however, only recently has the analysis of such prices been incorporated into the study of the demand for medical care.[2] It is now realized that such indirect prices as the opportunity costs of travel time and waiting time may have significant impacts on the demand for medical care. The importance of travel time is viewed as particularly germane for people living in rural areas due to the long distances that must often be traveled to receive care.

Few economists have studied the determinants of demand in rural areas, and the quantification of these factors is important for a number of reasons. Luft et al. (1976) point out that certain minorities are concentrated in rural areas and that rural residents are more likely to be poor, experience higher rates of accidents and disabilities, and travel further to reach physicians. Davis and Marshall (1979) indicate that improving rural medical services may also yield certain externalities such that regional development may be accelerated and migration from rural to urban areas slowed, if not reversed, thereby ameliorating urban problems. Furthermore, the neglect of rural health care needs has led to a disproportionately low share of benefits from public programs being directed toward rural areas.

The data used in this study were collected by the Department of Community Health Sciences (CHS) at Duke University and represent a virtual population survey of 665 families living in a rural community north of Durham, North Carolina. Among other variables, information was collected on the health status and utilization of health care by each family member. It is therefore expected that the results of this study will identify the determining factors of medical care utilization and aid health care planners and policy makers in their attempt to meet the medical care needs of the community.

A household utility model of the demand for medical goods and services is developed in Section II, and emphasis is placed on deriving testable implications from the model—especially with regard to interpersonal cross-price changes and the effects of indirect prices on demand. Tobit analysis is used in Section III to estimate individual and family medical care demand curves. In the concluding section I summarize my results, discuss the policy implications of my findings, and propose several issues for future research.

II. A HOUSEHOLD MODEL OF THE DEMAND FOR MEDICAL GOODS AND SERVICES

Whereas earlier studies have typically focused on the individual's demand for medical care, this model places emphasis on the family and the interaction effects that exist among household members.[3] The model employs a household utility maximization framework in which household utility is a function of the family members' utilization of medical goods and services and a composite bundle of other goods. The budget constraint utilizes Becker's (1965) concept of "full income" and particular attention is paid to the "full price" of medical care.

In the following subsection I present the general household utility model. In the next subsection (II.B) cross-price elasticities of demand and other comparative static results are examined, and in Section II.C a test of the substitutability of medical care between the husband and wife (in a two-person household) is developed. A summary is presented in the final part of this section and the testable hypotheses obtained from the model are reviewed.

A. The Household Utility Model

In view of the fact that one's stock of health is directly affected by other family members, an argument can be made for viewing the demand for medical goods and services as a family, decision process.[4] The health status of individual family members may be interrelated due both to hereditary factors and the communicability of diseases. The demand for medical care visits by individual family members may be influenced by household structure due to a redistribution of income from the head to other household members (e.g., see Becker, 1974) and the necessity for an adult (usually the wife) to accompany young progeny on medical care visits. The demand for medical visits by various household members may therefore be closely related to the opportunity cost of time and hence the wage and labor force participation rates of the husband and wife. For this reason, changes in the wage rate of one family member may not only influence that person's utilization of medical services but also the demand of other family members.

More formally, the family can be viewed as maximizing a utility function given by

$$U = U (M_j, N_j, D, Z) \qquad (j = 1, ..., n) \qquad (1)$$

where M_j represents medical goods and services purchased and consumed outside the household by the jth individual family member. Examples of M_j include private physician visits, group-practice or clinic visits, and visits to hospital outpatient departments. It should be pointed out that hospital admissions and length of stay could also be entered as arguments in the utility function. However, no adequate cost data (either monetary or opportunity) are available for inpatient care. Also, fewer than 5 percent of the people in the community were hospitalized during the survey. It is expected that the demand for hospital inpatient care is much less price-and-income elastic than the demand for ambulatory medical care. For a comparison of the two types of settings see Karen Davis and Louise B. Russell (1972). N_j measures the individual's utilization of medical goods and services solely within the houehold (examples of N_j include nonprescription drugs and remedies, and home care); D is a composite good reflecting sanitary conditions within the home; and Z is a vector of all other goods and services consumed by the household.[5] In a production function framework, individual health status, H_j, could be viewed as a commodity produced by some combination of M_j, N_j, and D. However, the production function approach is not needed to develop individual demand functions and as De Vany (1970) points out, the use of commodity production functions may lead to illogical results. While earlier researchers have recognized the need for also incorporating medical goods and services other than health care visits into the utility function, it has generally not been possible to implement such approaches empirically. The data used in this study include information on individual utilization of nonprescription drugs and medicines (N_j) and on the overall condition of the family's dwelling unit (D), and it is expected that these goods will also have a significant impact on health status and utility. The final good in the utility function, Z, represents a vector of other goods and services in the family utility function such that

$$Z = [Z_1, ..., Z_m]. \tag{2}$$

It should also be pointed out that family size (n) ranges from 1 to 18 household members, even though the majority of households (93 percent) have less than 7 members.

In the analysis that follows it will be assumed that the household utility function is separable between medical goods and services and Z_k, k = 1, ..., m. The assumption of weak separability implies that the marginal rates of substitution between any two medical goods is independent of Z_k. However, this does not imply that the demand equations for medical goods are entirely independent of Z_k. Changes in the price and consumption of Z_k will affect the income allocated to medical goods and services. Hence the effect of a change in Z_k is analogous to an income effect when one is considering its influence on the demand for medical goods and services. Phlips (1974), however, has demonstrated that the stronger assumption of additivity (strong separability), while imposing greater restrictions on the demand equations, is not unreasonsale when considering broad aggregates of goods.

The household maximizes utility subject to two constraints: an expenditure constraint and a time constraint. The expenditure constraint is

$$\sum_{j=1}^{n} P_j M_j + \sum_{j=1}^{n} Q_j N_j + P_D D + P_Z Z = \sum_{j=1}^{n} L_j T_j^L + Y. \tag{3}$$

The P_j and Q_j represent the market or monetary prices of medical care visits and household medicines, respectively, for each household member. Here P_D and P_Z indicate the respective (monetary) prices of D and Z; L_j is the individual's market wage rate and T_j^L measures time sold in the labor market; Y represents unearned household income. The left-hand side of Eq. (3) represents total household expenditures on goods and services, whereas the right-hand side indicates total (observed) family income. The time constraint (for an individual household member) is

$$T_j = T_j^L + T_j^M + T_j^N + T_j^D + T_j^Z + T_j^S. \tag{4}$$

Individuals allocate their total time (T_j) in the following ways: in selling their services in the labor market (T_j^L), in consuming extrahousehold and intrahousehold medical goods and services (T_j^M and T_j^N, respectively), in consuming or maintaining the household dwelling unit (T_j^D), in consuming Z, the composite commodity (T_j^Z), and in being sick (T_j^S).

The time constraint indicates that the cost of obtaining medical care involves more than the monetary price. In particular there are time costs involved with receiving health care. Equation (4) indicates that an increase in the amount of time spent receiving medical care must reduce labor market participation and/or the time available for other activities. Therefore the amount of time involved with receiving care is expected to be an important determinant of the demand for M_j by both nonlabor force participants and wage earners. Earlier studies in the economics literature (Acton, 1973a,b, 1975, 1976; Holtmann, 1972; Holtman et al., 1976) and public health literature (Shannon et al., 1969; Fetter and Thompson, 1966) indicate that these time costs are substantial. It should be pointed out that T_j^S, the time lost due to illness or injury, is different from T_j^M, the time input necessary to complete a medical care visit. Grossman (1972, p. 3) indicates that as one receives more medical care, health status may improve and thereby establish a negative correlation between these two variables. Equally plausible is the assumption that the deterioration in one's health necessitates the utilization of medical services. The assumption remains to be verified (or refuted) at the empirical level.

Due to the potentially large opportunity cost of time involved in receiving medical care, it is worthwhile to combine both constraints in order that the full cost of medical care (and other goods) can be seen. The cost of any commodity therefore will include both a direct and an indirect price. Understanding the role of indirect or time prices on the demand for medical care is particularly important if one wishes to assess variations in demand among alternative types of care. Clinics and hospital outpatient departments are typically lower priced than private physician office visits; however, the time prices involved with receiving care are usually higher. Health insurance coverage decreases the consumer's responsiveness to changes in money price and thereby increases the relative importance of nonmonetary prices to the patient. These reasons, coupled with the fact that members of many households in rural communities must travel long distances to reach a doctor, highlight the importance of time to the consumer in the medical care market. From Eqs. (3) and (4), the household's full income is

$$\sum_{j=1}^{n} [L_j (T_j^L + T_j^M + T_j^N + T_j^D + T_j^Z + T_j^S)] + Y = \sum_{j=1}^{n} L_j T_j + Y. \quad (5)$$

By considering individual sick time as a loss of full income, Eq. (5) can be rewritten as

$$\sum_{j=1}^{n} [L (T_j^L + T_j^M + T_j^N + T_j^D + T_j^Z)] + Y = \sum_{j=1}^{n} L_j(T_j - T_j^S) + Y. \quad (6)$$

Combining Eqs. (3) and (6) we obtain the household's full income budget constraint

$$\sum_{j=1}^{n} (P_j + L_j t_j^M)M_j + \sum_{j=1}^{n} (Q_j + L_j t_j^N)N_j$$

$$+ (P_D + \sum_{j=1}^{n} L_j t_j^D)D + (P_Z + \sum_{j=1}^{n} L_j t_j^Z)Z \quad (7)$$

$$= \sum_{j=1}^{n} L_j(T_j - T_j^S) + Y,$$

where the time inputs per unit of consumption are given as t_j.[6] Since the consumption (or use) of D pertains to the family unit as a whole, the relevant wage and time varibles are some combination of the inputs of individual household members.[7] It is also recognized that in many instances children and other family members may not be in the labor force. Therefore the relevant time cost of a child's medical visit may be more accurately represented by the mother's wage rate. In summary, Eq. (7) tell us that the family's full income (adjusted for sick time) is spent on medical goods and services both outside and within the household, maintenance of the dwelling unit, and the composite bundle Z.

To find the first-order conditions for a local maximum, we can now form the Lagrangian function

$$\Lambda = U (M_j, N_j, D, Z) - \lambda[\sum_{j=1}^{n} (P_j + L_j t_j^M)M_j$$

$$+ \sum_{j=1}^{n} (Q_j + L_j t_j^N)N_j + (P_D + \sum_{j=1}^{n} L_j t_j^D)D \quad (8)$$

$$+ (P_Z + \sum_{j=1}^{n} L_j t_j^Z)Z - \sum_{j=1}^{n} L_j (T_j - T_j^S) - Y]$$

where λ is a Lagrange multiplier. Differentiating with respect to M_j, N_j, D, Z, and λ we obtain

$$\frac{\partial \Lambda}{\partial M_j} = U_{M_j} - \lambda(P_j + L_j t_j^M) = 0 \ (j = 1, ..., n), \tag{9}$$

$$\frac{\partial \Lambda}{\partial N_j} = U_{N_j} - \lambda(Q_j + L_j t_j^N) = 0 \ (j = 1, ..., n), \tag{10}$$

$$\frac{\partial \Lambda}{\partial D} = U_D - \lambda(P_D + \sum_{j=1}^{n} L_j t_j^D) = 0, \tag{11}$$

$$\frac{\partial \Lambda}{\partial Z} = U_Z - \lambda(P_Z + \sum_{j=1}^{n} L_j t_j^Z) = 0, \tag{12}$$

and

$$\frac{-\partial \Lambda}{\partial \lambda} = \sum_{j=1}^{n} [(P_j + L_j t_j^M) M_j + (Q_j + L_j t_j^N) N_j]$$

$$+ (P_D + \sum_{j=1}^{n} L_j t_j^D) D + (P_Z + \sum_{j=1}^{n} L_j t_j^Z) Z \tag{13}$$

$$- \sum_{j=1}^{n} L_j (T_j - T_j^S) - Y = 0.$$

The utility function is assumed to be continuous, strictly quasi-concave, and twice differentiable with positive (and decreasing) marginal utilities. These assumptions are sufficient to ensure that the bordered Hessian formed by totally differentiating Eqs. (9)–(13) is negative definite, with principal minors that alternate in sign. The solution of such a system of first-order conditions yields a global maximum.[8]

Using this basic model we can examine the effect of income (both earned and unearned) and prices (both own and cross) on the demand for medical goods and services. It is also desirable to determine—if possible—the degree of substitutability (or complementarity) of medical visits between household members. These and other comparative static results will be discussed in turn.

B. Price and Wage Elasticities of the Demand for Medical Care

The purpose of this subsection[9] is to evaluate the effects of changes in the independent variables on the demand for medical care. Particular emphasis is placed on income-and-price changes and the cross-elasticities of demand between household members.[10] If we let J equal the bordered Hessian matrix formed by totally differentiating Eqs. (9)–(13), then the effect of a change in nonwage income on the demand for visits is given as

$$\frac{\partial M_j}{\partial Y} = \frac{J_{\lambda j}}{|J|} \qquad (j = 1, ..., n) \tag{14}$$

where $J_{\lambda j}$ is the cofactor formed by deleting the λth row and the M_jth column of J. Assuming that M_j is a normal commodity, an increase in nonwage income will increase the demand for visits.[11] To ensure that Eq. (14) is positive, the numerator and denominator must have the same sign. With the aid of this information the effects of an own-price change on the demand for a good can be determined.

$$\frac{\partial M_j}{\partial P_j} = \frac{\lambda J_{jj}}{|J|} - \frac{M_j J_{\lambda j}}{|J|}. \tag{15}$$

The latter expression on the right-hand side of Eq. (15) is the income effect premultiplied by $-M_j$. Hence Eq. (15) can be rewritten as

$$\frac{\partial M_j}{\partial P_j} = \frac{\lambda J_{jj}}{|J|} - M_j \frac{\partial M_j}{\partial Y}. \tag{16}$$

As long as M_j is not an inferior good, the latter expression on the right-hand side of Eq. (16) will be negative. An increase in price is tantamount to a reduction in real income; and as real income declines, so does the demand for normal goods and services. The first term on the right-hand side of Eq. (16) is the substitution effect, and it relates to the difference between the consumer's initial equilibrium and his equilibrium after a compensated price change (i.e., holding satisfaction, or the consumer's level of utility constant). Pfouts (1972), as well as others, has clearly demonstrated that the substitution effect is the same as a compensated change in demand. Therefore we have

$$\frac{\partial M_j}{\partial P_j} = \frac{\partial M_j}{\partial P_j}\bigg|_{\bar{U}} - M_j \frac{\partial M_j}{\partial Y}. \tag{17}$$

In the event of an own-price change, it is possible to sign Eqs. (15)–(17) negative. Since the principal minors of J alternate in sign, and since J_{jj} represents the next largest minor of J, the numerator and denominator of the substitution effect must have opposite signs. Hence, Eqs. (15)–(17) are unambiguously negative. However, in the event of a cross-price change we have

$$\frac{\partial M_j}{\partial P_i} = \frac{\lambda J_{ij}}{|J|} - \frac{M_i J_{\lambda j}}{|J|} \tag{18}$$

which is not signable a priori. It is unfortunate that the effects of cross-price changes are not clearly defined, since the direction of the effect determines whether the goods in question are substitutes (a positive cross-price effect) or complements (a negative cross-price effect). In the next subsection an attempt is made to construct a test of the substitutability (or complementarity) of medical visits between the husband and wife.

It should be recalled that the full cost of obtaining care involves a nonpecuniary as well as a pecuniary price. Therefore it is worthwhile to examine the effects of time prices as well as money prices on the demand for medical care. Acton (1972a) has shown that the effect of a change in the time input on the demand for visits is equal to a change in the monetary price, weighted by the wage rate, which is after all the price of time. It is also interesting to note that the elasticity of demand for visits with respect to changes in the nonpecuniary price is the same whether or not the time variable is weighted by the wage rate. Since the elasticity measures the percentage rate of change, we should expect its value to be invariant with respect to a scale factor, such as the wage rate.[12] Hence indicidual j's elasticity of demand for medical care, with respect to a change in the time input necessary for individual i to complete a visit, can be expressed equivalently as

$$\eta_{M_j t_i^M} = \eta_{M_j(L_i t_i^M)}. \tag{19}$$

The cross-price elasticities of demand with respect to monetary and full prices are given as

$$\eta_{M_j P_i} = \frac{\partial M_j}{\partial P_i} \frac{P_i}{M_j} \tag{20}$$

and

$$\eta_{M_j(P_i + L_i t_i^M)} = \frac{\partial M_j}{\partial (P_i + L_i t_i^M)} \frac{P_i + L_i t_i^M}{M_j} = \frac{\partial M_j}{\partial P_i} \frac{P_i + L_i t_i^M}{M_j}. \tag{21}$$

If we successively multiply Eq. (21) by the fraction of full price attributable to nonpecuniary and pecuniary prices we have

$$\eta_{M_j t_i^M} = \eta_{M_j(P_i + L_i t_i^M)} \frac{L_i t_i^M}{P_i + L_i t_i^M} \tag{22}$$

and

$$\eta_{M_j P_i} = \eta_{M_j(P_i + L_i t_i^M)} \frac{P_i}{P_i + L_i t_i^M}. \tag{23}$$

Therefore we can say that

$$\left| \eta_{M_j t_i} \right| \begin{array}{c} > \\ = \\ < \end{array} \left| \eta_{M_j P_i} \right| \quad \text{as} \quad L_i t_i^M \begin{array}{c} > \\ = \\ < \end{array} P_i. \tag{24}$$

Equation (24) is important for evaluating cross-price changes as well as own-price changes in demand. Equation (24) indicates that for families facing comparatively low monetary prices, ceberis paribus, the elasticity of demand with respect to nonmonetary prices is relatively large. There-fore we expect that individuals receiving medical care at clinics and other "free" sources of care should have a relatively larger response, ceteris paribus, to changes in time–price variables than other individuals. Consider the situation in which the wife (or other family member) receives care at a zero monetary price clinic, and consider another household in which the wife visits a private physician. Then, we would expect, a priori, that the elasticity of demand for visits by the husband with respect to a change in the nonpecuniary price of the wife would be absolutely greater in the former case. It is expected that the estimation of these elasticities will yield policy implications pertaining to a more efficient distribution of medical services. For example, if the time costs of the wife (or any other household member) are found to have a significant impact on the husband's demand for care, the implication is that studies which analyze the determinants of demand solely from the individual's point of view have a somewhat myopic perspective and that the household and the prices that other family members pay for medical care are important variables that should be included in the analysis—even when we are considering the demand for medical care by an individual family member. Programs aimed at increasing the utilization of medical services should consider not just the individual[13] but the household and the prices it pays as the unit of analysis.

Although changes in the wage rate create a substitution and an (off-setting) income effect, it is possible to compare the effects of changes in the wage rate between those individuals who receive "free" care and those who pay (a money price) for it. The effect of a change in the individual's wage rate, L_j, on his or her demand for medical care, M_j, is given as

$$\frac{\partial M_j}{\partial L_j} = \frac{T_j^L J_{\lambda j} + \lambda t_j^M J_{Mj} + \lambda t_j^N J_{Nj} + \lambda t_j^D J_{Dj} + \lambda t_j^Z J_{Zj}}{|J|}$$

$$= T_j^L \frac{\partial M_j}{\partial Y} + \frac{\lambda t_j^M J_{Mj}}{|J|} + \frac{\lambda t_j^N J_{Nj}}{|J|} + \frac{\lambda t_j^D J_{Dj}}{|J|} + \frac{\lambda t_j^Z J_{Zj}}{|J|} , \tag{25}$$

which is unsignable. However, the effects of changes in the wage rate can be more easily analyzed if we assume that only one household member receives care and if we exclude the composite goods Z and D from the analysis. These assumptions are not as restrictive as they may first appear. Due to the large number of small families and generally good health status of our population, the assumption of only one household member receiving care does not seem unreasonable.[14] The composite good Z can be eliminated due to our earlier assumption of separability;

and while the omission of D is not as defendable, it could be argued that consumption or utilization of sanitary conditions in the household dwelling unit relates to other goods and services as well as health and therefore the effect of D on M_j, due to a change in L_j, may be tenuous at best. In any event, it should be recalled that all that is desired here is to compare the effects of changes in the wage rate between those who pay no money price for care and those who do.

Given the foregoing assumptions, the bordered Hessian formed by totally differentiating Eqs. (9)–(13) can be presented as

$$J^* \equiv \begin{bmatrix} U_{M_jM_j} & U_{M_jN_j} & P_j + L_jt_j^M \\ U_{N_jM_j} & U_{N_jN_j} & Q_j + L_jt_j^N \\ P_j + L_jt_j^M & Q_j + L_jt_j^N & 0 \end{bmatrix} \tag{26}$$

and the partial derivative of M_j with respect to L_j is given as

$$\frac{\partial M_j}{\partial L_j} = T_j^L \frac{\partial M_j}{\partial Y} - \frac{\lambda t_j^M (Q_j + L_jt_j^N)(Q_j + L_jt_j^N)}{|J|}$$
$$+ \frac{\lambda t_j^N (P_j + L_jt_j^M)(Q_j + L_jt_j^N)}{|J^*|}. \tag{27}$$

In order for the substitution effect (from N_j to M_j) to be positive we need

$$\frac{t_j^N}{Q_j + L_jt_j^N} > \frac{t_j^M}{P_j + L_jt_j^M}, \tag{28}$$

that is, the time component in the full price of N_j must be greater than the time component in M_j. Multiplying both sides of the inequality by the wage rate yields

$$\frac{L_jt_j^N}{Q_j + L_jt_j^N} > \frac{L_jt_j^M}{P_j + L_jt_j^M}. \tag{29}$$

However, in the face of a zero monetary price for medical care (and not for household drugs and medicines), Eq. (29) becomes

$$\frac{L_jt_j^N}{Q_j + L_jt_j^N} > 1. \tag{30}$$

This implies that $L_jt_j^N > Q_j + L_jt_j^N$. Therefore, barring nonnegative money prices for N_j, Eq. (30) cannot hold. Hence, if medical care is "free," the substitution effect between N_j and M_j must be negative. Of course, it is still possible that the income effect may swamp the substitution effect and cause an increase in the demand for M_j as a result of a higher wage. Nevertheless, we expect the substitution effect of an increase in

L_j to be more negative (or the overall effect smaller) when an individual receives "free" care than when he pays for it. This implies that programs aimed at increasing the utilization of medical care services should perhaps attempt to provide a more time-efficient[15] (from the patient's point of view) distribution of health care facilities and/or initiate lump-sum income subsidies to the consumer, rather than support legislation to increase the (minimum) wage rate. And, what is more important, policy makers must realize the (potential) significance of nonpecuniary costs as well as monetary costs when evaluating programs to improve the consumer's access to medical care.

C. A Test of the Substitutability or Complementarity of Medical Care Visits

It was pointed out earlier [see Eq. (18)] that although the effect of a cross-price change on the demand for medical care was unsignable, it was desirable to test if medical visits by two (or more) household members substituted for or complemented each other. It should be mentioned that this test can be developed for other goods and services, as well as for other household members; however, we are primarily interested in determining the degree of substitutability between medical visits by the husband and the wife. Not only is this the most general test to construct (since most households in the sample had at least these two members), but it may also be the most relevant since it is ultimately the visit decisions of the parents and their relationship that determines the family's overall attitude toward obtaining health care. Moreover, if intrafamily medical visits tend to be related (either as substitutes or complements), it implies that programs formulated to increase health care contacts by a particular household member (say, the wife) should consider the demand by the husband (and other household members) as well. For purposes of simplicity it is assumed that the household contains two members (husband and wife) and that changes in the composite vector of other goods and services, Z, are ignored.[16] The total differential of the first-order conditions [Eqs. (9)–(13)] can now be presented as

$$
\overset{\text{A}}{\begin{bmatrix}
U_{M_wM_w} & U_{M_wM_h} & U_{M_wN_w} & U_{M_wN_h} & U_{M_wD} & F_w \\
U_{M_hM_w} & U_{M_hM_h} & U_{M_hN_w} & U_{M_hN_h} & U_{M_hD} & F_h \\
U_{N_wM_w} & U_{N_wM_h} & U_{N_wN_w} & U_{N_wN_h} & U_{N_wD} & G_w \\
U_{N_hM_w} & U_{N_hM_h} & U_{N_hN_w} & U_{N_hN_h} & U_{N_hD} & G_h \\
U_{DM_w} & U_{DM_h} & U_{DN_w} & U_{DN_h} & U_{DD} & F_D \\
F_w & F_h & G_w & G_h & F_D & 0
\end{bmatrix}}
\overset{\text{B}}{\begin{bmatrix}
dM_w \\
dM_h \\
dN_w \\
dN_h \\
dD \\
-d\lambda
\end{bmatrix}}
\qquad (31)
$$

$$
\begin{array}{c}
C \\
= \begin{bmatrix}
\lambda \ dF_w \\
\lambda \ dF_h \\
\lambda \ dG_w \\
\lambda \ dG_h \\
\lambda \ dD \\
-\Sigma M_j \ dF_j - \Sigma N_j \ dG_j - D \ dF_D \\
-\Sigma(T_j^S - T_j) \ dL_j - \sum L_j \ dT_j^S + dY
\end{bmatrix}
\end{array}
$$

where $F_j = P_j + L_j t_j^M$, $G_j = Q_j + L_j t_j^N$, and $F_D = P_D + L_j t_j^D$ ($j = h$, w).[17] Considering the situation in which the wife demands no medical visits ($dM_w = 0$), the system of equations can be rewritten as

$$
\underset{A^*}{\begin{bmatrix}
U_{M_hM_h} & U_{M_hN_w} & U_{M_hN_h} & U_{M_hD} & F_h \\
U_{N_wM_h} & U_{N_wN_w} & U_{N_wN_h} & U_{N_wD} & G_w \\
U_{N_hM_h} & U_{N_hN_w} & U_{N_hN_h} & U_{N_hD} & G_h \\
U_{DM_h} & U_{DN_w} & U_{DN_h} & U_{DD} & F_D \\
F_h & G_w & G_h & F_D & 0
\end{bmatrix}}
\underset{B^*}{\begin{bmatrix}
dM_h \\
dN_w \\
dN_h \\
dD \\
-d\lambda
\end{bmatrix}}
\tag{32}
$$

$$
\underset{C^*}{= \begin{bmatrix}
\lambda \ dF_h \\
\lambda \ dG_w \\
\lambda \ dG_h \\
\lambda \ dD \\
-M_h dF_h - \Sigma N_j \ dG_j - D \ dF_D \\
-\Sigma(T_j^S - T_j) \ dL_j - \Sigma L_j \ dT_j^S + dY
\end{bmatrix}}
$$

By applying Cramer's rule to Eq. (31) we can evaluate a change in nonwage income, Y[18]

$$
\frac{\partial M_i}{\partial Y} = \frac{A_{\lambda i}}{|A|} \qquad (i = h, w) \tag{33}
$$

where $A_{\lambda i}$ is the cofactor formed by deleting the λth row and ith column of A. Similarly a change in the full price of a medical visit can be expressed as

$$
\begin{aligned}
\frac{\partial M_i}{\partial F} &= \frac{\lambda A_{ji}}{|A|} - \frac{M_j A_{\lambda i}}{|A|} \\
&= \frac{\lambda A_{ji}}{|A|} - \frac{M_j \ \partial M_i}{\partial Y} \\
&= \frac{\partial M_i}{\partial F_j}\bigg|_{\bar{U}} - \frac{M_j \ \partial M_i}{\partial Y}
\end{aligned}
\tag{34}
$$

where $(\partial M_i/\partial F_j)|_{\bar{U}}$ is the substitution effect and $M_j \; \partial M_i/\partial Y$ is the income effect.

Kniesner (1976), in a recent *Econometrica* article, has shown that the husband's (wife's) demand for leisure, in response to a change in nonwage income, will differ depending upon the substitutability or complementarity of leisure between the wife and husband. Following Kniesner, a similar procedure can be used to determine the effect of unearned household income on the demand for visits by the husband and wife.[19] We will find that the response will vary, depending on the degree of substitutability between M_h and M_w.

A theorem by Jacobi (see Yamane, 1968) on determinants states that for an $n \times n$ matrix, Θ, with Θ^{adj} as the matrix of the cofactors of Θ, the following relationship holds

$$\Omega r = \bar{\Omega}_{n-r} \, |\Theta|^{r-1} \tag{35}$$

where $\Omega_r \equiv$ a minor of order r of $|\Theta^{adj}|$, and $\bar{\Omega}_{n-r} \equiv$ the complementary minor of Ω, but in $|\Theta|$. Applying Eq. (35) to Eqs. (31) and (32), we obtain

$$\begin{vmatrix} A_{M_wM_w} & A_{M_wM_h} \\ A_{M_hM_w} & A_{M_hM_h} \end{vmatrix} = A_{M^{\cdot_h}M_h} |A|, \tag{36}$$

or

$$A_{M_wM_w} \quad A_{M_hM_h} = A_{M^{\cdot_h}M_h}|A| + A_{M_hM_w}A_{M_wM_h},$$

and

$$\begin{vmatrix} A_{M_wM_w} & A_{M_wM_h} \\ A_{\lambda M_w} & A_{\lambda M_h} \end{vmatrix} = A_{M^{\cdot_h}}|A|, \tag{37}$$

or

$$A_{M_wM_w}A_{\lambda M_h} = A_{\lambda M^{\cdot_h}}|A| + A_{\lambda M_w}A_{M_wM_h}.$$

From Eq. (33) we know that

$$\frac{\partial M_h}{\partial Y^*} = \frac{A_{\lambda M^{\cdot_h}}}{|A^*|}. \tag{38}$$

Using Eqs. (31) and (32) we can say that

$$|A^*| = A_{M_wM_w}. \tag{39}$$

Substituting Eqs. (37) and (39) into Eq. (38) yields

$$\frac{\partial M_h}{\partial Y^*} = \frac{-A_{\lambda M_w}A_{M_wM_h}}{|A|A_{M_wM_w}} + \frac{A_{M_wM_w}A_{\lambda M_h}}{|A|A_{M_wM_w}}$$

$$= -\left[\frac{A_{\lambda M_w}}{|A|} \; \frac{A_{M_wM_h}}{|A|} \right] \frac{|A|}{A_{M_wM_w}} + \frac{A_{\lambda M_h}}{A} \tag{40}$$

$$= \frac{-\dfrac{A_{\lambda M_w} A_{M_w M_h}}{|A| \quad |A|}}{\dfrac{A_{M_w M_w}}{|A|}} + \frac{A_{\lambda M_h}}{|A|}$$

or

$$\frac{\dfrac{A_{\lambda M_w} A_{M_w M_h}}{|A| \quad |A|}}{\dfrac{A_{M_w M_w}}{|A|}} = \frac{A_{\lambda M_h}}{|A|} - \frac{\partial M_h}{\partial Y^*}. \tag{41}$$

From Eq. (34) and the symmetry of the bordered Hessian, A, we know that

$$\left.\frac{\partial M_h}{\partial F_w}\right|_{\dot{U}} = \frac{\lambda A_{M_w M_h}}{|A|} = \frac{\lambda A_{M_h M_w}}{|A|} = \left.\frac{\partial M_w}{F_h}\right|_{\dot{U}}; \tag{42}$$

$$\left.\frac{\partial M_w}{\partial F_w}\right|_{\dot{U}} = \frac{A_{M_w M_w}}{A}; \tag{43}$$

and

$$\frac{\partial M_w}{\partial F_h} = \frac{\lambda A_{M_h M_w}}{|A|} - \frac{M_h A_{\lambda M_w}}{|A|}. \tag{44}$$

Substituting Eqs. (42) and (43) into Eq. (41) gives

$$\frac{\dfrac{\partial M_w}{\partial Y}\left.\left(\dfrac{\partial M_h}{\partial F_w}\right)\right|_{\dot{U}}}{\left.\dfrac{\partial M_w}{\partial F_w}\right|_{\dot{U}}} = \frac{\partial M_h}{\partial Y} - \frac{\partial M_h}{\partial Y^*}. \tag{45}$$

Assuming that M_h and M_w are both normal goods, then $\partial M_w/\partial Y$ is greater than zero, $(\partial M_w/\partial F_w)|_{\dot{U}}$ is less than zero, and we can say that

$$\frac{\partial M_h}{\partial Y} \underset{>}{\overset{<}{=}} \frac{\partial M_h}{\partial Y^*} \quad \text{as} \quad \left.\frac{\partial M_h}{\partial F_w}\right|_{\dot{U}} \underset{<}{\overset{>}{=}} 0. \tag{46}$$

Equation (46) indicates that if there is a greater response of M_h to changes in unearned income when the wife is receiving care as compared to when she is not, then $(\partial M_h/\partial F_w)_{\dot{U}}$ is less than zero, which implies that M_h and M_w are complements. Similarly if $\partial M_h/\partial Y$ is less than $\partial M_h/\partial Y^*$, then M_h and M_w are substitutes. Hence we have a simple test, which can be verified empirically, to determine whether medical visits of the husband and wife are substitutes or complements. Moreover, the results of this test should coincide with those obtained by examining the (Slutsky) decomposition of a change in price. Recall that the effect of a (cross-)

price change on demand can be broken down into substitution and income effects such that

$$\frac{\partial M_h}{\partial F_w} = \left.\frac{\partial M_h}{\partial F_w}\right|_{\bar{U}} - M_w\frac{\partial M_h}{\partial Y} \tag{47}$$

Therefore, examination of the compensated price change (substitution effect) and income coefficients (along with M_w) will also determine whether M_h and M_w are substitutes or complements. The two approaches will, we hope, yield similar results.

There are however several caveats which should be mentioned. First, is that the decision to see a doctor may be influenced to a large extent not only by the health status of other family members but also by other epidemiological factors which cannot be controlled for. It is possible that the sample may have a high incidence of illness due to the proximity of a pollutant or be susceptible to some virus such that any evidence of substitutability or complementarity within the household cannot be singled out. Second, it should be mentioned that the accuracy of the unearned income variable used in the study is somewhat suspect, since the only income variable available from the survey was total household income. However, a proxy for earned income was constructed from the 1970 Public Use Sample, thereby enabling estimation of nonwage income.[20] Nevertheless, it is worthwhile to examine empirically the response of M_h (M_w) to changes in unearned income. If the response is greater when the wife (husband) is receiving care, as compared to when she (he) is not, then M_h and M_w are complements.

D. Summary of Theoretical Results

In this section a family model of the demand for medical goods and services is constructed. The inclusion of all household members and the family's use of household medical goods and services in the analysis represent an extension of existing demand models. Although the discussion and comparative static results are presented for two-person households, the results may be extended to n family members. Household utility is maximized subject to a full-income constraint, and emphasis is placed on both the pecuniary and nonpecuniary costs of obtaining care. The principal theoretical results are reviewed below.

Assuming that medical care is a normal good,

$$\frac{\partial M_j}{\partial Y} > 0 \qquad (j = 1, ..., n) \tag{48}$$

and

$$\frac{\partial M_j}{\partial P_j} < 0 \qquad (j = 1, ..., n). \tag{49}$$

The effects of cross-(monetary)price changes are unsignable a priori; however, we are able to test indirectly whether the medical visits by various household members substitute or complement each other. If $\partial M_h / \partial Y$ when the wife is receiving care is greater (*less*) than $\partial M_h / \partial Y$ when the wife is not receiving care, then medical visits by the husband and wife are complements (*substitutes*).

Changes in the amount of time required to receive medical care act in the same direction as monetary price changes, and when the time input necessary to receive care is weighted by the individual's wage rate (the price of time), its effect on the demand for care is analogous to a money price change

$$\frac{\partial M_j}{\partial (L_i t_i^M)} = \frac{\partial M_j}{\partial P_i} = \frac{\partial M_j}{\partial (P_i + L_i t_i^M)} . \tag{50}$$

A comparison of the elasticities of demand with respect to time and (money) price verifies the increase in relative importance of time costs to the consumer as money price approaches zero. Furthermore, the (time) price that one family member pays for care, may effect the demand for visits by other household members.

$$\left| \eta_{M_j T_i} \right| \begin{array}{c} > \\ = \\ < \end{array} \left| \eta_{M_j P_i} \right| \qquad \text{as} \qquad L_i t_i^M \begin{array}{c} > \\ = \\ < \end{array} P_i . \tag{51}$$

The effects of changes in the wage rate, $\partial M_j / \partial L_j$, on the demand for medical visits are expected to be smaller (more negative) for those individuals receiving free care.

In summary, the theoretical results suggest that the effects of income and prices—both pecuniary and nonpecuniary, as well as own and cross—on the demand for medical care may be substantial. In the next section we examine these hypotheses empirically.

III. EMPIRICAL RESULTS

Having developed a theoretical model of the demand for medical care, the next step is to test the theoretical results and relationships empirically. In the following subsections I present empirical results from the estimation of my model. In Section III.A, I outline the (Tobit) estimating technique and discuss why ordinary least-squares estimation leads to inefficient results. In Section III.B the data and the variables used in the econometric analysis are described, and in Section III.C, I review the main theoretical results and specify the form of the estimating equations. In the remainder of this section, empirical results for both individual family members and the household unit are discussed. The results are summarized in Section III.H and policy implications are suggested.[21]

A. Estimation Technique

Although the theoretical model does not establish an explicit functional form (linear, nonlinear, etc.) for the estimating equations, the nature of the data suggests that ordinary least squares (OLS) is an inefficient estimating procedure. When a model is estimated by OLS it is assumed that the full ideal conditions hold. In particular, it is assumed that the random disturbance term, ε_i, is normally distributed, has a mean of zero, and constant variance; ε_i is assumed to be continuous in the range from minus infinity to plus infinity and is distributed symmetrically around its mean. The distribution of ε_i is fully determined by the mean and variance. This implies that the expected value of the dependent variable is determined partly by a vector of nonstochastic independent variables and partly by the random disturbance term ε_i.[22] In this case however, the dependent variable—the number of medical care visits—is bounded by zero for a substantial number of observations, and under OLS it is (very) possible for the independent variables to take on values which yield an expected value of the dependent variable beneath its limiting value.[23] As long as the dependent variable is bounded (either above or below) for a large number of observations, the assumption of normality of disturbance terms—and hence of the estimated coefficients—is violated, and therefore the classical tests of significance are inappropriate.

Tobin (1958) has developed a technique for estimating limited or bounded dependent variables and argues convincingly that the special nature of the dependent variable should be preserved. When a dependent variable is bounded or limited, explanatory variables may be expected to influence both the probability of limit responses and the magnitude of nonlimit observations. If we are interested in analyzing the probability of limit (or nonlimit) responses, probit analysis is an appropriate estimation technique; if, instead, we are interested in "explaining" the magnitude of the dependent variable, OLS is a suitable estimating procedure. However, neither approach is adquate for accounting for both types of behavior in the dependent variable; each involves a loss in information and, therefore, in efficiency as well. Probit analysis cannot control for a (wide) range of observations not at the limit, whereas multiple regression analysis cannot adjust for a large number of bounded observations. Hence, the procedure developed by Tobin is a hybrid of the probit and multiple regression techniques. If the sum of the linear combination of explanatory variables and the disturbance term is positive, the dependent variable is set equal to this sum. Otherwise the dependent variable is sct cqual to zcro.[24] Following Tobin then, a Tobit (maximum-likelihood) estimation technique is employed in the empirical analysis.[25]

B. Data

The data that are used were obtained from the Department of Community Health Sciences at Duke University.[26] During a twenty-one month period this department conducted an extensive household survey in two rural communities north of Durham, North Carolina.[27] The communities studied were Rougemont/Bahama and Bragtown; however, only data from the Rougemont/Bahama survey are analyzed in this study. Although the survey consisted of five visits—an initial health survey, followed up by four panel-study visits—only data from the initial survey and the first and third panel studies are used in this project.[28] To ensure continued community acceptance of the project, at least $2\frac{1}{2}$ months were permitted to elapse between each individual household visit. Every household in the community was visited, and the completion rate was extraordinarily high—94.4 percent. The number of households interviewed was 665, and the estimated number of persons living in the community is 2,275.

Before describing the variables used in the current analysis, a word or two should be said about the organization of the data and the form of the estimating equations. The survey was conducted by a team of interviewers which made personal visits to each household in the community. The primary purpose of the initial household survey was to gather demographic and background health data on the community. Due both to budget limitations and the project's concern with the health care needs of middle- and lower-income households, 53 households with total incomes of at least $16,000 were dropped from the panel study visits. Each panel study visit provides a detailed monitoring of health status and medical care utilization during the preceding 3 months. Information was collected on the monetary cost of obtaining care as well as the opportunity cost of time associated with completing medical care visits.

Information was collected on the head of household, as well as on all other family members. In most circumstances the head of household (or primary income earner) was male (83%), and in virtually all cases the spouse of the head was female.[29] However, all households with two or more members did not necessarily have a spouse (or wife) present. Of the 582 households with two or more members, there were 91 without a spouse. Needless to say, in all circumstances one household member was designated as the head. Other household members include sons and daughters of the head, other relatives, and boarders; however, in most households (85%), family members other than the head and spouse were progeny of the head of household. Demand for medical care equations are estimated for the head of household, for the spouse of the head, for the family as a unit, and for a subset of the family which excludes both the head and spouse.

A glossary of the varibles used in the econometric analysis is presented at the end of the chapter; means and standard deviations are contained in Tables 1 and 2. Table 1 includes those variables that are related to health and medical care, while in Table 2 those variables which are economic or demographic in nature are listed.[30] The visit (VISTH, VISTW) and fee (FEEH, FEEW) information in Table 1 indicates that heads of households have fewer medical care visits than their wives, and on the average, tend to pay less for them. Medical care visits include visits to private physicians, hospital outpatient departments, and clinics. The information on fees reflects the amount that the respondent indicated was his/her typical fee at his/her usual source of care. Data were also collected on total household medical visit expenditures; however, due to the high multicolinearity between visits and expenditures and the lack of individual expenditure data, the "usual fee" variable is used as the (monetary) price of receiving medical care.[31]

Table 1. Means and Standard Deviations of Health Related Variables

Variable	Mean	Standard Deviation	No. of Observations
VISTH	2.06	3.82	567
VISTW	2.94	4.21	419
AFAMV	1.96	2.68	663
AKIDV	1.34	2.45	396
FEEH	8.07	10.65	534
FEEW	12.32	12.00	413
AVFFE	8.75	9.61	663
AVKFE	5.99	7.16	396
TRAVL	0.44	0.21	546
WAIT	0.92	1.43	523
APPT	10.46	18.63	511
INSPM	96.12	108.11	557
DRUGH	0.52	—[a]	663
DRUGW	0.63	—[a]	491
DRUGA	0.70	—[a]	663
SICKH	0.30	—[a]	663
SICKW	0.26	—[a]	491
SICKF	0.40	—[a]	663
PHYCH	0.57	—[a]	663
PHYCW	0.67	—[a]	491
DWELL₁	0.76	—[a]	663
MCARH	0.23	—[a]	663
MCARW	0.10	—[a]	491
MCAID	0.15	—[a]	663

Note: [a]Standard deviations are not presented for binary variables.

Table 2. Means and Standard Deviations of Economic and
Demographic Variables

Variable	Mean	Standard Deviation	No. of Observations
EARNH	2.31	1.18	606
EARNW	1.44	0.50	478
WORKH	0.72	—[a]	663
NWRKH	0.28	—[a]	663
WORKW	0.45	—[a]	491
NWRKW	0.55	—[a]	491
INC	66.17	42.06	512
UNINC	19.61	32.59	512
LFEH	2.54	1.15	452
NLFEH	1.63	0.99	154
LFEW	1.50	0.51	217
NLFEW	1.39	0.48	261
TVLEH	0.96	0.66	495
TVLEW	0.61	0.32	394
LFTEH	1.05	0.65	360
NLTEH	0.74	0.64	135
LFTEW	0.64	0.33	170
NLTEW	0.58	0.31	224
COUNT	3.41	2.09	663
RACE	0.28	—[a]	663
SEXH	0.17	—[a]	663

Note: [a]Standard deviations are not presented for binary variables.

In addition to the individual data on visits and prices, two other pairs of variables measure these values for the household as a unit and for household members other than the head and wife. The respective household and other household member visit variables are AFAMV and AKIDV, while the fee variables are AVFFE and AVKFE.[32] In each case, these variables are created on a per household member basis, since it is expected that larger households will have both more visits and higher total fees due solely to the larger number of potential patients living in the household.

The three time–price variables that are used are travel time from the home to the usual source of care (TRAVL), time spent waiting in the waiting room (WAIT), and the number of days it takes to get an appointment at the usual source of care in nonemergency situations (APPT). Data on these time–price variables were collected on a household rather than an individual basis; however, when weighted by the individual's wage rate these variables can be used as estimates of the individual's opportunity cost of time.

Although most households either receive free ambulatory care or pay for it out-of-pocket, a health insurance variable (INSPM) is included in the regression equations to estimate the effect of health insurance on the demand for medical care.[33] Admittedly this variable is very imprecise; there are no data available on the amount or extent of coverage for specific ailments or on deductibles or coinsurance rates.[34] Information on health insurance premiums was collected for the household as a unit and in no way identifies the degree of coverage for individual family members.

Three different binary variables are used to estimate the utilization of medical goods and services within the household. During the panel study visits, questions were asked regarding the utilization of drugs and medicines by various household members. If the head, wife, or either parent used any drugs, medicines, or remedies, and it was not prescribed by a doctor, the appropriate dummy variable (DRUGH, DRUGW, DRUGA) is set equal to 1. In an attempt to quantify the level of sanitation in the household another binary variable (DWELL$_1$) is set equal to 1 if the interviewer rated the dwelling unit as being in excellent condition. The omitted reference group includes those households that are in deteriorating (18 percent) and dilapidated (6 percent) condition.

Various measures of illness and disability were available from the survey, e.g., number of acute and chronic conditions, number of bed days; however, the individual's subjective evaluation of his/her own health status is used here. Earlier estimates of the model that included the number of acute and chronic conditions as independent variables yielded estimates which were highly significant; it is unclear, however, to what extent the reporting of such conditions is influenced in turn by the physician's diagnosis of the actual visit. The number of bed days due to illness or injury, while generally significant, was not as powerful as either the number of acute and chronic conditions, or the individual's self-evaluation in "explaining" the demand for visits.

Two other binary variables are used in an attempt to control for quality differences in the various types of medical visits. PHYCH (PHYCW) is set equal to one if the head's (wife's) usual source of care is a private physician. The omitted reference group includes those individuals who usually attend clinics and hospital outpatient departments (approximately 31 percent of heads and wives) and those who have no usual source of care (approximately 9 percent).

The last group of health-related variables measures whether or not the head or wife is eligible for Medicare benefits (MCARM, MCARW) and whether or not the household is eligible for Medicaid (MCAID). An individual is considered eligible for Medicare if he/she is at least 65 years old; eligibility requirements for Medicaid are determined by household size, income, and geographic location.[35]

The economic and demographic variables are listed in Table 2. The earnings variables measure estimated hourly wage rates for the head of household (EARNH) and the wife (EARNW). Since no information is available from the Rougemont/Bahama survey to permit us to measure individual wage rates (and hence the opportunity cost of time), county data from the Public Use Samples from the 1970 Census are used to calculate proxy wage variables.

Geographically, the commumities of Rougemont and Bahama are located in the northernmost tip of Durham County. The comparable county group, available from the Public Use Samples, includes Durham, Wake, and Orange counties. These counties are among the most urban and populous in the state of North Carolina.[36] Preliminary comparisons of the demographic characteristics of the people in (rural) Rougemont/Bahama with those in this Public Use Sample county group indicate that there are substantial differences between the two populations.[37] Rather than use the Wake, Durham, Orange County group, it was decided to use the 10-county group that borders Durham County to the north and east.[38] The available demographic and economic variables indicate that the population in this group is highly comparable with that of Rougemont/Bahama.

Although the census data do not contain an explicit wage variable, it is possible to construct one by dividing the individual's total earned income by weeks and hours worked. Total earned income includes wage and salary income as well as earnings from self-employed enterprises (businesses, farming, private practices, etc.) during the preceding calendar year (i.e., 1969). Weeks worked is the number of weeks that the respondent reported as being employed in 1969. The hours worked variable measures the number of hours that the respondent worked in the week prior to the census. Unfortunately there is no guarantee that the number of hours worked during this reference week is an accurate estimate of the individual's hourly employment per week for the preceding year. With this caveat in mind, two different wage variables were computed: one by dividing weekly earnings by the house variable, and the second by dividing weekly earnings by 40, under the (somewhat heroic) assumption that the respondent was fully employed for the weeks he/she reported as having worked. The regression results obtained from the latter variable were preferable to the former (lower standard errors on the coefficients, and higher $\bar{R}^2$ and F values) and they are the ones used to construct the wage variable for the Rougemont/Bahama data.

Mincer (1974) and Mincer and Polachek (1974), as well as others, have provided both a theoretical and empirical foundation for the form of the wage-estimating equation, and it need not be developed in detail here. There is, however, one additional issue which should be considered before we consider the wage-regression estimates. The wage regression from the Public Use Sample is estimated for persons who were employed (at least part time) in 1969 and whose computed wage was greater than zero. Since an estimate of the value of time is desired for all members of the community and not just those who work, the analysis must be modified to construct a wage variable for those not in the labor force.

Gronau (1973, 1974), Heckman (1974, 1977), and others have grappled with the theoretical and empirical issues associated with measuring the opportunity cost of time for those not at work and they have been successful in developing procedures for estimating the value of time for those not employed.[39] Newhouse and Phelps (1976), in an article dealing with the demand for medical care services, attempt to estimate the value of time by using Heckman's (1974) procedure. Unfortunately, they are unable to obtain reliable estimates.[40] As an alternative they estimate a wage equation for those employed and use the resulting estimates to construct a wage variable for those unemployed by setting the weeks worked variable to zero. Newhouse and Phelps recognize that their estimates are biased; however, they point out (like Gronau, 1973) that the direction of the bias is not obvious, and they suggest that any bias in their price elasticity estimates is likely to be small (1976, pp. 269–270). The procedure used here is similar to the one employed by Newhouse and Phelps.[41]

If we compare the means of the computed wage variables for working and nonworking wives (LFEW and NLFEW in Table 2) we see that the wage rate for nonworking wives is less than that for working wives but well within Gronau's (1973) suggested 20-percent interval.[42] There is a much larger difference between the earnings of employed and nonworking heads (LFEH, NLFEH); however, this group is much less homogeneous than that of the wives. At any rate it should be reiterated that the wage variables used here are at best proxies for the opportunity cost of time— due both to the construction of the wage variable in the census data and the use of regression coefficients to create a wage variable for people in Rougemont/Bahama—and care should be exercised in interpreting their effect on the demand for medical care.

It is worthwhile to mention several of the other variables included in Table 2. The binary variables for labor force participation indicate that nearly three-quarters of all the heads of households are employed (WORKH) whereas slightly less than half of the wives (WORKW) are working in the labor force. Mean household income is $6,617; however it should be recalled that households with incomes greater than $16,000 have been omitted from the analysis.[43] Since wages and unearned income exhibit different effects on the demand for medical care, it is desirable to separate total household income into its earned and unearned components. By using the proxy wage variable for household members who are currently employed, an estimate of total earned household income can be obtained.

Subtracting this estimate from total household income yields unearned household income (UNINC).[44] The race and sex binary variables indicate that 28 percent of all households are black and that 17 percent of the heads of households are female. Average household size is about 3.4 people. Finally, there are three pairs of wage–travel time interaction terms. TVLEH and TVLEW measure the cost of travel time for the head and wife, respectively, while LFTEH (LFTEW) and NLTEH (NLTEW) provide separate estimates of this variable for working and nonworking heads (wives).

C. Review of the Theoretical Results and Format of the Empirical Model

Having discussed the data to be used at some length, it is worthwhile to recapitulate the main theoretical results before presenting the empirical model.

1. The comparative static results developed in Section II indicate that monetary price has a negative effect on the demand for medical care (assuming that medical care visits are a normal good).
2. Changes in the amount of time required to receive care act in the same direction as monetary price changes; and when the time input necessary to receive care is weighted by the individual's wage rate, its effect on the demand for care is analogous to a change in money price. Furthermore, the absolute value of the elasticity of demand with respect to time should be greater than *(less than, equal to)* the absolute value of the price elasticity of demand, if the time price of receiving care is greater than *(less than, equal to)* the money price.
3. Although cross-price changes are not signable a priori, a test is developed which indicates that medical care visits by the husband and wife are complements *(substitutes)* if the effect of unearned income on the husband's demand for medical care when the wife is receiving care is greater *(less)* than when she is not. While an alternative estimate of the income compensated cross-price term can be obtained by examining the estimated coefficients of cross-price and income (weighted by the spouse's visits), the two procedures should provide a useful check for one another.
4. Finally, the effect of a change in the wage rate on the demand for medical visits is expected to be smaller (more negative) for individuals receiving free care. This is due to the increased relative importance of opportunity costs as monetary costs get smaller.

Although the aforementioned theoretical results emphasize the effect of economic variables on the demand for medical care, the model suggests that other variables should be included in the empirical analysis as well.

Since the utility model developed earlier includes both extrahousehold and intrahousehold medical services, it is desirable to estimate demand equations for both ambulatory medical visits and medical goods and services used solely within the household. Unfortunately the price and quantity data available for intrahousehold medical care are not (statistically) robust enough to allow for separate estimates. Household members were asked if they took any of a series of medicines and whether or not it was prescribed by a physician.

There is no information available pertaining to the amount of medicines taken or the price that was paid.[45] In an attempt to test for any substitutability or complementarity that may exist between the two types of medical goods, a binary variable corresponding to the individual's utilization of nonprescription medicines is included in the estimating equations.[46] Although the utilization of nonprescription drugs and household remedies may substitute for medical care visits, it is also possible that the two goods may serve as complements.[47]

The influence of other household members on the demand for medical care is implicitly considered above in the cross-price term; however, family size is also included as an explanatory variable in the individual demand equations.[48] Even though larger households should, on the average, have more visits than smaller households, the effect of family size on an individual's demand for care may be negative. Holding income constant, as household size increases each individual's share of any available good or service decreases.[49]

Since medical visits are by no means homogeneous, a binary variable corresponding to the individual's usual source of care is included in the estimating equations. Although the type of visit and extensiveness of treatment may vary within as well as among given medical care settings, it is expected that this variable will control for quality (or taste) differences among alternative sources of care. Health status is expected to have a significant effect on the demand for medical care, and it is controlled for as well in the empirical analysis.[50] Finally, the effects of health insurance, medicare, and medicaid are adjusted for. Coverage by any (or all) of these variables should both increase the demand for care, and reduce the influence of price and income on demand.

The general format of the demand for medical care equation can be specified as

$$\text{visits} = \beta_0 + \beta_1 \overset{-}{\text{price}} + \beta_2 \overset{+}{\text{income}} + \beta_3 \overset{?}{\text{other medical}}$$
$$\text{goods} + \beta_4 \overset{-}{\text{family size}} + \beta_5 \overset{+}{\text{quality}} + \beta_6 \overset{+}{\text{ill}} \qquad (52)$$
$$\text{health} + \beta_7 \overset{+}{\text{health insurance}} + \varepsilon$$

where the expected signs of the coefficients are given above the variables.[51]

The empirical results are presented by household member, and in the next subsection the results for the head of household are discussed. The basic demand model is considered first, and then the effects of cross-price changes are examined. In the subsections that follow, results for the wife, the household as a unit, and other family members are analyzed.

D.   The Demand for Medical Visits by the Head of Household

The Tobit estimation results for the head of household are presented in Tables 3 and 4. In Table 3 travel time is weighted by the head's estimated wage rate; in Table 4 travel time is unweighted. It should be pointed out that the reported t statistics are not exact but rather are asymptotically normal variables; the estimated elasticities are of the expected value locus of the dependent variable, with respect to the independent variables, calculated at mean values.

Equation (53) in Table 3 includes only the economic variables from the model and the place of care dummy variable (PHYCH). Two different measures of the opportunity cost of travel time are used: one for employed heads of households (LFTEH), and one for unemployed heads (NLTEH). Separating the time-cost variable in this way allows its effect to vary with labor force status. Given the imprecision of the estimated wage variable (especially for individuals not in the labor force), this approach may yield more meaningful estimates of the opportunity cost of time.[52] Similarly, in Eq. (57) in Table 4, one wage variable is included for employed heads of households (LFEH) and another variable is included for nonworking heads (NLFEH).

Recall that due to contrasting income and substitution effects, the effect of a change in the wage rate on the demand for medical visits is not signable a priori. It now appears that the substitution effect may dominate for employed individuals whereas the income effect may control the demand for care for those who are unemployed.[53] Although a nonworking head of household may have a higher value of time than an employed head, employed individuals actually sacrifice money income by taking time to consume goods and services rather than working in the market place. Therefore, it does not seem unreasonable that the substitution effect should dominate the income effect for employed heads.[54]

The other nonmonetary price variables (waiting time and appointment time) were included along with travel time in earlier estimating equations; however, their effect on the demand for medical visits never attained significance. Appointment time, we recall, measures the days spent waiting for an appointment; and while it may be inconvenient for the consumer to have to wait for an appointment, the time spent waiting does

Table 3. The Demand for Medical Visits by the Head of Household: Travel Time Weighted by the Cost Time[a]

Independent Variables	53			54			55			56		
	Coef	t	η	Coef	t	η	Coef	t	η	Coef	t	η
FEEH	−0.031	−0.90	−0.054	−0.033	−0.96	−0.058	−0.028	−0.81	0.050	−0.025	−0.73	−0.045
LFTEH	−0.932	−1.74	−0.149	−0.814	−1.52	−0.131	−0.495	−0.92	−0.081	−0.309	−0.52	−0.051
NLTEH	1.896	2.23	0.078	2.011	2.36	0.083	1.381	1.60	0.058	1.106	1.28	0.047
UNINC	0.015	1.44	0.066	0.015	1.36	0.063	0.014	1.32	0.062	0.021	1.83	0.093
PHYCH	0.980	1.31	0.118	0.841	1.13	0.102	0.536	0.72	0.066	0.147	0.19	0.018
SICKH							2.206	2.96	0.139	1.957	2.53	0.123
DRUGH				1.637	2.31	0.216	1.453	2.07	0.195	1.585	2.24	0.214
COUNT							−0.337	−2.08	−0.253	−0.313	−1.86	−0.235
MCAID										1.560	1.48	0.058
MCARH										0.514	0.50	0.022
INSPM										0.005	1.63	0.114
CONSTANT	−0.021	−0.03		−1.076	−1.27		−0.443	−0.39		−1.445	−1.12	

Note: [a]364 observations.

113

Table 4. The Demand for Medical Visits by the Head of Household: Unweighted Travel Time[a]

Independent Variables	57			58			59			60		
	Coef	t	η	Coef	t	η	Coef	t	η	Coef	t	η
TRAVL	-1.456	-0.91	-0.135	-1.513	-0.94	-0.141	-1.880	-1.18	-0.179	-1.976	-1.23	-0.189
FEEH	-0.034	-0.98	-0.060	-0.037	-1.04	-0.064	-0.029	-0.85	-0.052	-0.025	-0.73	-0.045
LFEH	-0.463	-1.38	-0.168	-0.346	-1.02	-0.126	-0.043	-0.12	-0.016	0.168	0.40	0.063
NLFEH	0.942	1.94	0.090	1.075	2.20	0.103	0.890	1.81	0.087	0.820	1.65	0.081
UNINC	0.012	1.13	0.052	0.011	1.04	0.048	0.012	1.08	0.051	0.021	1.74	0.091
PHYCH	1.070	1.43	0.129	0.919	1.23	0.112	0.572	0.76	0.071	0.170	0.22	0.021
SICKH							2.273	2.98	0.144	2.090	2.68	0.132
DRUGH				1.680	2.36	0.223	1.537	2.18	0.207	1.675	2.37	0.227
COUNT							-0.329	-2.02	-0.248	-0.303	-1.79	-0.228
MCAID										1.860	1.71	0.069
MCARH										0.511	0.47	0.022
INSPM										0.005	1.43	0.101
CONSTANT	0.687	0.62		-0.509	-0.42		-0.106	-0.07		-1.369	-0.79	

Note: [a]364 observations.

114

not preclude the possibility of concurrent economic or noneconomic activities. As such, it is difficult to place a monetary weight on the appointment time variable. It is also possible that patients associate long delays in receiving appointments with higher-quality sources of care and, therefore, may be willing to wait for appointments rather than receive treatment in lower-quality settings.[55] This latter influence of appointment time on demand tends to offset the negative effect described earlier.

The lack of significance of the waiting time variable also runs against my theoretical expectations; however, Acton (1976, p. 175), provides several explanations for the dominance of travel time over waiting time. In the first place, Acton points out, travel time entails additional monetary outlays—either explicit or implicit; waiting time, however, rarely involves an additional pecuniary expense. Secondly, waiting time, ceteris paribus, may be more pleasant than traveling for the patient and, hence, preferred. For both reasons Acton (1976, p. 175) expects "a greater elasticity of demand for travel time than for waiting time."

Although the waiting time and appointment time variables do not have a significant impact on the demand for medical care, the effect of waiting time is considerably increased when travel time is omitted from the estimating equation.[56] Appointment time, however, never had a significant impact on demand. The model was also estimated with a combined travel and waiting time variable; the results were comparable to those in Tables 3 and 4.

Considering the results in Tables 3 and 4 we see that the alternative specifications of travel time have little effect on the other coefficients. The monetary cost variable (FEEH) has the expected negative sign throughout; however, it is never significant. The opportunity cost of travel time for working heads (LFTEH) is significant only at low levels of confidence, and only in Eqs. (53) and (54). The travel time cost variable for nonworking heads (NLTEH), though, is positive and significant.

The results from the basic model are presented in Eqs. (56) and (60) in Tables 3 and 4, respectively. Of the economic variables in Eq. (56), unearned income (UNINC) and the opportunity cost of travel time for unearned heads have a positive influence on the demand for visits.[57] In Eq. (60) travel time (TRAVL) has a negative effect on demand, whereas increases in unearned income and the estimated value of time for unemployed heads (NLFEH) tend to be associated with increases in the demand for care. Two of the three insurance variables are significant; however, their effect on the price and income variables is not as clearcut as I had anticipated. The coefficient on price decreases as expected (although not significantly), when insurance premiums are included in the analysis. However, since the price variable remains insignificant, little more can be said about it. The estimated effect of unearned income on demand increases both in magnitude and significance when the insurance variables are added to the model.[58]

The noneconomic variables in Eqs. (56) and (60) generally behave as expected, and—with the exception of the binary quality variable (PHYCH)—they are significant. Sicker people have more visits, and increases in family size tend to diminish the demand for care by the head. Increases in the utilization of nonprescription drugs and remedies by the head of household (DRUGH) are associated with a higher utilization of medical visits, indicating that the two goods are complements. It should also be pointed out that the condition of the household dwelling unit (DWELL₁) never had a significant impact on demand.

The results in Tables 3 and 4 are generally supportive of the theoretical model, although the evidence is far from overwhelming. Price behaves in the expected fashion, but it is insignificant. The unimportance of the price variable may be due in part to a discrepancy between the reported usual fee and the actual fee at the respondent's source of care. It should also be pointed out that when household members were asked what improvements they would like to see made in their medical care facilities only 24 (3.6 percent) responded that the cost of obtaining care was too expensive. The majority of households (56 percent) replied that no improvements were needed. Even though price does not have a significant effect on demand, it is worthwhile to point out that the estimated elasticities are comparable with those obtained in other studies of the demand for ambulatory medical care.

The results of several other demand for health care studies are presented in Table 5.[59] Notice that in only one case (Holtmann et al., 1976) are both price and travel elasticities included in the analysis. However, Holtmann and Olsen's findings are not directly comparable to mine since they consider the demand for dental care.[60] Acton's research (1973a, 1975, 1973b, 1976) provides us with the most prolific estimates of time prices, yet he has no information on money price.[61] The results presented here, while not unilaterally significant, are more complete in the sense that both monetary and nonmonetary prices are controlled for.

The price elasticities reported in Tables 3 and 4 are generally smaller than those in Table 5, yet they do not seem to be vastly different from what other researchers have found. The estimated travel time elasticities in Tables 3 and 4 are greater (in absolute value) than the money price elasticities of demand and are generally more significant. However, a comparison of Acton's travel elasticities with these indicates that Acton's population is relatively more responsive to changes in the price of time; this is especially true if we consider the unweighted travel time variable. It should be pointed out though, that Acton uses the mean amount of time for those observations with missing values and thereby decreases

Table 5. Elasticities of the Demand for Ambulatory Medical Care: A Summary of Other Findings.

Author(s)	Price	Wage Income	Nonwage Income	Total Income	Travel Time	Travel Time × W	Waiting Time	Waiting Time × W	Working
Acton (1973a)[e]		−0.15[a]	0.08[a]		−2.07[b,d]		−0.17[a]		0.09[a]
Acton (1973a)[f]		0.12[a]	0.06[a]		0.05[c,d]		−0.03[a]		−0.01[a]
Acton (1976)[e]		−0.04[c]	0.04[c]		−0.62[b]	−0.16[b]	−0.12[c]	−0.33[b]	
		−0.11[b]	0.25[b]		−0.96[b]	−0.20[b]			
Acton (1976)[f]		0.08[b]	−0.14[b]		−0.25[b]	−0.03[c]	−0.05[c]	−0.11[b]	
		0.17[b]	0.05[b]		−0.34[b]	0.002[c]			
Phelps and Newhouse (1972)	−0.14[b,g]								
Newhouse and Phelps (1974)	−0.10[b]	0.03		0.08[b]					
Newhouse and Phelps (1976)	−0.08[b,h]		−0.004[c]						
Holtmann, et al. (1976)	−0.03[b]			0.12[b]	−0.08[b]		−0.05[b]		
	−0.12[b]			0.28[b]			−0.20[b]		

Notes:
[a] No significance level is reported.
[b] Variable is significant at the 90 percent level or higher using a one-tailed test.
[c] Variable is not significant.
[d] The travel time variable is the distance to the outpatient department where the interview was conducted.
[e] The dependent variable is the number of visits to a hospital outpatient department or clinic.
[f] The dependent variable is the number of visits to a private physician.
[g] The price elasticity is calculated for the 0–25 percent range of coinsurance. The estimated total price are elasticity varies from −0.93 to −0.32 depending on the assumed price of time.
[h] The price variable is the physician's office visit coinsurance rate multiplied by the price.
[i] The dependent variable is the number of dental visits.

117

the efficiency of his time estimates, and he may bias the estimated coefficients of the other variables in his equation as well: "It was necessary to use the mean value for about three-fourths of the times associated with free care and about one-fourth of the times associated with non-free care in both samples" (Acton, 1976, p. 204). Furthermore, his treatment of the price of time for individuals not in the labor force may impart further bias to his results. Acton (1976, p. 174) uses a value of 1 cent per minute if the person is not working or if earned income is not reported for the household. Acton is fully aware of these inadequacies in the data (and points them out to the reader as well); they are not repeated here to criticize his results but to point out that Acton's findings (like mine) should be interpreted with care.

Comparing the elasticities in Eqs. (56) and (60) in Tables 3 and 4, we find that the travel time elasticity (TRAVL) is larger than any other price variable. Recall that one of the results of the theoretical model is that the (absolute value of the) elasticity of demand with respect to travel time is greater than *(less than, equal to)* the price elasticity of demand, if the time cost of receiving care is greater than *(less than, equal to)* the monetary cost. What I find is that, even when time costs are less than monetary costs (a comparison of the means indicates that this is the case), the time price elasticity exceeds the monetary price elasticity of demand. This may be due in part to an underestimate of the wage variable, yet this result lends further support to the theory that travel time is more important to the consumer than money price.

The remaining elasticities in the model substantiate the importance of ill health and insurance on the demand for care (although neither effect is as great as travel time); and it should be noted that the family size (COUNT) and household medicine (DRUGH) elasticities are also relatively important. The family size elasticity is very similar to that reported by Newhouse and Phelps (1976, p. 276), and in their analysis too the relative magnitude of the family size elasticity is high. The positive effect of household drugs and remedies on demand suggests that visits and non-prescription medicines are complements, but it is possible that a simultaneous relationship may exist between the two variables. To the extent that physicians prescribe household care and remedies to patients, the utilization of household drugs and remedies is a result rather than a cause of physician visits.

A chi-square test statistic is computed for Eqs. (56) and (60) to test if the estimated coefficients are significantly different from zero, and the results indicate that the null hypothesis of $\beta_1 = \beta_2 = \cdots = \beta_k = 0$ can be rejected with a 95 percent level of confidence.[62] In the following chart the predicted or expected values of Y (the dependent variable), as calculated from regression equation (56) are compared with the actual mean values from the sample.

Predicted probability of Y
greater than the limit:
0.52

Observed frequency of Y
greater than the limit:
0.59

Expected value of Y for entire
sample:
1.85

Observed mean value of Y for
entire sample:
2.25

Expected value of Y for
nonlimit observations:
3.60

Observed mean value of Y for
nonlimit observations:
3.83

Although no overall measure of goodness of fit is available from the Tobit estimating technique, the statistics above indicate that the regression model does an adequate job of accounting for the variation in the number of visits.

It should be mentioned that in other specifications of the model demographic characteristics such as age, race, sex and education were also controlled for. Age was entered both linearly and squared to allow for nonlinear variations in demand, and the signs of the estimated coefficients indicate that a U-shaped relationship exists between visits and age (a high volume of visits at young ages, a decrease in demand during midlife, and a positive relationship between age and visits as one gets old).[63] The coefficients on age are statistically significant, but only when MCARH (head's eligibility for Medicare) is excluded from the regression equation. Race and sex were insignificant determinants of demand, and interacting these binary variables with the other explanatory variables in the equation did little to increase their power.[64] Education did not have a significant impact on demand; this may be due to the importance of education in constructing the proxy wage variable.

Having considered the basic model of the demand for medical care, the next step is to expand the analysis to include the effects of cross-price changes and allow for substitutability among visits. Following these results, the discussion focuses on the demand for care by other household members.

The influence of the wife's wage rate and usual price of care on the head's demand for medical visits is considered in Table 6. The price of care for the wife (FEEW) has an insignificant effect on demand by the head, although it is interesting to note that the effect is always negative and that the estimated elasticities are much higher than the head's own-price elasticities.[65] Participation in the labor force by the wife (WORKW) has a negative influence on the head's demand, whereas increases in her wage rate effect demand positively. The positive effect of the wife's

Table 6. The Effect of Cross-Price Changes on the Demand for Medical Visits by the Head of Household[a]

Independent Variables	61			62			63		
	Coef	t	η	Coef	t	η	Coef	t	η
FEEH	-0.008	-0.17	-0.017	-0.008	-0.17	-0.017	-0.008	-0.17	-0.017
LFEH	0.107	0.23	0.054	-0.348	-0.63	-0.176	-0.325	-0.59	-0.164
NLFEH	0.969	1.68	0.079	0.525	0.81	0.043	0.545	0.84	0.044
TRAVL	-1.109	-0.46	-0.117	-0.826	-0.34	-0.088	-1.016	-0.42	-0.108
UNINC	0.016	1.21	0.075	0.018	1.35	0.084	0.018	1.39	0.086
INSPM	0.005	1.53	0.150	0.004	1.18	0.119	0.004	1.17	0.118
SICKH	2.817	2.96	0.179	2.949	3.10	0.189	2.960	3.12	0.189
DRUGH	1.013	1.22	0.143	1.113	1.34	0.158	1.129	1.36	0.160
MCAID	-0.897	-0.51	-0.016	-0.466	-0.26	-0.008	-0.582	-0.33	-0.010
COUNT	-0.093	-0.49	-0.089	-0.021	-0.11	-0.020	-0.031	-0.16	-0.029
FEEW	-0.030	-0.70	-0.088	-0.034	-0.78	-0.099	-0.034	-0.80	-0.101
WORKW	-2.042	-2.43	-0.223	-2.131	-2.54	-0.234			
EARNW				1.973	1.46	0.669			
LFEW							1.108	0.81	0.170
NLFEW							2.494	1.81	0.461
CONSTANT	-1.056	-0.49		-3.064	-1.20		-3.812	-1.49	

Note: [a]242 observations.

120

wage indicates that it operates like an income effect; however, the negative effect of her labor force participation is somewhat unsettling. Married men are expected to demand fewer medical visits than their single counterparts due to the provision of care in the household by their spouses,[66] and I therefore anticipated that an increase in labor force participation by the wife would tend to decrease the amount of care supplied in the household and increase the demand for extrahousehold medical visits by the head. However, a further examination of the data may provide an explanation for this result. The partial correlation coefficient between the wife's labor force participation and level of education is high (approximately 0.63) and Grossman (1976, p. 176) finds that the wife's level of education is significantly (and positively) related to the health status of her husband. At any rate, given the degree of significance of the cross-price term, there is only tentative support of complementarity between medical visits of the husband and wife.[67,68]

The results in Eqs. (64) and (65) in Table 7 give further support to the notion of complementarity between medical visits of the husband and wife. The test developed earlier predicts that if the effect of unearned income on demand is greater when the wife is receiving care [Eq. (65)] than when she is not [Eq. (64)], then the two visits are complements. The unearned income coefficient (UNINC) in Eq. (64) is negative and insignificant, whereas in Eq. (65) UNINC has a positive and significant influence on demand. This result is supportive of the findings in Table 6, but like before, must be considered tentative.[69]

Finally, in Eqs. (66) and (67) in Table 7 the model is reestimated for heads whose usual fee is greater than zero and for those who usually pay nothing. I expect that the wage rate will have a more pronounced effect on individuals receiving "free" care since nonmonetary costs (i.e., time) become relatively more important as money price gets smaller. The results in Eqs. (66) and (67), however, indicate that neither wage variable (EARNH) is significant. This may be due in part to inaccuracies in the computed wage term.[70] Yet, if we consider the work status variable, we find that WORKH has a much larger effect on heads who usually pay nothing and the estimated elasticity is nearly twice that for those who pay. This suggests that the costs involved with taking time off from work may be greater for individuals receiving free care.[71]

E. The Demand for Medical Visits by the Wife

The estimation results for the wife of the head of household are presented in Table 8. The specifications of the equations are similar to one another, except with regard to the wage and time cost variables. The fee and travel variables have the expected negative signs but are not

Table 7. Factors Influencing the Demand for Medical Visits by the Head of Household When:
(64) The Wife is Not Demanding Any Visits
(65) The Wife Is Also Demanding Visits
(66) The Usual Fee Is Greater Than Zero
(67) The Usual Fee Is Equal to Zero

Independent Variables	64^a			65^b			66^c			67^d		
	Coef	t	η	Coef	t	η	Coef	t	η	Coef	t	η
FEEH	-0.052	-0.27	-0.071	-0.025	-0.62	-0.048						
UNINC	-0.026	-0.66	-0.121	0.038	2.64	0.162	0.014	1.08	0.066	-0.001	-0.05	-0.003
LFTEH	1.026	0.37	0.190	-1.634	-1.76	-0.307						
NLTEH	1.950	0.22	0.019	-0.021	-0.02	-0.001						
SICKH	0.999	0.32	0.045	3.177	2.89	0.182	2.713	2.75	0.145	1.289	1.07	0.114
DRUGH	4.664	1.51	0.629	1.069	1.10	0.129	2.404	2.64	0.322	-0.081	-0.08	-0.012
COUNT	-0.263	-0.53	-0.237	-0.223	-0.96	-0.716	-0.376	-1.75	-0.264	-0.254	-1.04	-0.231
INSPM	0.026	1.88	0.495	0.002	0.54	0.053	0.003	0.66	0.059	0.006	0.91	0.009
EARNH							-0.027	-0.06	-0.013	0.024	0.04	0.012
TRAVL							-5.873	-2.26	-0.551	0.165	0.09	0.017
WORKH							-1.498	-1.37	-0.227	-2.818	-2.15	-0.492
CONSTANT	-7.989	-1.38		0.022	0.01		2.785	1.36		1.670	0.80	

Notes:
[a] 60 observations.
[b] 203 observations.
[c] 238 observations.
[d] 123 observations.

122

Table 8. Factors Influencing the Demand for Medical Care by the Wife[a]

Independent Variables	68			69			70		
	Coef	t	η	Coef	t	η	Coef	t	η
FEEW	−0.003	−0.13	−0.009	−0.004	−0.16	−0.001	−0.004	−0.17	−0.011
LFTEW	−1.154	−0.99	−0.071						
NLTEW	−0.369	−0.31	−0.026						
UNINC	0.009	0.98	0.040	0.009	0.94	0.040	0.010	0.98	0.041
INSPM	0.001	0.45	0.028	0.001	0.40	0.026	0.001	0.40	0.026
SICKW	2.479	3.60	0.146	2.385	3.49	0.141	2.398	3.51	0.141
DRUGW	0.013	0.02	0.002	−0.012	−0.02	−0.002	0.007	0.01	0.001
PHYCW	1.542	2.18	0.215	1.423	2.02	0.199	1.443	2.05	0.202
MCARW	−0.991	−0.76	−0.013						
COUNT	−0.095	−0.65	−0.081	−0.056	−0.38	−0.048	−0.059	−0.40	−0.050
TRAVL				−1.441	−0.85	−0.137	−1.476	−0.88	−0.140
WORKW				−0.659	−1.06	−0.063			
EARNW				0.069	0.09	0.020			
MCAID				−0.172	−0.15	−0.003	−0.146	−0.12	−0.003
LFEW							−0.152	−0.19	−0.020
NLFEW							0.242	0.29	0.039
CONSTANT	0.977	0.68		1.306	0.65		1.010	0.51	

Note: [a]286 observations.

123

significant.[72] Unearned income (UNINC) and insurance premiums (INSPM) have a positive influence on demand but are also insignificant. In fact, the only significant variables are health status (SICKW) and the quality of care (PHYCW). Wives tend to go to the doctor more often (than husbands) when they are sick and are more likely to go if their usual source of care is a private physician. The unimportance of the economic variables does not support the results of my theoretical model, although it is worthwhile to note that the factors that influence demand differ across household members. The basic model was also reestimated using wage and fee variables for the head of household, as well as other household members, but none of these variables were significant.

F. The Demand for Medical Care by the Household as a Unit

The results in Table 9 extend the basic demand model by estimating demand for medical care equations for the household as a unit. The results support the basic model presented earlier for the heads of households but are generally much stronger. Monetary price (AVFEE) is significant [at least in Eqs. (72) and (74)] and the estimated elasticities are very close to those reported by other researchers.[73] The travel time elasticities are roughly twice the size of the fee elasticities, but are still smaller than those reported by Acton (1976).[74] The higher time price elasticities in Acton's study may be attributed, in part, to the higher percent of patients having private physician office visits (and hence higher money prices) in my data set. Recall that the time price elasticity of demand becomes relatively more important to the consumer, ceteris paribus, as money prices get smaller. To the extent that the monetary, out of pocket, cost of medical care is higher in Rougemont/Bahama, than for the people in Acton's study, I would expect to find lower time price elasticities in my data. Unfortunately, there is no way of comparing money prices between the two studies since Acton's data do not include any variables to measure the money price of medical visits. However, a comparison of the travel times in the two data sets indicates that travel time is longer for Acton's sample;[75] this provides an additional rationale for the discrepancy in the time price elasticities.[76]

Unearned household income (UNINC) and insurance premiums (INSPM) have a significant impact on demand, and (family) health status (SICKF) and household remedies (DRUGA) continue to be important determinants of utilization.

The head's wage rate (EARNH) has a significant impact on household demand when the wife's wage rate (EARNW) is omitted from the estimating equation [Eq. (73) in Table 9]; however, when EARNW is included [Eq. (74)], EARNH is insignificant. The importance of EARNW, rather than EARNH,

Table 9. Factors Influencing the Demand for Medical Care by the Household

Independent Variables	71[a]			72[b]			73[b]			74[b]		
	Coef	t	η	Coef	t	η	Coef	t	η	Coef	t	η
AVFFE	-0.008	-0.55	-0.021	-0.024	-1.54	-0.075	-0.017	-1.11	-0.053	-0.025	-1.63	-0.079
TRAVL	-0.973	-1.49	-0.128	-1.001	-1.23	-0.142	-0.973	-1.18	-0.137	-0.906	-1.11	-0.129
UNINC	0.011	2.41	0.062	0.016	3.16	0.096	0.013	2.56	0.080	0.014	2.72	0.086
INSPM	0.002	1.78	0.067	0.002	1.34	0.068	0.002	1.51	0.076	0.002	1.32	0.066
DRUGA	0.656	1.77	0.159	0.587	1.42	0.153	0.718	1.72	0.185	0.638	1.54	0.167
SICKF	1.240	4.31	0.159	1.128	3.37	0.144	1.174	3.29	0.149	1.130	3.23	0.145
WORKW				-0.280	-0.84	-0.040				-0.277	-0.84	-0.040
EARNW				1.194	3.00	0.528				1.067	2.14	0.475
WORKH							-0.880	-1.62	-0.230	-0.930	-1.72	-0.247
EARNH							0.310	1.83	0.237	0.008	0.04	0.006
MCARW				1.585	2.35	0.034				2.438	2.84	0.053
MCARH							-0.391	-0.65	-0.015	-1.534	-1.99	-0.061
MCAID				0.294	0.46	0.008	0.003	0.01	0.000	0.054	0.08	0.001
CONSTANT	1.203	2.34		-0.278	-0.32		1.226	1.32		0.758	0.73	

Notes:
[a] 458 observations.
[b] 314 observations.

suggests that the utilization of medical care visits may be a luxury, financed to a considerable extent by secondary or added worker incomes.

G. The Demand for Medical Care by Other Household Members

Finally, in Table 10, results for household members other than the husband and wife are presented. Since the majority of other family members are children, the wife's wage (EARNW) and labor force participation status (WORKW) are included in Eq. (76) to estimate the time price of receiving medical care. An earlier specification of the model included the family head's wage and labor force participation status, but both variables were insignificant. One interpretation of the negative coefficient on WORKW in Eq. (76) in Table 10 is that working wives are less able to accompany other household members (especially children) on medical care visits and therefore demand is reduced. The positive coefficient on EARNW, however, indicates (as in Table 9) an increased ability to pay for medical care outside the home as earned income rises.

It is worthwhile to point out that for the first time the health status binary variable, SICKF, is insignificant. Since health status was usually reported by the respondent (i.e., the wife, and occasionally the husband) for the entire household, it is possible that the information obtained is most accurate for the wife and head and less precise for other family members. This may explain why SICKF has a significant impact on the demand by the entire household (see Table 9) but has no effect on the utilization by progeny and other household members.[77]

AVKFE, the average price of a medical visit per "other" household member, has a negative effect on the demand for visits. Its influence on

Table 10. Factors Influencing the Demand for Medical Care by Other Household Members

Independent Variables	75[a]			76[b]		
	Coef	t	η	Coef	t	η
AVKFE	−0.016	−0.57	−0.032	−0.045	−1.54	−0.097
TRAVL	−0.720	−0.70	−0.104	0.114	0.11	0.017
UNINC	0.009	1.46	0.051	0.008	1.21	0.051
INSPM	−0.001	−0.48	−0.031			
DRUGA	1.171	2.11	0.318	1.081	1.94	0.350
SICKF	0.380	0.89	0.051	0.428	0.96	0.056
EARNW				0.626	1.22	0.291
WORKW				−0.560	−1.27	−0.094
CONSTANT	0.171	0.22		−0.517	−0.48	

Notes:
[a] 279 observations.
[b] 242 observations.

utilization is similar to that of AVFFE (the average price of a medical visit per household member) in Eqs. (72) and (74) in Table 9. These are the only times that the money price of medical care has any noticeable impact on demand. The degree of responsiveness to changes in money price may therefore be greater for groups of consumers than for single individuals. From the individual perspective, price is an insignificant determinant of demand; however, from the viewpoint of the household or central decision-making unit, demand is much more price elastic. Perhaps more options or alternative sources of medical care are available or brought into consideration when the household, rather than the individual, is the decision-making unit. At any rate, there appears to be some indication that the demand for ambulatory medical care by the family (or some subgroup of the household unit) differs from the demand by individual household members.[78]

H. Conclusion

The empirical results are briefly recapitulated in this subsection and several policy implications of the analysis are suggested. However, a detailed discussion of the policy implications and suggestions for future research is contained in Section IV.

1. The results from the basic demand model for heads of households indicate that for this rural community travel time and unearned income are more important determinants of the utilization of medical visits than is the money price. The utilization of household drugs and remedies is positively related to the demand for care, whereas family size is negatively related to demand.
2. An extension of the model that includes the usual medical fee for the wife is insignificant, although there is tentative support for the hypothesis that husband and wife medical visits act as complements.
3. The economic variables from the model have an insignificant effect on the demand for medical visits by the wife of the household, but individual health status and usual source of care are important determinants of demand.
4. When the household is considered as the unit of analysis, all of the variables in the model are generally significant. This may be due to the public nature of medical care goods (if one person receives care, other family members benefit as well), and it adds further support to the complementarity of individual visits suggested in point 2, above. (Obviously, it takes fewer resources for two or more individuals to go to the doctor at the same time, than it does for each to make separate visits.)

5. The demand for medical visits by household members other than the husband and wife is significantly affected by the wife's wage rate (positively) and her labor force status (negatively).
6. The other time–price variables—waiting time and appointment time—are insignificant determinants of demand.
7. The household's insurance premiums are typically a positive determinant of demand.
8. The results indicate that health status, as expected, has a significant impact on the demand for ambulatory medical visits.

These findings suggest that programs aimed at increasing the accessibility of medical care would achieve little by lowering monetary prices; a more effective way to increase utilization is to decrease travel time and perhaps give income subsidies to the needy.

The significance of the household results indicate that the family may be a more relevant unit of analysis than the individual. In any event, the findings suggest that studies focusing exclusively on the demand for medical care by individuals may be ignoring valuable information both on other family members and on the household as a decision-making unit.

IV. CONCLUSIONS, POLICY IMPLICATIONS, AND FUTURE RESEARCH

In the second and third sections of this chapter a household model of the demand for medical care was developed and tested using data from a southern rural community. Throughout, emphasis has been placed on the interaction effects that exist between household members and on the influence of both direct and indirect prices on the utilization of ambulatory medical services. Empirical results are presented for both individual family members and the household as a unit. Although I have attempted throughout to relate my results to the existing literature, it is worthwhile at this point to step back and see how these findings correspond to other demand for health care studies. It is also desirable to examine the suggestions this research has for health care policy and to consider its implications for future research. I begin by briefly recapitulating the main theoretical and empirical results of the study and reviewing the major differences between my results and those of other researchers. I then point out the policy implications of my work and propose several issues for future research.

Theoretically, this research is most closely related to that of Grossman (1972a) and Acton (1973a). While both Grossman and Acton recognize the importance of the family in determining the utilization of medical care,[79] their theoretical models are based on individual utility maximization. The approach taken here is somewhat different in that the analysis is couched in a household utility framework and comparative statics are used to emphasize the effects of cross-price changes (i.e., the price of medical care paid by other household members) on individual demand. My analysis of changes in the full (money and time) price of medical care is, however, related to Acton's theoretical model.

Although the household utility approach differs somewhat from earlier models of demand for medical care, it is perhaps the empirical analysis which contains the most important contributions of this research. The individual demand results vary considerably across family members and also vis-à-vis the household unit; I know of no other study which includes both individual and family results. The influence of the economic variables on demand is particularly interesting, especially with regard to the effects of cross-price changes and the relative magnitude of the money- and time-price elasticities.

Other researchers have attempted to weigh the effects of money and time prices on the demand for medical care; however, for the most part, such comparisons have been hampered by inadequate data. Acton's work (1973a,b, 1975, 1976), is perhaps the most notable in the time-price, demand-for-health literature; however, his studies are drawn from populations which pay a zero money price for medical care. Hence, Acton is unable to analyze the relative importance of direct and indirect price elasticities of demand. In a study of the demand for dental services, Holtmann and Olsen (1976) do estimate both money- and time-price elasticities of demand, but they provide no estimates of the opportunity cost of time (wage rates) and their price variable is not a precise measure of fee; rather, it is calculated by dividing total (dental care) expenditures by the number of visits. As such, the estimated price coefficients have a negative bias. Phelps and Newhouse (1972; also Newhouse and Phelps, 1976) talk about the importance of nonpecuniary prices on the demand for medical care; however, they do not have adequate data on either travel or waiting time.[80]

This study is distinctive in that both money and time prices are controlled for and the estimated elasticities reported in the last section verify the relative importance of indirect prices in determining medical care demand. The results, while not overwhelming in a statistical sense, consistently indicate that the patients in this rural sample are more responsive to changes in travel time than changes in fee. The general lack of significance of the fee variable can perhaps be attributed to Medicaid and Medicare eligibility and health insurance coverage;[81] nevertheless, the results imply that demand is very price inelastic. The coefficients on earned income further accentuate the opportunity or time cost of re ceiving medical care, especially for employed heads of households.

The results suggest that programs aimed at increasing the accessibility or utilization of ambulatory medical services in the community may well be advised to focus more attention on indirect rather than direct prices. One way of reducing travel costs is to locate health care facilities centrally in order to minimize the distance that patients must travel to receive care.[82] On strictly economic grounds, a nondiscriminatory solution would be reached when the full cost (both time and money price) of receiving a unit of (quality-adjusted) medical care was equal for all members of the community. However, some would strongly object to the use of full price as a rationing device on the grounds that access to medical care is a right that all individuals have, regardless of income—or availability of time. Perhaps, then, a rationing of medical services according to need would be more equitable. At any rate, when we are considering the barriers or costs of receiving medical care, the importance of time costs (vis-à-vis money costs) should not be overlooked.

Another economic variable which has a consistent impact on utilization is unearned household income. The results indicate that income subsidies or reductions in taxes would have a greater impact on utilization than a lowering of money prices. The effects of both unearned income and travel time corroborate Acton's results (1973a, 1976) and point to similarities between Acton's urban sample and these rural estimates. Both studies, however, deal with middle- and lower-income samples and therefore these conclusions may not be applicable to higher-income groups.

Other researchers (Acton, 1976; Newhouse and Phelps, 1976; Davis and Russell, 1972) consider the effects of cross-price changes on the demand for ambulatory medical care; however, the price changes considered are typically the prices paid at alternative sources of care (i.e., private physician versus clinic visits, inpatient versus outpatient care). Here, since the household is treated as an economic decision-making unit, the cross-price changes considered are the costs of medical visits paid by other household members. There is tentative support indicating that medical care visits by the husband and wife are complements, although the relationship is not symmetrical.[83] The demand for medical care by the husband is (somewhat) responsive to changes in the wife's price, but the wife's demand is not affected by her spouse's cost of receiving care. This asymmetry may be due to household priorities placed on the wife's health status, a greater desire by the wife for extrahousehold medical care, or differences in the relative cost of receiving care for the husband and wife.[84] At any rate, the demand for visits by the wife appears to be more (cross-)price inelastic than the demand by the family head.[85]

There is also evidence indicating that the wife's (estimated) opportunity cost of time has a significant influence on the demand for visits by the head, other family members, and the household as a unit. This positive influence is analogous to an income effect but is much stronger than either the effect of the head's proxy wage variable or unearned income on demand. Overall, the cross-price results indicate that the wife's (full) cost of receiving medical care is a significant determinant of utilization by both the head of household and other family members. This suggests that demand studies should take the presence of other household members and family structure into consideration when analyzing the determinants of individual medical care utilization.

The importance of the household unit becomes even more apparent when the family results are compared with the individual demand estimates. The increased significance of the household results lends support to Becker's (1974) concept of a central decision-making (or utility-maximizing) unit within the household which considers individual price differences and selects alternative sources of care and utilization rates for various household members. It is also possible that from the household perspective it is more expedient for certain family members (e.g., children) to schedule group rather than individual visits.[86] Group visits may provide certain "economies of demand" within the household and thereby lower the full cost of receiving care. This is especially true when a parent or other household member accompanies the group on medical care visits. In any event, the results indicate that the household unit is at least as responsive as individuals to changes in the economic and noneconomic variables in the model—and in some instances is even more responsive.

The household and cross-price change results indicate that other family members and household structure may be important determinants of medical care demand. At the very least, the findings imply that future researchers should consider family characteristics when analyzing the utilization of medical care services. The unearned income and time-price results substantiate Acton's findings and highlight the importance of economic factors other than money prices and health insurance when we are studying the demand for medical care.

In view of the conclusions and policy implications discussed herein, there are several directions in which this research should be extended. Since these results represent the first economic analysis of time prices in rural areas, more rural research is needed to substantiate these findings. It should also be recalled that the results reported here apply directly to only one rural community and may not be representative of other rural areas. It is especially important to collect complete household as well as individual data and to gather information across a wide range of income groups.

Alternatively, the model could be respecified in a household production function framework, and a simultaneous model of the production of health and the demand for medical care could be estimated. It would also be interesting to examine the joint production aspects of household behavior and to compare the estimates from such a model with those reported here.

The need for additional research notwithstanding, it is hoped that the findings reported here contribute to an understanding of the determinants of medical care and point to new areas of consideration for health care policy.

GLOSSARY

Section II

U	Household utility
M_j	Individual demand for extrahousehold medical goods and services (i.e., visits)
N_j	Individual demand for intrahousehold medical goods and services (i.e., nonprescription drugs and household remedies)
D	A composite good reflecting household sanitary conditions
Z	A vector of other goods and services in the family utility function
P_j	Pecuniary price of medical visits for individual j
Q_j	Pecuniary price of N_j
P_D	Pecuniary price of D
P_Z	Pecuniary price of Z
L_j	Individual market wage rate
Y	Total unearned household income
T_j	Total time available to the individual
T_j^L	Time spent in the labor force by individual j
T_j^M	Total time spent in the consumption of M_j
t_j^M	Time spent per unit of M_j
T_j^N	Total time spent in the consumption of N_j
t_j^N	Time spent per unit of N_j
T_j^D	Total time spent in the consumption of D by individual j
t_j^D	Time spent per unit of D by individual j
T_j^Z	Total time spent in the consumption of Z by individual j
t_j^Z	Time spent per unit of Z by individual j
T_j^S	Total sick time of individual j
F_j	Full price of M_j
G_j	Full price of N_j
F_D	Full price of D

Section III

AFAMV	Average number of medical care visits per household member
AKIDV	Average number of medical care visits per child in each household
APPT	Number of days it takes the household to get an appointment at its usual source of care when it is not an emergency
AVFFE[a]	Average medical visit fee per household member
AVKFE[a]	Average medical visit fee per child in the household
COUNT	Number of people in the household
DRUGA	Binary variable set equal to one if either the husband or wife uses any nonprescription drugs or remedies
DRUGH	Binary variable set equal to one if the head of household uses any nonprescription drugs or remedies
DRUGW	Binary variable set equal to one if the wife of the head of household uses any nonprescription drugs or remedies
DWELL$_1$	Binary variable set equal to one if the household's dwelling unit is in "sound condition;" the omitted reference group includes those households that were classified by the interviewer as "deteriorating" or "dilapidated"
EARNH	Estimated hourly wage rate for the head of household
EARNW	Estimated hourly wage rate for the wife of the head of household
FEEH[a]	Usual fee that the head of household pays at his/her usual source of medical care
FEEW[a]	Usual fee that the wife of the head of household pays at her usual source of medical care
INC[b]	Total household income measured in hundreds of dollars
INSPM	Total (semiannual) household expenditures for health insurance premiums
LFEH	WORKH $\times$ EARNH
LFEW	WORKW $\times$ EARNW
LFTEH	WORKH $\times$ TRAVL $\times$ EARNH
LFTEW	WORKW $\times$ TRAVL $\times$ EARNW
MCAID	Binary variable set equal to one if the household is eligible for Medicaid
MCARH	Binary variable set equal to one if the head of household is eligible for Medicare
MCARW	Binary variable set equal to one if the wife of the head of household is eligible for Medicare
NLFEH	NWRKH $\times$ EARNH
NLFEW	NWRKW $\times$ EARNW
NLTEH	NWRKH $\times$ TRAVL $\times$ EARNH
NLTEW	NWRKW $\times$ TRAVL $\times$ EARNW
NWRKH	Binary variable set equal to one if the head of household is not working
NWRKW	Binary variable set equal to one if the wife of the head of household is not working

PHYCH   Binary variable set equal to one if the head of households' usual place of care is a private physician; the omitted reference group includes heads who usually attend clinics, hospital outpatient departments and those who have no usual source of care

PHYCW   Binary variable set equal to one if the wife of the head of household usually receives care at a private physician; the omitted reference group includes wives who usually attend clinics or hospital outpatient departments and those who have no usual source of care

RACE   Binary variable set equal to one if the household is black

SEXH   Binary variable set equal to one if the head of household is female

SICKF   Binary variable set equal to one if anyone in the household is in fair or poor health

SICKH   Binary variable set equal to one if the head of household's health status is fair or poor; the omitted reference group includes heads with excellent or good health

SICKW   Binary variable set equal to one if the wife's health status is fair or poor; the omitted reference group includes wives with excellent or good health

TRAVL   Number of hours it takes to travel from home to the usual source of care

TVLEH   TRAVL × EARNH

TVLEW   TRAVL × EARNW

VISTH   Number of medical care visits by the head of household

VISTW   Number of medical care visits by the wife of the head of household

WAIT   Hours spent waiting in the waiting room at usual source of care

WORKH   Binary variable set equal to one if the head of household is working

WORKW   Binary variable set equal to one if the wife of the head of household is working

Notes:

[a]Continuous fee variables are computed by assigning midpoints to the following closed-fee intervals: $1–10; $11–20; $21–30; $31–40. Actual observations were available for those individuals who pay nothing; $50 is used as the price for individuals who pay more than $40

[b]A continuous income variable is computed by assigning midpoints to the following closed-income intervals: $2,000–3,999; $4,000–5,999; $6,000–7,999; $8,000–9,999; $10,000–11,999; $12,000–15,999. Here, $1,000 is used as the income for households reporting income less than $2,000.

ACKNOWLEDGMENTS

This study was funded by a dissertation support grant from the National Center for Health Services Research (No. 1 R03 HS 02417-01). I am extremely grateful to the National Center for this support. The data for this project were collected under a grant from the Robert Wood Johnson Foundation to the Department of Community Health Sciences (CHS) at Duke University and I would like to thank Eva Salber from CHS and Sandra Greene from Blue Cross–Blue Shield of North Carolina (formerly at CHS) for making these data available to me. I am also indebted to Richard Scheffler from the Department of Economics at George

Washington University for his lucid comments and criticisms of various drafts of this paper.

NOTES

1. The types of cross-price changes considered here are the prices paid for medical care by other household members.

2. The first theoretical and econometric analysis of the effects of time costs on the demand for medical care was done by Acton (1973).

3. The model developed here is most closely related to and relies most heavily on the work of Grossman (1972a,b) and Acton (1973a,b, 1975, 1976).

4. Throughout, the words *family* and *household* are used interchangeably. The family is a group of (related) individuals living together in the same dwelling unit. Most households consist of a head, wife, and offspring, although in many larger households additional family members include grandparents, aunts, and uncles as well. Only in rare circumstances do households contain members who are unrelated to the head.

5. A glossary of the symbols used is included at the end of the chapter.

6. It should be pointed out that the form of the budget constraint implies that the time per unit of good is fixed; however, given the data available to measure time prices, this does not seem to be an overly restrictive assumption. Questions were asked regarding the household's travel time, waiting time, and appointment time for its usual source of care. As such, the time variables obtained can be viewed more as average amounts than explicit time measures which may vary according to type of condition and place of care.

7. Another alternative is to treat D as a (household) public good which is paid for by the primary wage earner in the family. A similar argument applies to the utilization of the goods and services in Z, but it should be mentioned that it is the demand for medical goods and services in which we are primarily interested.

8. In the interest of minimizing space the system of totally differentiated equations is not presented here. The interested reader is referred to Miners (1979).

9. It should be pointed out that while the tests developed in this subsection pertain to the family, they are in many respects comparable to the individual tests constructed by Acton (1973a).

10. The analysis centers on the demand for visits, rather than N_j and D, not because the latter are unimportant but because no reliable price measure, either pecuniary or nonpecuniary, is available to estimate the price of medical goods used within the household.

11. The assumption of normality of the M_j may not hold if quality differences exist among visits. An attempt is made to control for quality differences in the empirical tests of the model by including (dummy) variables corresponding to the respondent's usual source of care.

12. The analysis assumes that the wage rate is not endogenous and that the same wage rate applies to all visits made by the individual.

13. In several previous studies, researchers have examined the relationship between individual health status and the allocation of time within the household—especially with regard to labor supply decisions. See, for example, Parsons (1977) and Scheffler and Iden (1974).

14. Sixty-nine percent of the heads of household and 74 percent of the wives reported that their health status was excellent or good (rather than fair or poor); 51 percent of the heads and 37 percent of the wives had no medical visits during the sample period.

15. By "time efficient" I mean that the opportunity cost or indirect price of receiving care is kept as low as possible for the consumer. Time costs may be reduced by locating

medical facilities in areas accessible to patients, arranging practice hours to complement working hours, and scheduling appointments to minimize waiting time. It should be pointed out, however, that medical settings or waiting times that are optimal from the patients' point of view may not be viewed as time-efficient from the physicians' or the practices' perspective. See Fetter and Thompson (1966) and White and Pike (1964).

16. The omission of Z from the analysis follows from the earlier assumption of separability of the utility function between all medical goods and services on the one hand, and Z on the other.

17. We now consider only full price changes in our analysis.

18. Several of the preliminary comparative static results presented in this section were discussed earlier but are included in the discussion here to maintain clarity and for ease of exposition.

19. It should be pointed out that this (indirect) test is strictly correct only if the sole difference between two households is in the demand for medical visits by the wife (i.e., $M_w \neq 0$ vs. $M_w = 0$).

20. This procedure is discussed in the next section.

21. For a more detailed discussion of the policy implications of this research, see Section IV.

22. For an indepth discussion of OLS and the full ideal conditions see Kmenta (1971).

23. Forty-three percent of all heads of households, 26 percent of all wives, and 60 percent of all other household members had no medical care visits.

24. For a more detailed discussion of the tobit estimation procedure the interested reader is referred to Tobin (1958) and Theil (1971, pp. 631–632).

25. The Tobit package used was developed by Charles Phelps of the Rand Corporation in Santa Monica, Calif. A word of thanks should also be extended to Frank Sloan for making this package available to Richard Scheffler, who subsequently made it available to me.

26. I am indebted to Dr. Eva Salber of the Department of Community Health Sciences (CHS), and Dr. Sandra Greene of Blue Cross–Blue Shield of North Carolina (previously at CHS) for making these data available to me.

27. The survey was funded by a grant from the Robert Wood Johnson foundation.

28. The initial survey was conducted from September 1973 to February 1974; follow-up visit 1 began June 3, 1974 and ended August 25, 1974; visit 3 took place between November 18, 1974 and March 2, 1975.

29. In three instances (out of 665) there were female heads of household with husbands; however, due to missing observations on other variables, these households are not included in the empirical analysis.

30. The description of the data focuses primarily on the variables used in the econometric analysis. For a more detailed description of the Rougemont/Bahama health survey the interested reader is referred to Salber et al. (1976).

31. Information on a third price variable was also collected—the amount the household expected to pay for chronic condition check-ups and minor condition visits; however, it too was not available on an individual basis. Preliminary estimates of the model that included this variable yielded insignificant coefficients of price.

32. The variables for other household members contain the word "KID" and the letter "K" since in most instances other household members are children. Eighty-three percent of all household members, other than the head and wife, are 18 years old or less.

33. Only 41 percent of all households responded that hospitalizations were paid primarily by health insurance. There are no data available to measure the extent that health insurance is used to pay for outpatient or ambulatory care visits.

34. The *deductible* is a fixed amount which the consumer must pay before receiving any health insurance benefits or reimbursement. The *coinsurance rate* is that percentage of the fee which the consumer must pay after the deductible has been exceeded. For example, if an insurance policy has a $100.000 deductible and a 20% coinsurance rate, the consumer must pay $140.00 of a $300.00 medical bill.

35. It is possible that some people who are less than 65 years old are eligible for Medicare due to medical disabilities; unfortunately no data are available to measure this occurrence. The regional income and family size cutoffs for medicaid are as follows: $1,700 for one-person households; $2,200 for two-person households; $2,500 for three-person households; and $2,800 for four-person households. For families with more than four members add $200 to the $2,800 income cut-off for each additional household member.

36. The city of Durham, the state capital, Raleigh, and the town of Chapel Hill are all located in this county group.

37. Among other variables, the two groups are dissimilar in location of employment, type of employment, years of education, and total household income.

38. The counties included in this group are Edgecombe, Franklin, Granville, Halifax, Nash, Northampton, Person, Vance, Warren, and Wilson.

39. For a more detailed review of this research, see Miners (1979, pp. 95–98).

40. When the starting point was changed, the maximum likelihood estimator converged to different values.

41. The census regression results, both for those employed and unemployed, are presented in Miners (1979).

42. A t-test performed on the two variables indicates however, that the two wage variables are significantly different. The confidence level is 98 percent.

43. Average household income for the entire community is 8309 dollars.

44. The plausibility of the mean value of the unearned income variable lends further support (albeit heuristic support) to the computed wage proxy variable.

45. Data pertaining to the household's overall expenditures for prescriptions and other medicines is available; however, it neither identifies individual expenditures nor does it differentiate between prescribed and nonprescribed medicines. Earlier estimates of the model that included this expenditure variable yielded coefficients which were generally insignificant.

46. Only the effect of nonprescription medicines is examined since it is assumed that prescription drugs and medical visits are complements.

47. Medical visits and nonprescription household remedies may serve as complements in the following ways: First, an individual with a particular ailment may receive preliminary care or treatment in the household, and if that is unsuccessful a professional medical care visit may be demanded. Secondly, as a consequence of a medical visit, a physician may "prescribe" rest and care in the household.

48. It is realized that in a broader framework, family size should be an endogenous rather than exogenous variable; however, modeling the determinants of family size is beyond the scope of the current project. See, for example, Willis (1974).

49. It is also possible that larger families may be relatively more susceptible to ill health or contagious conditions than small households; however, I know of no evidence to support this hypothesis.

50. In a production function framework, medical visits are viewed as an input in the production of health. Here, it is argued, the demand for visits is determined in part by one's level of health. An alternative model might include both individual medical visits and health as endogenous variables in a simultaneous framework. This, however, is beyond the scope of the current analysis.

51. It should be pointed out that in the empirical analysis an attempt is also made to control for certain demographic influences in demand (sex, race, age, education). The results are generally not significant, however, and are discussed below.

52. I am grateful to Dr. Michael Grossman of the National Bureau of Economic Research (NBER) and the Graduate School of City University of New York for suggesting this dichotomy to me. Although the coefficients on LFTEH and NLTEH explicitly separate the effect of travel time for working and nonworking heads, it should be pointed out that these estimates are comparable to the results obtained when TVLEH and TVLEH × WORKH are included in the regression equation instead.

53. Grossman (1972a, p. 22) points out that "a high wage rate induces an individual to substitute market goods for his own time in the production of commodities." Hence in Grossman's (investment) framework a higher wage increases the value of time to the individual and induces him (or her) to substitute medical visits for the now relatively higher priced home (or time) inputs. When Grossman formulates the demand for health as a consumption good he finds, like Acton and myself, that the effects of wage changes on demand are ambiguous. However, Grossman (1972a, p. 35) allows for the possibility that the overall effect on demand, due to a change in the wage rate, may be negative. "If time costs were relatively more important in the production of health than in the production of a typical nonmarket commodity, the relative price of health would rise with wage rate, which would reduce the quantity demanded."

54. In his empirical analysis Grossman (1972a, pp. 56, 57) finds that the wage rate has a positive and significant effect on the demand for health, but a negative and insignificant effect in his medical care expenditure equation.

55. Although sufficient data do not exist to measure differences in appointment time among providers of care within the same setting, the available statistics indicate that appointment time for whites is on the average about 17 days, whereas blacks wait approximately 8 days for an appointment. Seventy-four percent of white households reported private physicians as their usual source of care; the corresponding figure for black families is 28 percent.

56. The fact that the significance of the waiting time variable increases when travel time is omitted from the equation suggests that the two variables are correlated; however, the estimated correlation coefficient between the two time variables is only -0.20. For a more detailed presentation of the waiting time results, exclusive of the travel time variable, see Miners (1979, p. 156).

57. It should be pointed out that when total household income was included in the estimating equation, rather than unearned household income, the results were insignificant.

58. It should be pointed out, however, that when insurance premiums (INSPM) is the only included insurance term, the effect of UNINC on demand is diminished. When Medicaid eligibility (MCAID) is controlled for instead, the effect of unearned income is increased, presumably due to the negative correlation between Medicaid and income. The overall effect of insurance on UNINC, shown in Eqs. (56) and (60), suggests that unearned income is more highly correlated with MCAID than INSPM. The partial correlation coefficient between UNINC and INSPM is approximately 0.31; the correlation between UNINC and MCAID is -0.63.

59. It should be pointed out that in many previous demand studies (e.g., Grossman, 1972a; Rosett and Huang, 1973), the dependent variable is medical expenditures. For purposes of comparison, only studies with visits as the dependent variable are included in Table V.

60. It should also be pointed out that Holtman and Olsen (1976) do not have explicit data for the price of care but instead divide total expenditures by the number of visits.

61. Acton points out that since his research is conducted on low-income groups, many of which receive "free" care, the bias in his estimates is not severe (1976, p. 173).

62. The chi-square test statistics (and degrees of freedom) for Eqs. (56) and (60), respectively, are 20.37 (11) and 21.39 (12).

63. Using the estimated coefficients of age, the minimum point of the U-shaped curve is calculated to occur at approximately 41 years of age. Acton's results (1976, p. 180) indicate that the minimum point of the curve is at 35 years of age. (The mean age in Acton's study is 27 years; here the mean age for heads of households is 48 years.)

64. There were several exceptions. Medicaid eligibility was more important for black families, whereas health insurance premiums were more important for whites. Family size had a larger negative effect on demand for male heads of households, while unearned income had a larger positive effect for males.

65. These price elasticities are very similar to those reported in Table 5.

66. For a discussion of the effect of martial status on health see Fuchs (1974, pp. 50–51).

67. Recall that the effect of a cross price change can be written as

$$\frac{\partial M_h}{\partial P_w} = \frac{\partial M_h}{\partial P_w}\bigg|_{\bar{U}} - \frac{M_w \partial M_h}{\partial Y}.$$

Using the coefficients from Eq. (61) in Table 6 and the mean value of medical visits for the wife yields

$$\frac{\partial M_h}{\partial P_w} = -0.030 - (2.892)(0.016) = -0.080.$$

68. It should also be pointed out that neither the wife's cost of travel time nor the fee variable for the other household members had a significant effect on the head's demand for medical care.

69. I would have greater confidence in this result if income behaved in the proper fashion in Eq. (64) and if there were more than 60 useable observations.

70. When LFTEH and NLTEH were included in the regressions instead, the results were also insignificant.

71. It is also possible that people who usually pay for medical care are more likely to be salaried and may therefore be less responsive to time costs.

72. The other time measures, WAIT and APPT, were also insignificant.

73. See Table 5.

74. The other time variables still have no effect on demand, but it should be pointed out that the coefficient on appointment time was positive throughout and significant in several cases, suggesting that some families may be willing to wait to receive higher quality care.

75. See Acton (1976, p. 195), and (my) Table 1.

76. It should be pointed out that if there were a positive correlation between money price and travel time, the omission of money price from the estimating equation would bias the coefficient on travel time away from zero (i.e., more negative) and make the time-price elasticity of demand appear larger (in absolute value) than it is.

77. Note too, that a comparison of the means in Table 1 indicates that the majority of household visits were received by the wife and the head of household.

78. One caveat is in order. In light of the lack of overwhelming significance of the price (and other) variables in the "subgroup" estimating equations in Table 10, one should be cautious not to put too much confidence in these results.

79. Both researchers include family size in their empirical analysis and find that it has a negative impact on the demand for medical care.

80. In their first study Phelps and Newhouse (1972) have grouped information on the distance to the provider of medical care but no data on wage rates, travel, or waiting times.

In the second study, Newhouse and Phelps (1976) construct a proxy wage variable; however, they lack adequate travel and waiting time data.

81. It should be recalled that relatively few households are eligible for Medicare or Medicaid benefits and that the insurance variable only measures gross household insurance expenditures.

82. A further reduction in the opportunity cost of receiving medical care could be achieved by rescheduling practice hours to shorten patient queues and to offer services during periods of consumer slack (nonemployment) time. However, in view of the low levels of significance of the waiting time estimates, little weight can be placed on this alternative.

83. Other tests of complementarity between other household members' medical visits and those of the husband and wife were not significant.

84. Heads and wives report virtually the same health status, yet wives have more medical visits and pay, on the average, four dollars more per visit than heads. See Table 1.

85. The estimates in Section IV also indicate that for the wife the full price elasticity of demand is very low.

86. When one household member contracts a communicable disease (e.g., the flu), the entire household may go to the doctor (for flu shots). It may also be convenient to schedule checkups for family groups rather than individual household members.

REFERENCES

Acton, Jan Paul (1973a), *Demand for Health Care When Time Prices Vary More Than Money Prices.* The Rand Corporation, R-1189-OEO/NYC (May).

————(1973b), *Demand for Health Care Among the Urban Poor with Special Emphasis on the Role of Time.* The Rand Corporation, R-1151-OEO/NYC (Apr.).

————(1975), "Nonmonetary Factors in the Demand for Medical Services: Some Empirical Evidence," *Journal of Political Economy 83*(2), 595–614.

————(1976), "Demand for Health Care Among the Urban Poor, with Special Emphasis on the Role of Time," in *The Role of Health Insurance in the Health Services Sector,* Richard N. Rosett (ed.). New York: National Bureau of Economic Research.

Becker, Gary S. (1965), "A Theory of the Allocation of Time," *Economic Journal 75*(299), 493–517.

————(1974), "A Theory of Social Interactions," *Journal of Political Economy 82*(6), 1063–1093.

Davis, Karen, and Russell, Louise B. (1972), "The Substitution of Hospital Outpatient Care for Inpatient Care," *Review of Economics and Statistics 54*(2), 109–120.

Davis, Karen, and Marshall, Ray (1979), "New Developments in the Market for Rural Health Care" in *Research in Health Economics* (Richard M. Scheffler, ed.), Vol. 1. Greenwich, Conn: JAI Press.

De Vany, Arthur (1970), "Time in the Budget of the Consumer: The Theory of Consumer Demand and Labor Supply Under a Time Constraint," Ph.D. dissertation, University of California, Los Angeles, 1970. (Ann Arbor, Mich.: University Microfilms, 1971.)

Fetter, Robert B., and Thompson, John D. (1966), "Patients' Waiting Time and Doctors' Idle Time in the Outpatient Setting," *Health Services Research 1*(1), 66–90.

Fuchs, Victor R. (1974), *Who Shall Live?* New York: Basic Books.

Fuchs, Victor R., and Newhouse Joseph P. (1978), "The Conference and Unresolved Problems," *Journal of Human Resources 13*(Suppl.), 5.

Gronau, Reuben (1973), "The Measurement of Output of the Nonmarket Sector: The Evaluation of Housewives' Time," in *The Measurement of Economic and Social Performance,* Milton Moss (ed.). New York: National Bureau of Economic Research, pp. 163–190.

_____(1974), "The Effect of Children on the Housewife's Value of Time," in *Economics of the Family,* Theodore W. Schultz (ed.). Chicago: University of Chicago Press, pp. 457–488.

Grossman, Michael (1972a), *The Demand for Health: A Theoretical and Empirical Investigation.* New York: National Bureau of Economic Research.

_____(1972b), "On the Concept of Health Capital and the Demand for Health," *Journal of Political Economy 80*(2), 223–255.

_____(1976), "The Correlation Between Health and Schooling," in *Household Production and Consumption,* Nestor E. Terleckyj (ed.). New York: National Bureau of Economic Research, pp. 147–211.

Heckman, James (1974), "Shadow Prices, Market Wages, and Labor Supply," *Econometrica 42*(4), pp. 679–694.

_____(1977), "Sample Selection Bias as a Specification Error," Working Paper No. 172, National Bureau of Economic Research Working Paper Ser. (Mar.).

Holtmann, A. G. (1972), "Prices, Time, and Technology in the Medical Care Market," *Journal of Human Resources 7*(2), 179–190.

Holtmann, A. G., and Olsen, E. Odgers, Jr. (1976), "The Demand for Dental Care: A Study of Consumption and Household Production," *Journal of Human Resources 9*(4).

Kmenta, Jan (1971), *Elements of Econometrics.* New York: Macmillan.

Kniesner, Thomas J. (1976), "An Indirect Test of Complementarity in A Family Labor Supply Model," *Econometrica 44*(4), 651–669.

Luft, Harold S., Hershey, John C., and Morrell, Joan (1976), "Factors Affecting the Use of Physician Services In a Rural Community," *American Journal of Public Health 66*(9), 865–871.

Mincer, Jacob (1974), *Schooling, Experience, and Earnings.* New York: National Bureau of Economic Research.

Mincer, Jacob, and Polachek, Solomon (1974), "Family Investments in Human Capital: Earnings of Women," *Economics of the Family* (Theodore W. Schultz, ed.). Chicago: University of Chicago Press, pp. 397–429.

Miners, Laurence A. (1979), "The Family's Demand for Health: A Rural Investigation," Ph.D. dissertation, University of North Carolina, Chapel Hill.

Newhouse, Joseph P. (1978), *The Economics of Medical Care.* Reading, Mass.: Addison-Wesley, pp. 1, 2.

Newhouse, Joseph, and Phelps, Charles (1974), *Price and Income Elasticities for Medical Care Services.* The Rand Corporation, R-1197-NC/OEO (June).

_____(1976), "New Estimates of Price and Income Elasticities of Medical Care Services," in *The Role of Health Insurance in the Health Services Sector.* (Richard N. Rosett, ed.). New York: National Bureau of Economic Research, pp. 261–313.

Parsons, Donald O. (1977), "Health, Family Structure, and Labor Supply," *American Economic Review 64*(4), 703–712.

Pfouts, Ralph W. (1972), *Elementary Economics: A Mathematical Approach.* New York: Wiley, pp. 159–161.

Phelps, Charles, and Newhouse, Joseph (1972), *The Effects of Coinsurance on the Demand for Physician Services.* The Rand Corporation, R-976-OEO (June).

Phlips, Louis (1974), *Applied Consumption Analysis.* New York: American Elsevier, p. 70.

Rosett, Richard N., and Huang, Lien fu (1973), "The Effect of Health Insurance on the Demand for Medical Care," *Journal of Political Economy 81*(2), Pt. 1, 281–305.

Scheffler, Richard M., and Iden, George (1974), "The Effect of Disability on Labor Supply," *Industrial and Labor Relations Review 28*, Oct., 122–132.

Salber, Eva J., Greene, Sandra B., Feldman, Jacob J., and Hunter, Georgia (1976), "Access to Medical Care in a Southern Rural Community," *Medical Care 14*(12), 971–986.

Shannon, Gary W., Bashshar, Rashid L., and Metzner, Charles A. (1969), "The Concept of Distance as a Factor in Accessibility and Utilization of Health Care," *Medical Care Review 26*, 143–161.

Theil, Henri (1971), *Principles of Econometrics*. New York: Wiley.

Tobin, James (1958). "Estimation of Relationships for Limited Dependent Variables," *Econometrica 26*(1), 24–36.

White, M. F. Blanco, and Pike, M. C. (1964), "Appointment Systems in Out-patients' Clinics and the Effect of Patients' Unpunctuality," *Medical Care 2*(1), 133–144.

Willis, Robert J. (1974), "Economic Theory of Fertility Behavior," in *Economics of the Family*. Theodore W. Schultz (ed.). Chicago: University of Chicago Press, pp. 25–75.

Yamane, Taro (1968), *Mathematics for Economists*, 2nd ed. Englewood Cliffs, N.J.: Prentice-Hall, pp. 396–397.

THE DEMAND FOR DENTAL CARE SERVICES, BY INCOME AND INSURANCE STATUS

Teh-wei Hu

I. INTRODUCTION

This study analyzes the demand for dental care services among different income classes as well as the effects of dental insurance coverage. The demand for dental care services is defined as the number of dental visits per year, using dental expenditures as a supplemental dependent variable. The demand models are estimated from the 1970 National Opinion Research Center (NORC) health survey data with a total of 11,376 individuals. Among them, 589 individuals had free dental care, 811 had dental insurance, and 9,976 had no dental insurance. By income classification, excluding the free dental care sample, 6,336 individuals belonged to the above-poverty sample and 4,454 belonged to the below-poverty sample (annual income less than $4,700, with family size of four).

Advances in Health Economics and Health Services Research, Vol. 2, pgs. 143–195.
(Volume 1 published as Research in Health Economics)
Copyright © 1981 by JAI Press Inc.
All rights of reproduction in any form reserved.
ISBN: 0-89232-100-8

There are a number of estimates of total consumer dental expenditures (Social Security Administration, the American Dental Association (ADA); and the NORC). Among these, only the Social Security Administration estimates provide systematic annual expenditures. The Social Security Administration estimated that consumer dental expenditures totalled about $8.1 billion in 1976 (Gibson and Mueller, 1977), an increase of more than 50 percent in real terms since 1955, after adjustments for price and population increases are made. In fact, in the 2-year period between 1974 and 1976, consumer dental expenditures increased by $1.6 billion, a substantial amount.

In terms of dental visits, a NORC survey indicates that the percentage of the population seeing a dentist increased from 34 percent in 1953, to 38 percent in 1965, and to 45 percent in 1970. Although the NORC data do not show an increase in per capita dental visits between their 1963 and 1970 surveys (1.5 visits in 1963 vs. 1.4 visits in 1970), the ADA estimated that the mean patient visits per dentist has increased slightly— from 1.51 in 1955 to 1.81 in 1971 and to 1.90 in 1975 (ADA Survey of Dental Practice, 1956, 1971, 1976).

Compared to hospital and physician services, demand for dental services is considered to have low priority. In the past, dental care for anything other than dental disease was regarded primarily as a "luxury" or "cosmetic" service and is still so considered by many persons. Many needed dental care services, however, fall within the area of preventive health care. The differences in utilization among hospital, physician, and dental services can be seen by comparing the NORC survey data for 1958, 1963, and 1970, reported in Table 1. Table 1 shows that 66 percent of the population saw a physician in 1958, 65 percent in 1963, and 68 percent in 1970. No data are available on the percentage of the population admitted to hospitals prior to 1970, but data on hospital admissions per 100 person-years are available in the survey. Table 1 shows relatively

Table 1. Physician Visits, Hospital Admissions, and Dental Visits, By Percent of Population in the NORC Survey, 1958, 1965, and 1970

Type of Survey	1958	1965	1970
Physician visits (percent seeing)	66	65	68
Hospital admissions (per 100 person-years)	12	13	14
Dental visits (percent seeing)	35	38	45

Source: Ronald Andersen, Joanna Kravits, Odin Anderson, and Joan Daley, *Health Service Use: National Trends and Variations.* U.S. Department of Health, Education, and Welfare Publ. No. (HSM) 73-3004 (1972), Tables 4, 12, and 16.

stable figures for hospital admissions also: 12 persons per 100 person-years in 1958, 13 persons per 100 in 1963, and 14 persons per 100 in 1970. Dental visits, however, have increased rapidly—34 percent of the population visited dentists in 1958, 38 percent in 1963, and 45 percent in 1970.

As shown in the NORC survey (Andersen et al., 1972), between 1963 and 1970, the percentage of persons visiting dentists increased slightly for most income classes. However, dental visits among low-income families increased more rapidly than among higher-income groups. Sixteen percent of the NORC survey respondents with family incomes under $2,000 had visited a dentist in 1963. The number rose to 23 percent in 1970. Despite this increase in dental visits by low-income families, in 1970 a person in the highest income group ($17,500 and over) was three times as likely (67 percent vs. 23 percent) to see a dentist than a low-income person. It is obvious, then, that the level of utilization for dental care among low-income families is quite low as compared to high-income families.

It has often been argued that because utilization of dental services is less essential and more voluntary than other types of medical care, the demand for dental care services is somewhat more income and price elastic than other types of medical services. Income and prices may be barriers to the demand for dental care, especially preventive care for the poor. The introduction of Medicaid coverage for dental care may have removed these barriers, as suggested by Andersen et al. (1972). The 1970 NORC survey reported that, among low-income families actually seeing a dentist, mean visits per person were 3.2 per year, as high as the figure for other income groups (Andersen et al., 1972). For families with incomes under $5,000, about 30 percent of dental expenses are paid by Medicaid or other welfare payments, as compared to 5–10 percent paid by insurance programs for other income groups (Andersen et al., 1973). All of the various ways of financing dental care (voluntary insurance, Medicaid, Medicare, cash welfare payments, etc.) have differing effects on the demand for dental care services.

Several questions can be raised about the factors responsible for the magnitude of change in these dental care statistics. These questions are as follows:

1. What factors affected the increase in demand for dental care ser-vices among low-income families during recent years? Is third party dental coverage the only major factor?
2. Even though dental visits among low-income families have risen rapidly, a large gap still exists in utilization of dental care services by high- and low-income families. Is income the most important

explanatory variable here? What are the effects of other sociodemographic variables on dental services utilization among these
two income groups?

3.   To what extent have the supply of dentists and water fluoridation
     programs affected the utilization of dental services?

To answer these questions, it is necessary to study the demand for dental
services among low- and other-income-level families so that comparisions
can be made. This study also places particular emphasis on the effects
of dental insurance on the demand for dental care.

Two major policy implications are directly related to an understanding
of the demand for dental services. First, an effective design for dental
insurance coverage can be recommended for the more comprehensive
coverage envisaged in various National Health Insurance (NHI) plans
if the factors affecting the utilization or nonutilization of dental services
are clearly understood. For instance, the possible different price and
income effects on dental care for different races, ages, sexes, and income
and educational groups may require different designs to achieve the
objectives of NHI. In addition, the problems of possible overutilization
and nonfinancial barriers (such as the supply factor) among different
population groups should be examined in a study of the demand for
dental care services. Secondly, knowledge of the demand parameters for
dental care services will permit more effective planning of dental care
resources. Based on the effects of increased third-party dental care payment on the demand for dental care services, policy makers can rec-
ommend or design schemes to increase or redistribute dental care
manpower.

The plan of this study is as follows: a review of the literature is
presented in Section II; Section III provides the specification models;
Section IV contains the data description; methods of estimation and
empirical results are discussed in Section V; and policy implications and
concluding remarks are presented in Section VI.

II.   LITERATURE REVIEW

For a better understanding of the status of research on the utilization
of and demand for dental care services, a brief literature review follows.
A number of studies have been made on the demand for dental care,
based either on time-series or cross-sectional data, using individuals,
households, individual dentists, states, or the nation as units of observation. The studies are presented in chronological order.

Andersen and Benham (1970) used the 1964 NORC survey data on
2,367 families to estimate demand for health services, including dental
care services. Expenditures, rather than quantity, were used as the de-

pendent variable, and various aspects of health insurance were used as proxies for price, together with extensive breakdowns of quality and demographic variables as independent variables.

Several hypotheses were tested in this study. The first was that the income elasticity for dental expenditures would be lower if price and quality of care, as well as some other demographic characteristics, were introduced into the expenditures model. The results showed that when the income variable alone was used, income elasticity was .83; adding price and other variables, income elasticity was reduced to .61. The researchers suggested that the price component, which is a proxy measure including health insurance premiums and type of health insurance enrollment, is more important than other variables in reducing elasticity.

As a test of the second hypothesis—that dental expenditures are more sensitive to permanent or expected lifetime income than to measured income—a two-stage instrumental variable analysis was performed. The result of the permanent income equation is basically the same as for the observed income equation, although the income elasticity rises from .61 to .99, providing support for the permanent income hypotheses.

Interestingly enough, this permanent income hypothesis is not supported by data on expenditures for physicians' services, which Andersen and Benham (1970) also tested using the same data source. Income elasticities for physicians' services are generally known to be significantly below dental service elasticities. The differing effects of expenditures on physicians' and dentists' services on permanent income elasticities provide further evidence of the fundamental differences between these types of health services.

Silver (1970) included dental expenses as one of the health expenditure variables in his study, based on 1961 to 1962 interview data from 22,000 households. Silver found income and sex to be important determinants of dental expenditures. Income elasticities (ranging from 2.4 to 3.3 depending on the specification) were unusually high when compared with other studies. Fein (1970) has suggested that these elasticities are overstated due to the omission of variables that capture the effects of price discrimination, free care, and insurance expenditures.

Upton and Silverman (1972) estimated the effect of fluoridation on the future demand for dental services. The data were collected from dentists' records on the number and types of treatment performed in 15 Midwestern towns for a week. They found an income elasticity of demand for dentists of 2.2, which is higher than other estimates. Their work showed the use of fluoride reduces the demand for dental care, a finding that is consistent with dental clinical studies (McClure, 1962).

Feldstein (1973) studied the demand for dental care using both time-series and cross-sectional national data. The time-series models used Census Bureau data on per capita income, as well as U.S. Department

of Commerce data on personal expenditures for dental care and ADA
data on price per visit. Two time series equations were estimated for
1929 to 1970. The first, employing per capita income as an independent
variable, showed an excellent fit in predicting per capita dental expenditures. The income elasticity so estimated was 1.022. The second equation
was estimated as part of a simultaneous supply–demand model. Using
two-stage regression least-squares analysis, with dental visits per thousand population as the dependent variable, Feldstein found price and
income elasticities to be strongly significant, with values of -1.43 and
1.71, respectively.

Also estimated were cross-sectional equations of per capita and family
dental expenditures by state and city, respectively. Both equations provide explanatory variables measuring income and extent of fluoridation.
The per capita expenditure was estimated for 1960 and 1967; however,
only the 1967 equation was reported. The inclusion of the fluoridation
variable (in this case, percentage of population using fluoridated water)
shows a significant negative correlation relative to dental visits. The
income elasticity is 1.03.

The family dental expenditure equation in Feldstein's study, based on
data from 38 U.S. cities, shows a somewhat better fit than the per capita
equation. The income elasticity thus estimated is equal to a significant
and relatively large value of 1.82. As noted by Feldstein, this result is
not surprising, due to the use of expenditures as the dependent variable.
Feldstein correctly points out that dental expenditures, as compared to
dental visits, are sensitive not only to an increased quantity of dental
service but also to higher quality. This sensitivity to quality provides an
additional explanation for the very high elasticity estimates of Silver
discussed previously.

Phelps and Newhouse (1974) estimated the effects of price on the
demand for dental care using data from dental insurance plans. Based
on data from coinsurance plans, they found that the demand for dental
care would be 30 percent higher with full coverage than with a 20 percent
coinsurance payment. They also compared data from a New York City
voluntary, prepaid group practice plan with dental utilization for the U.S.
population as a whole. The voluntary enrollment group showed about
180 percent higher utilization of dental services than the U.S. population,
the difference reflecting the effect of self-selection into dental insurance
plans. Phelps and Newhouse also found that demand for children's dental
services was more responsive to price than was demand for dental services for adults.

Maurizi (1975) used the 1961 state data to estimate the impact of a
national dental insurance program on the dental care market. He formulated a demand and supply two-equation linear model using the two-
state least-squares technique to estimate the equilibrium quantity and

price of dental care. He estimated price elasticity to be −1.76 and income elasticity to be 1.06, but the price elasticity of supply was lower, i.e., .79, which nevertheless was greater than the figure of .29 estimated by Feldstein (1973). Maurizi (1975) concluded that with a 20 percent co-payment the total expenditures could increase to more than twice the level that they would be otherwise.

A basic shortcoming in all of the preceding studies is the omission of factors that would account for the effect of waiting time on the demand for dental services. This problem has been considered and given extensive treatment by Holtmann and Olsen (1976). Their analysis is based on data collected by means of 923 household interviews in a five-county area of New York and Pennsylvania during 1971 and 1972. The sample generally encompassed the middle class, with relatively limited coverage of low-income families.

Data were collected on the number of dental visits made by the house-hold in the past year, the educational level of the head of the household, the time spent traveling to the dentist, the waiting time at the dentist, the number of children and adults in the family, annual income, and total dental expenditures of the household during the last year. In addition, variables on the stock of dental health were constructed from the per-centage of households visiting the dentist in the prior year, and in the previous 2- to 5-year period.

Holtmann and Olsen base their empirical work on the theory originally developed by Becker (1965). This theory allows for the production of goods by the consumer which increase his well-being. In the case at hand, the consumer produces dental hygiene by (among other things) using his time in traveling and waiting for dental care, thereby foregoing wages or other benefits. Thus, in this model, both time and price act as rationing agents. For the empirical analysis, Holtmann and Olsen fit both linear and log-linear regression equations of dental visits to the data variables given above. They also include several taste variables, such as "no need," "no money," "dentist not available," and "no time" in their models.

Their findings indicate that income is highly significant, although its effect on dental visits is inelastic. The estimated income elasticity is only .29, which is considerably lower than in other studies. The price elasticity is negative as expected, but it is not significant at the .1 level. Although the travel time variable is not significant and of the wrong sign, the waiting time variable is of the correct sign (negative) and statistically significant.

To test the relationships between money price, waiting time, and in-come, a log-linear model including interaction variables was estimated. The price interaction terms were created by multiplying price by a 0–1 dummy variable for four income classes. The waiting time interaction variables were constructed similarly. This interaction model indicates that both money prices and waiting time are significant factors in the demand for dental care, although the elasticities are rather small. However, for the lowest income class (under $4,400), the price and waiting time elasticities are significantly larger than those of other income classes. The estimated values are 0.57 and 0.29, respectively.

Manning and Phelps (1977) used NORC 1970 health survey data to estimate the demand for various dental services. A sample of 8,145 individuals was used in the study. Individuals who received free dental care or those with dental insurance were excluded. The prices for visits were constructed by using the 1971 retail prices published by the Bureau of Labor Statistics and matching them city-by-city with the NORC sample cities. Both income and prices were deflated into real terms. Fluoridation data for each city were obtained from a telephone survey of water departments in sample cities. Estimation of the demand for dental care was made using the nonlinear limited dependent variable (Tobit) regression technique. Estimation of the demand for individual types of dental care (cleaning, examination, extractions, orthodontia, etc.) relied on discriminant analysis.

Detailed breakdowns of subsamples, such as adult white male, adult white female, white children, and their corresponding nonwhite counterparts, were analyzed. Their nonwhite results are statistically less satisfactory, thus they concentrate their discussion on results for whites. First, they present various price and income elasticities of the demand for types of dental services for whites. For cleaning services, the price elasticities are $-.79$ for women, $-.14$ for men, and -1.34 for children. The magnitude of income elasticities of cleaning service for these three groups are similar, ranging from .74 to .80. For filling services, the price elasticities are $-.58$ for women, $-.73$ for men, and $-.95$ for children. The income elasticities for filling are .54 for women, .88 for men, and .28 for children. There were no detailed explanations for reasons of relative difference in value among these estimated elasticities.

Manning and Phelps also estimated the price and income elasticities with respect to dental visits. The price elasticities are -65 for men, $-.78$ for women, and -1.40 for children, while income elasticities are .61 for men, .55 for women, and .87 for children. These estimates are all highly statistically significant.

Manning and Phelps finally presented the effect of insurance (by the price reduction of 25 percent and at zero price) on the demand for dental visits. They concluded that demand for dental visits appears roughly to double for adults and triple for children, when they are removed from paying the full price to paying nothing for dental care.

A summary of the findings of the studies reported above appears in Table 2, so that the ranges of estimates can be compared. Table 2 in-

Table 2. Summary of Selected Estimates of Price and Income
Elasticities of Demand for Dental Visits

Study	Data	Price Elasticity	Income Elasticity
Anderson and Benham (1970)	1964 NORC Survey	—	.61 to .99
Silver (1970)	1961 and 1962 Household Survey	—	2.4 to 3.3
Upton and Silverman (1972)	1965 Dentist Survey	—	2.2
Feldstein (1973)	1929–1970	−1.43	1.02 to 1.71
Maurizi (1975)	1961 Dental Survey	−1.76	1.06
Holtmann and Olsen (1976)	1971–1972 Household Survey	−.03	.29
Manning and Phelps (1977)	1970 NORC	−.65 to −1.40	.55 to .87

dicates that the estimated income elasticities range from .1 (Holtmann
and Olsen, 1976) to 2.2 (Upton and Silverman, 1972) whereas the estimated price elasticities range from −.03 (Holtmann and Olsen, 1976) to
−1.76 (Maurizi, 1975). The wide range of estimates also shows that
knowledge of the demand for dental care is either inconsistent or incomplete. This is not due to shortcomings of the aforementioned researchers but to the basic differences in data sources (time periods and
units of observation), statistical estimation methods (ordinary least-
squares, instrumental variable technique, two-stage least-squares, Tobit
analysis, and discriminant analysis), and specification of the models
(single equation vs. simultaneous equation, omitted variables, and the
definition of variables).

While the foregoing studies have provided useful information on the
demand for dental care services in general, there is a need for further
study of the demand for dental care services at the low-income level and
the effects of third-party dental coverage on the demand for dental care.
The differences between the present study and previous studies can be
discussed in terms of model specification, statistical estimation, or data
base. For instance, the studies by Andersen and Benham (1970) and
Silver (1970) used dental expenditures instead of number and type of
visits. Upton and Silverman (1972) used number and type of dental visit
variables and they estimated the effects of income and fluoridation on
dental care demand, but they ignored the price effect. Feldstein (1973)
and Maurizi (1975) have made important contributions to the economic

literature on dental health and financing, but their empirical estimations omitted sociodemographic and insurance variables in their demand functions. Holtmann and Olsen (1975) emphasized the time variable, but their price variable is questionable and less than 10 percent of their sample (77 families) are low-income families (having income of less than $5,000). Manning and Phelps (1976) excluded families with dental insurance or free dental care; thus it is difficult to determine the effect of insurance on the demand for dental care services from their study. The present study estimates the demand function for dental care services among low-income families by incorporating the dental insurance variable into the model.

III. SPECIFICATIONS OF MODEL

Utilizing a formal demand function under the assumption of utility maximization subject to income constraints, one can devise an equation that expresses that the demand for dental care, like the demand for other types of health care services, is influenced by the price of dental services, the individual's income, dental insurance coverage, and sociodemographic variables such as race, sex, education, age and location. In addition, other exogenous factors are particularly relevant to the demand for dental care—such as water fluoridation and supply of dentists.

The demand for dental care services in this study can be expressed in two ways. One is the number of dental visits per unit of time. The other is the amount of money spent on dental services per unit of time. Neither of these is a perfect measure. The number of dental visits does not indicate the quality or intensity of dental services rendered, such as the number and technical difficulty of fillings, extractions, cleanings, dentures, or gum treatment. Dental expenditures *may* capture some of the difference in quality and intensity of dental care, but variations in expenditures may be due to variation in prices as well as to quality differences. The ideal demand variables would be various types of dental visits, instead of a total number of dental visits, which involves the "case-mix" problem. However, these ideal variables are not available. This study uses both number of dental visits and total dental expenditures as alternative demand variables. The dental expenditures variable may capture some of the case-mix problems in the analysis.

The price of dental services and the demand for dental services should be inversely related. Since the data does not contain this price variable, it is necessary to construct one. Holtmann and Olsen (1976) used the total out-of-pocket dental expenditures divided by total number of visits in a family (in families with no dental visits, the price variable was approximated from the mean price paid by all dental patients). This type of price variable has two limitations. First, the created price variable is itself an endogenous variable in the demand analysis, so that correlation occurs between this variable and the error term of the demand function. The correlation between endogenous regression and error terms causes biased estimates of the estimated regression coefficients. Although this difficulty can be resolved by means of the instrumental variable technique, it is not an ideal price variable. The second limitation is that the quality difference in relation to number of dental visits is not clearly revealed in the created price variable, since it is assumed that each visit will cost the same price regardless of the type of services. This second limitation cannot be resolved.

The price variable used in this study was obtained from a 1971 Bureau of Labor Statistics (BLS) survey of retail prices of dental visits. A weighted dental price was constructed based on various types of dental services, such as cleaning, filling, extraction, etc. These prices are matched city-by-city to the NORC sample cities. These prices, as well as family incomes, were deflated in real terms by using the BLS cost-of-living index for a family of four persons among these sample cities. For individuals not located in those cities, prices are approximated by nearby cities or rural area cost-of-living index. It should be noted that this price variable has no simultaneous equation bias, since the price data are macrodata, while the demand figures are individual microdata. It implicitly assumes that consumers are price takers in dental care service.

Recent studies by Acton (1975) and Holtmann and Olsen (1976) suggest that waiting time or travel time is a nonmonetary price for receiving health care services, the so-called time price. However, the NORC data do not contain specific time information for dental services. The data contain travel time and waiting time information for "regular source of medical care" which may not be relevant for dental care services. For instance, on the average the waiting time for seeing a dentist is about 50 percent less than it is for seeing a physician, according to Holtmann and Olsen (1976). Therefore, no waiting time variable is included in this demand for dental analysis.

Population per dentist can serve as an approximation of travel time and time waiting to have an appointment with a dentist. The population per dentist variable is also a supply factor which suggests that lower population per dentist increases availability of dental services and also reflects lower access times and waiting times. Since the supply of dentists is macrodata and the demand data are individual microdata, no simultaneous equation bias is involved.

In addition to the variables, price, income, and supply of dentists, which are included in the demand function, variables such as age, race, sex, education, location of residence, and the health status of the individual also reflect differences in demand for dental care services. For instance, age and dental visits may have an "inverse-U" relationship such that the youngest and oldest age groups see less of their dentists than do teen- or middle-aged groups. The white population visits dentists more often than does the nonwhite population. More educated persons see dentists more often than do less educated persons, and the urban population visits dentists more frequently than the rural population. Health status is measured by the individual. It seems that a person in poor health may be less concerned about his dental care than a healthy person, who may be more likely to seek preventive dental services.

The availability of fluoridated water or the amount of fluoridation in the water has some negative effects on the need for dental care, as shown by Feldstein (1973), Ast et al. (1970), and McClure (1962). On the other hand, the recent Manning Phelps (1977) study shows a mixed effect of fluoridation on dental visits. In this study the fluoridated water variable is coded in the form of a dummy variable. If a community has more than 1.0 part per million fluoridation in the water, a value of 1 is coded, otherwise a value of 0 is coded. Data were obtained from the National Institutes of Health (1969).

Since the present study is particularly interested in the effects of dental care insurance on the demand for dental care services, dental insurance coverage is also an important variable in the model. A number of past studies have not included dental insurance as a separate variable. They attempt to approximate the effects of insurance by changing the net price and ignoring the possible shift in demand that may result from the provision of dental insurance. In this study dental insurance is explicitly introduced to examine its effect on dental visits. The NORC survey does not provide clear information of the copayment structure of dental coverage for each individual. The survey presents dental expenditures broken down by source of payment (voluntary insurance, Medicare, out of pocket, and other sources), but these are ex post facto results and do not reveal insurance information for those who use no dental services. The only difficulty in creating a special category of dental insurance coverage is that it does not capture free dental care, such as Medicaid, Veteran's Administration insurance coverage, workmen's compensation, or individuals covered by someone else's liability insurance. These individuals can be picked up by comparing their out-of-pocket dental expenditures and total dental payments. If total dental payments are positive while out-of-pocket dental expenditures are zero, then these individuals must have free care. Therefore, this study divides the dental insurance variable into three categories: individuals with no dental insurance, individuals with dental insurance coverage, and individuals with free dental care services. Since individuals who have free dental care face zero price, their dental consumption may be different from that of other groups, and requires separate analysis.

Based on previous discussions, the demand for dental visits among individuals with or without dental insurance (excluding those who have free care), is specified in Eq. (1).

$$D_v = f (P, Y, R, S, A, E, L, H, I, PD, F, U_1) \qquad (1)$$

where D_v = number of dental visits of the individual;
P = weighted price of dental visits in the city or country;
Y = disposable family income;
R = 1 for white, 0 for nonwhite;
S = 1 for male, 0 for female;
A = dummy variables for age groups;
E = dummy variables for years of education;
L = 1 for urban area, 0 for rural area;
H = dummy variables for personal health status;
I_1 = 1 for dental insurance coverage, 0 for otherwise;
PD = population per dentist in the area;
F = 1 if water has 1.0 or more than 1.0 part per million fluoridation, 0 for otherwise;
U_1 = error terms in the equation.

A supplemental equation for dental visits is individual dental expenditures, which is an approximation of the intensity or the case mix of dental care. In Eq. (2), which represents individual dental expenditures, the education variable is expressed in terms of the status of the head of household, and income is expressed in terms of total household income. Specification in Eq. (2) is very similar to Eq. (1), except for the deletion of the price variable, and addition of a family size variable.

$$E_d = f (Y, R, S, A, E, L, I, PD, F, N, U_2) \qquad (2)$$

where E_d = individual dental expenditures;
N = family size;
U_2 = error terms in the equation.

Finally, dental insurance itself is an endogenous variable. Individuals may have dental insurance because they anticipate extensive use of dental care services. Therefore, the insurance variable and the number of dental visits may be interrelated. Thus, a dental insurance equation is specified, as shown in Eq. (3).

$$I = f (Y, R, S, E, O, U_3) \qquad (3)$$

where O = dummy variables for various occupations;
U_3 = error terms in the equation.

The occupation variable is introduced into the equation in order to capture the possible differences in fringe benefits and dental insurance status that exist among different occupations. Given the endogenous assumption of the insurance variable, the proper estimation procedure is the two-stage least-squares with the Probit technique for Eq. (3) as the first-stage estimation. The model has three equations with three endogenous variables (D_v, E_d, and I) and is overidentified.

One way to avoid the simultaneity problem of the insurance variable is to separate the sample into three groups as noted above: free dental care, dental insurance, and no dental insurance. In each group, Eqs. (1) and (2) will be estimated (obviously the insurance variable is deleted from the equation). In the free dental care group, the price variable is not included as it is in the other two groups. A comparison of these estimates should reveal the possible differences in the demand for dental visits.

Since this study focuses on the demand for dental care among low-income families, separate analyses will be performed for below- and above-poverty-level groups and for whites and nonwhites.

IV.   DESCRIPTION OF DATA

The data on dental visits, dental expenditures, income, and other sociodemographic variables are based on a 1970 Health Care Survey conducted by the National Opinion Research Center (NORC) during 1971. A report prepared by Ronald Andersen et al. (1972) provides a detailed description and summary of this survey. As compared to the Health Expenditures Interview conducted by the National Center for Health Statistics, the NORC survey reports in greater detail the various sources of dental care services and methods of payment. Furthermore, the NORC data oversampled the inner city poor, the aged, and rural residents. This design allows for more detailed analyses of the demand for dental care services among disadvantaged populations than do other data sources.

The 1971 survey includes 3,880 families comprising 11,822 individuals. One or more members of each family provided information regarding the use of dental services, the cost of dental services, and the method of payment utilized for the calendar year 1970. Of the 11,822 individuals, about 4,700 are low-income ($0–$5,999), 3,700 are middle-income ($6,-000–$10,999), and 2,850 individuals are high-income ($11,000 and over). Poor and near-poverty-level families were identified based upon the Bureau of Labor Statistics' definitions. A family was considered near poverty level or below if it reported an income less than the amounts shown in the accompanying tabulation for a given family size.

Family Size	Annual Income
1	$2,600
2	$3,700
3	$4,500
4	$5,700
5	$6,600
6	$7,500
7+	$9,100

Since different income classes have different sampling weights in the survey, the descriptive data are adjusted by these weights. The unit of analysis for dental visits and dental expenditures is the individual, while the unit of analysis for dental expenditures is the family.

Among the 11,822 individuals in the sample, there are 446 individuals with missing data; these are deleted from the analyses. Among the remaining observations, 589 individuals used dental services but did not pay dental care expenditures. In other words, these 589 individuals faced zero price, so that their dental consumption may differ from that of other groups and deserves a separate analysis. Since the present study is especially interested in the demand for dental care among low-income families, the remaining 10,787 individuals are further divided into below-poverty (4,454 individuals) and above-poverty groups (6,336 individuals). The *below-poverty-level group* is defined as comprising those individuals who are members of families with incomes under $6,000.

Table 3 provides the means and standard errors of the basic socio-demographic, economic, and dental utilization variables of the total study sample and for the above- and below-poverty level subgroups.

Table 3.   Means and Standard Errors of Selected Variables
Total Sample and By Income, 1970 NORC Data

	Sample		
Variable	*Total Sample*	*Above Poverty*	*Below Poverty*
Dental visit	.99	1.34	.52
	(.03)	(.04)	(.02)
Dental payment[a]	$ 18.60	$ 25.05	$ 8.39
(out-of-pocket)	(.69)	(1.06)	(.63)
Family Income[a]	$8,345.79	$11,389.01	$3,950.79
	(76.65)	(49.78)	(34.08)
Price[a]	$ 9.77	$ 9.63	$ 9.96
	(.02)	(.02)	(.02)

Table 3.   (Cont.)

Variable	Total Sample	Above Poverty	Below Poverty
		Sample	
Dental insurance	.07	.11	.03
	(.003)	(.002)	(.001)
Male	.48	.50	.44
	(.01)	(.01)	(.01)
White	.69	.79	.53
	(.01)	(.01)	(.01)
Urban	.65	.62	.69
	(.01)	(.01)	(.01)
Education (none)	.01	.00	.01
	(.01)	(.01)	(.01)
Education (1–7 years)	.49	.15	.25
	(.01)	(.01)	(.01)
Education (8–12 years)	.37	.40	.31
	(.01)	(.01)	(.01)
Education (>12 years)	.13	.18	.05
	(.01)	(.01)	(.01)
Age (less than 5 years)	.09	.08	.11
	(.01)	(.01)	(.01)
Age (5–15 years)	.24	.23	.25
	(.01)	(.01)	(.01)
Age (16–44 years)	.35	.36	.33
	(.01)	(.01)	(.01)
Age (>45 years)	.32	.33	.31
	(.01)	(.01)	(.01)
Health (excellent and good)	.78	.82	.72
	(.01)	(.01)	(.01)
Health (fair)	.14	.13	.17
	(.01)	(.01)	(.01)
Health (poor)	.04	.03	.07
	(.01)	(.01)	(.01)
Water fluoridation	.42	.44	.38
	(.01)	(.01)	(.01)
Population per dentist	2,241.56	2,183.74	2,325.31
	(12.71)	(11.20)	(13.25)
Sample size	10,787	6,336	4,454

Note: [a] Adjusted by the 1970 cost-of-living index.

For the total sample, individuals had an average of one dental visit per year with an $18.6 out-of-pocket dental payment. The average family income for the total sample was $8,346. The average weighted dental visit price was $9.8 during 1970. It should be noted that all of these monetary figures are deflated by the cost-of-living indices in their areas.

Among the total sample, 7 percent had dental insurance. Among the above-poverty sample, 11 percent had dental insurance; only 3 percent of the below-poverty sample had such insurance.

About 48 percent of the sample are male, 69 percent are white, and 65 percent reside in urban areas. Thirty-three percent of the individuals are children under 15 years old, and about 50 percent had less than 8 years of schooling. Forty-two percent of the individuals reside in fluoridated water areas. In the total sample, the population–dentist ratio is 2,142.

Table 3 also provides the income difference between the above-poverty and below-poverty samples. The mean family income is $3,950 for the low-income group and $11,389 for the above-poverty group. Below-poverty individuals averaged .5 dental visits per year and paid $8.40 out-of-pocket; the above-poverty group averaged 1.3 visits and paid $25.

The weighted dental fees are similar: $9.96 per visit for below-poverty and $9.63 for above-poverty. There are fewer males in the below-poverty group (44 percent) than in the above-poverty group (50 percent). The above-poverty level group had more education and included more whites than did the below-poverty group.

The below-poverty-level group also includes more children than the above-poverty group. Fewer people in the lower income group resided in areas with fluoridated water, and they had less access to dentists (2,325 persons/dentist) than the higher-income group (2,183 persons/dentist).

Table 4 presents the means and standard errors of variables by sample under three subgroups: no dental insurance, dental insurance, and free dental care. It can be seen that the average family income for the no dental insurance group is $8,094, or about $2,340 less than that of the insurance-covered group, and the free dental care group has the lowest average income: $5,772. By definition, the no dental insurance group pays their total dental care expenditures of $18.25 per person out-of-pocket. The dental insurance group has a higher average dental bill of $29.75 per person, of which $22.61 is paid out-of-pocket. (In other words, dental insurance covers, on the average, about $7 per person within the dental insurance sample.) The free dental care group pays no dental bills at all; among this group a third party has paid an average of $58 per person.

Table 4   Means and Standard Errors of Variables Included in the
Study, by Dental Insurance (1970 NORC Data)

	Sample		
Variable	*No Dental Insurance*	*Dental Insurance*	*Free Dental Care*
Dental visit	.96	1.39	3.26
	(.03)	(.09)	(.14)
Dental payment[a]	$18.25	$22.61	
(out-of-pocket)	(.72)	(2.31)	—
Total dental expenditure	$18.71	$29.75	$58.02
	(.72)	(3.26)	(4.54)
Family income	$8,094.56	$11,436.13	$5,772.61
	(74.32)	(212.68)	(174.18)
Price	$9.78	$9.74	$10.01
	(.02)	(.08)	(.08)
Male	.45	.49	.45
	(.01)	(.02)	(.02)
White	.68	.82	.49
	(.01)	(.01)	(.02)
Urban	.66	.64	.85
	(.01)	(.02)	(.01)
Education (none)	.01	.001	.003
	(.002)	(.001)	(.002)
Education (1–7 years)	.49	.40	.58
	(.004)	(.01)	(.015)
Education (8–12 years)	.37	.41	.34
	(.005)	(.02)	(.02)
Education (>12 years)	.13	.81	.07
	(.003)	(.01)	(.01)
Age (less than 4 years)	.09	.10	.02
	(.003)	(.01)	(.005)
Age (5–15 years)	.24	.27	.34
	(.004)	(.02)	(.02)
Age (16–44 years)	.34	.43	.55
	(.005)	(.02)	(.02)
Age (>45 years)	.32	.20	.10
	(.005)	(.01)	(.01)
Health (excellent and	.80	.85	.76
good)	(.006)	(.01)	(.02)
Health (fair)	.15	.10	.16
	(.004)	(.01)	(.01)

Table 4. (Cont.)

	Sample		
Variable	No Dental Insurance	Dental Insurance	Free Dental Care
Health (poor)	.05	.02	.07
	(.002)	(.005)	(.01)
Water fluoridation	.40	.54	.56
	(.005)	(.02)	(.02)
Population per dentist	2,264.15	2,020.61	1,841.86
	(13.37)	(39.61)	(40.38)
Sample size	9,976	811	589

Note: ᵃ Adjusted by the 1970 cost-of-living index.

These differences in dental expenditures are also reflected in the average number of dental visits during 1970. The no dental insurance sample visited the dentist about once a year (.96); the dental insurance sample visited dentists more than once a year (1.39); and the free dental care sample visited more than three times a year (3.26). The differences among these three groups in terms of dental visits, dental expenditures, and income levels implies that the free dental care that is available mainly to the low-income group leads to much more utilization of dental services than among higher-income individuals.

It is also interesting to note that both the no dental insurance and dental insurance groups face a similar price for dental services, but the free dental care group faces higher dental prices (although they do not have to pay by themselves). This difference in price could be due to the higher percentage of urban residents in the free dental care group, where prices may be higher, as shown in Table 4. Eighty-five percent of the free dental care group resides in urban areas.

Among the free dental care group, whites and nonwhites are about equally represented in the sample, whereas 82 percent of those who have dental insurance are white. Education level is higher among the dental insurance group, while the free dental care group has the lowest education level among the three sample groups.

Population per dentist is lowest among the free dental care group (1,842 persons per dentist), followed by that for the dental insurance group (2,021 per dentist), and the no dental insurance group (2,264 per dentist). These differences, too, could be explained by reference to urban and rural location.

Table 5 relates the dental price and income variables to dental insurance and race differences. Dental prices are the weighted average of

Table 5. Means and Standard Errors of Dental Price and Income in Relation to Insurance and Race (in 1970 dollars)

	Above Poverty		Below Poverty		White		Nonwhite	
	Income	Price	Income	Price	Income	Price	Income	Price
Have dental insurance	12,414 (233)	9.60 (.10)	5,466 (166)	10.09 (.11)	11,662 (238)	9.60 (.09)	9,442 (514)	10.03 (.22)
No dental insurance	11,283 (124)	9.64 (.03)	3,909 (34)	9.96 (.03)	9,001 (111)	9.61 (.02)	6,158 (78)	10.13 (.04)

prices deflated by the cost-of-living index in the area of residence. It can be seen that persons with dental insurance have higher incomes within the same income category (above poverty or below poverty) or race group.

It is striking that nonwhites and below-poverty groups face higher dental prices than whites and above-poverty groups do, as shown in Table 5. Possibly, as noted earlier, more nonwhites and poor individuals reside in urban areas, where dental care prices are higher than in non-urban areas.

Previous studies indicate that insurance, income, and race are important variables associated with the amount of dental services utilization. A simple mean value comparison is shown in Table 6. Table 6 suggests that for persons who have no dental insurance and are either poor or nonwhite, the average number of dental visits per year is almost half that of their counterparts who have dental insurance. In other words, on the average, a nonwhite person or poor person visits a dentist once a year when he has dental insurance, but when he has none he visits a dentist only once every 2 years. On the other hand, a white person or a person who has an above-poverty-level income visits the dentist just about as often regardless of whether he is insured or not.

It should be noted that these associations between dental visits, insurance, income level, and race are gross in nature and that the differences between the number of dental visits and (a) insurance, (b) income level, and (c) race could be due to location, education, and many other factors. In order to properly estimate the net relations between dental visits and insurance or dental visits and income, a regression model should be used to include all these relevant factors as explanatory variables. Section V provides the results of econometric estimations.

V. EMPIRICAL ESTIMATIONS AND RESULTS: DENTAL VISITS

Since the dependent variable "dental visits" is a discrete dichotomous variable with a large number of values concentrated at zero, the classical

Table 6. Means and Standard Errors of Dental Visits in Relation to Insurance, Income, and Race

Dental Insurance	Above Poverty	Below Poverty	White	Nonwhite
Have dental insurance	1.39	1.07	1.17	.87
	(.05)	(.24)	(.09)	(.21)
No dental insurance	1.29	.50	1.17	.46
	(.04)	(.03)	(.03)	(.04)

least-squares approach is not an appropriate method of estimation. The dichotomous dependent variable will cause heteroskedasticity of the error term and thus inefficient estimation of regression coefficients. Furthermore, the classical least-squares method will overestimate sample observations at both zero and one values. Therefore, Tobit estimation technique is used for the dental visit and dental insurance equations.

In Section III, the model assumes that dental insurance is an endogenous variable, i.e., that individuals have dental insurance because they anticipate using dental care services. Therefore, the insurance variable and the number of dental visits may be interrelated. To avoid bias in the dental visit equation, we estimated the insurance equation by Probit technique and then used the predicted probability of having dental insurance as an instrumental variable in estimating the dental visit equation. The resulting coefficients for the dental insurance variable were unduly large, however (two digit values). Thus, we decided to estimate the dental visits equation using the straightforward Tobit technique and actual coding of dental insurance as the explanatory variable instead of the predicted probability of dental insurance. This technique may cause bias of estimated coefficients in the model if the insurance variable is endogenous and the error terms of the dental visits equation and the insurance equation are correlated. On the other hand, it can be argued that dental insurance is not endogenous. Most individuals who have dental insurance are covered by Medicaid, Medicare, or industry fringe benefits. Such individuals are covered by dental insurance regardless of their anticipation of future dental services utilization. Dental insurance, therefore, is not an endogenous variable in the demand equation. The Appendix presents the empirical estimation of the dental insurance equation.

A.   Total Sample, Above Poverty, and Below Poverty Samples

The results of the Tobin estimation of dental visits among the total sample and among above-poverty and below-poverty individuals are presented in Table 7. Chi-squares show that the characteristics included in the estimation contribute significantly to the explanation of the utilization of dental visits.

Income and Price Variables.   As theory predicted, income has a positive effect on dental visits. In fact, income is one of the most important of the variables that (in terms of the level of significance) affect the demand for dental visits. The price variable has a statistically significant negative effect on the demand for dental visits in the total sample and below-poverty group, but has no significant effect on the demand for dental

Table 7. Individual Demand for Dental Visits, by Income Level,
Tobit Results

Variable	Sample[a]		
	Total Sample	Above Poverty	Below Poverty
Constant	−6.55 (.58)	−5.48 (.68)	−7.30 (1.02)
Male	−.79*** (.14)	−.79*** (.17)	−1.15*** (.26)
Urban	−.04 (.18)	.52** (.21)	−1.26*** (.33)
White	3.24*** (.19)	2.96*** (.24)	2.63*** (.30)
Family income	.000089*** (.000008)	.000048*** (.000008)	.00025*** (.00006)
Education (none = 0)			
Education (1–7 years)	.16 (.35)	−.10 (.45)	.63 (.56)
Education (8–12 years)	1.68*** (.34)	1.25*** (.44)	2.03*** (.55)
Education (>12 years)	3.63*** (.38)	3.17 (4.80)	3.71*** (.72)
Health (Excellent = n; good = 0)			
Health (fair)	−.25 (.21)	−.07 (.26)	−.39 (.37)
Health (poor)	−1.36*** (.38)	−1.32*** (.54)	−.72 (.55)
Age (<5)	−4.32*** (.53)	−4.27*** (.63)	−4.66*** (.98)
Age (5–17)	2.10*** (.34)	2.40*** (.42)	1.89*** (.57)
Age (18–45)	.58*** (.18)	.31 (.21)	1.29** (.37)
Age (>45 = 0)			
Price	−.075** (.037)	−.040 (.041)	−.096* (.057)
Pop/dentist	−.00022*** (.00006)	−.00026*** (.00008)	−.00014* (.00008)
Fluoridation	.23 (.15)	.18 (.18)	−.05 (.29)

Table 7. (Cont.)

	Sample[a]		
Variable	Total Sample	Above Poverty	Below Poverty
Dental insurance	.71***	.14	2.40***
	(.25)	(.26)	(.65)
$\hat{\sigma}$	5.67	5.56	5.74
Sample size	10787	6346	4441
Chi-square	1355	987	358

Notes: [a] Values in parentheses are standard errors of coefficients.
  * Indicates the 10 percent level of significance (at two-tailed test).
  ** Indicates the 5 percent level of significance (at two-tailed test).
  *** Indicates the 1 percent level of significance (at two-tailed test).

visits among the above-poverty group. To evaluate the effects of income and price on the demand for dental visits, it is necessary to assume a given sociodemographic status of an individual in the Tobit model. Based on the mode of these dichotomous sociodemographic variables [male, urban, white, high school education, good health, and age range (18–45)] and on the sample means of continuous variables (income, price, and pop/dentist), the estimated income elasticities for those who have dental insurance are .20 for the total sample, .14 for the above-poverty group, and .25 for the below-poverty group. The estimated income elasticities for those who do not have dental insurance are .21 for the total sample, .15 for the above poverty group, and .29 for the below-poverty group, as shown in Table 8. The estimated price elasticities are −.19 for the total sample (insurance or without insurance), −.10 for above poverty (insurance or without insurance), −.23 for below poverty with insurance, and −.28 for below poverty without insurance.

The results presented in Table 8 have several implications:

First, both income and price elasticities are relatively low in comparison with those of Manning and Phelps (1977). They are also lower than the general belief that the demand for dental services is income and price elastic would lead one to believe. The difference in magnitude between this study and others may be attributable to the introduction of the dental insurance variable into the equation. Other possible explanations for the relatively low values are the relatively small budget proportion of the budget allotted for dental care within families and the negative attitudes (pain aversion) toward dental care that may induce people to avoid it.

Table 8. Estimated Income and Price Elasticities of Demand for Dental Visits[a]

		Sample		
Variable		Total Sample	Above Poverty	Below Poverty
Income	Insurance = 1	.20***	.14***	.25***
	No insurance = 0	.21***	.15***	.29***
Price	Insurance = 1	−.19**	−.10	−.23*
	No insurance = 0	−.20**	−.10	−.28*

Source: Data from Table 7.
Notes: * Indicates the 10 percent level of significance (at two-tailed test).
       ** Indicates the 5 percent level of significance (at two-tailed test).
       *** Indicates the 1 percent level of significance (at two-tailed test).
       [a] A simple dichotomous dependent variable is specified that

$$Y = a + bM + cp + e,$$

where M is income and p is price. The Tobit model specified that an index I can be generated such that

$$Y_j = 0 \qquad \text{for} \quad I_j \le e_j$$

and

$$Y_j = I_j - e_j \qquad \text{for} \quad I_j > e_j$$

where Y is the value of the dependent variable, I is a linear combination of the independent variables to which Y is hypothetically related, and e is a $N(0\sigma^2)$ variable. The predicted expected value of the dependent variable given the index I is given by

$$\hat{Y}_j = \hat{I}_j F\left(\frac{\hat{I}_j}{\sigma}\right) + \dot{\sigma} \, f\left(\frac{\hat{I}_j}{\sigma}\right),$$

where F and f are the standard normal cumulative distribution and standard normal density functions, respectively.
The definition of income elasticity is that

$$E_m = \frac{\partial \hat{Y}_j}{\partial M} \cdot \frac{M}{\hat{Y}_j}.$$

However,

$$\frac{\partial \hat{Y}_j}{\partial M} = \left[\hat{Y}_j \frac{\partial F\left(\frac{\hat{I}_j}{\sigma}\right)}{\partial M} + F\left(\frac{\hat{I}_j}{\sigma}\right) \frac{\partial Y_j}{\partial M} \right] + \left[\sigma \frac{\partial f\left(\frac{\hat{I}}{\sigma}\right)}{\partial M} + f\left(\frac{\hat{I}}{\sigma}\right) \frac{\partial \delta}{\partial p} \right]$$

$$= F\left(\frac{\hat{I}_j}{\sigma}\right) \cdot \frac{\partial \hat{I}}{\partial M} = F\left(\frac{\hat{I}_j}{\sigma}\right) \cdot b.$$

Thus

$$E_m = F\left(\frac{\hat{I}_j}{\sigma}\right) \cdot b \cdot \frac{M}{\hat{Y}_j}.$$

Second, the magnitudes of income and price elasticities are comparable, although the income elasticities are slightly higher than the price elasticities within each respective sample group. It can also be seen that income and price elasticities are higher for below-poverty individuals than for above-poverty individuals. This finding contradicts the conclusion reached by Manning and Phelps (1977). They concluded that the price elasticity of demand for dental visits becomes larger with larger income. This is true when the elasticities are estimated from the same demand curve (with positive sign of the income coefficient and negative sign of the price coefficient in the same demand equation) and we assume that the parallel upward shift of the demand curve is due to the increase in income. However, there is no guarantee that high-income and low-income individuals have the same slope of demand curve. This study indicates that a demand curve for dental visits is much more price responsive for low-income individuals than for high-income individuals.

Third, individuals without dental insurance have higher income elasticities than individuals with dental insurance, especially among the below-poverty sample. There is no difference in terms of price elasticity among insurance and noninsurance above-poverty individuals. However, the price elasticity is higher for noninsured individuals than for insured individuals among the below-poverty sample.

Dental Insurance Variable. For both the total sample and the below-poverty sample, dental insurance is highly positively significant in affecting the demand for dental visits. The magnitude of these insurance coefficients indicates that dental insurance has a much stronger effect for the below-poverty sample than for the other group. The statistical results indicate no significant difference in dental visits among the insured or uninsured above-poverty sample.

Holding other factors constant, Table 9 provides the estimated probabilities and expected number of dental visits for insured and uninsured individuals and other sociodemographic classifications. As Table 9 indicates, the probability of dental visits is .39 for an insured individual as compared to .34 for an uninsured individual, among the total sample. For the above-poverty sample, the probabilities are .40 and .39 for insured and uninsured individuals, respectively. Thus, the difference among the above-poverty sample is minimal. On the other hand, the insured below-poverty individual has a probability of dental visits of .39, while the uninsured below-poverty individual has a much lower probability of .24. Again, it can be seen that a below-poverty individual having dental insurance will visit dentists as often as an above-poverty insured individual. The pattern of difference in the expected number of dental

Table 9. Estimated Probabilities and Expected Number of Dental Visits 1970 NORC Sample

Variable	Estimated Probability $\left[F\left(\frac{\hat{I}}{\sigma}\right) \right]$			Expected Number of Dental Visits ($\hat{Y}$)		
	Total Sample	Above Poverty	Below Poverty	Total Sample	Above Poverty	Below Poverty
Dental insurance[a]	.39	.40	.39	1.49	1.58	1.54
No dental insurance[a]	.34	.39	.24	1.30	1.48	.81
High income ($11,389)[b]	.36	.39	—	1.33	1.48	—
Average income ($8,346)[b]	.34	—	—	1.30	—	—
Low income ($3,951)[b]	.31	—	.24	1.13	—	.81
White, male, age 18–45[b]	.34	.39	.24	1.33	1.48	.81
Nonwhite[c]	.16	.21	.13	.46	.59	.28
Female[d]	.39	.46	.31	1.54	1.77	1.11
Children (5–17 years old)[e]	.45	.53	.28	1.83	2.45	.94

Source: Data from Table 7.

Notes: [a] Assuming one is a healthy male between the ages of 18 and 45 who resides in an urban area with average income levels in the sample, and given the mean values of dental fees and population/dentist ratio.

[b] Assuming one is a healthy male between the ages of 18–45 who resides in an urban area with no dental insurance and with average income levels in the sample, and given the mean values of dental fees and popultion/dentist ratio.

[c] Same assumption as in footnote b, except this person is nonwhite.

[d] Same assumption as in footnote b, except this person is female.

[e] Same assumption as in footnote b, except this person is between 5 and 17 years of age.

visits among insured and uninsured individuals is similar to that for the estimated probabilities of dental visits.

Sociodemographic Variables. Table 7 shows that in the total sample and the above- and below-poverty samples, males visit dentists significantly less than do females. The difference is especially large in the below-poverty population. Whites visit dentists more often than nonwhites— a pattern similar to that for other health care utilizations (physicians and hospital visits).[1]

Table 9 estimates the probabilities and expected number of dental visits for female and nonwhite individuals. A white female has a probability of .39 of visiting a dentist in the total sample, with an expected number of dental visits of 1.54, as compared to a .34 probability of visiting a dentist for a white male, with an expected number of dental visits of 1.33. A nonwhite male has only a .16 probability of visiting a dentist, with .46 as the expected number of visits. Table 9 indicates that a nonwhite male in the below-poverty group has a probability of visiting a dentist of only .13.

While there is no significant difference between the urban and rural populations in terms of dental visits among the total sample, the above-poverty urban sample visited dentists more often than their rural counterparts and the below-poverty urban population visited dentists less frequently than the rural below-poverty population.

Level of education has a positive effect on dental visits: the higher the level of education, the more frequent the dental visits. In terms of health status, the results indicate no significant difference between excellent and fair health status populations in the number of dental visits, but individuals in poor health made fewer dental visits. Presumably, individuals in poor health have other priorities in health care utilization.

Among the age classification, individuals older than 45 constitute the omitted category. As shown in Table 7, children less than 5 years old visit dentists less often than do other age groups, whereas children between 5 and 17 years old have more dental visits than any other age group. As shown in Table 9, a white male child between 5 and 17 has a probability of .45 of visiting a dentist in the total sample, with an expected number of dental visits of 1.83, the highest value among the total sample equation.

Supply of Dentists and Water Fluoridation. The supply or accessibility of dentists is a significant factor in the demand for dental visits. The higher the population per dentist, the fewer dental visits made by individuals in the area. This variable is more statistically significant for the above-poverty sample than for the below-poverty sample.

Water fluoridation appears to have no significant effect on the demand for dental care services. Although the clinical literature has established the positive effect of fluoridation on dental health and thus implies less need for dental care, the present study does not provide positive evidence. The fluoridation variable reflects the degree of flouridation in the water but contains no information about the duration of fluoridation in an area. Manning and Phelps (1977) used both classifications but did not find fluoridation to be related to lowered dental visits either.

In summary, Table 9 shows that dental insurance has a greater effect on low-income individuals than on high-income individuals, although it has positive effects on the demand for dental services among both groups. Assuming no dental insurance for both whites and nonwhites, nonwhite individuals have a much lower probability (about half that of white individuals) of visiting a dentist. For below-poverty nonwhite individuals, the probability of seeing a dentist is about .13; the expected number of dental visits is .28.

B. Dental Insurance, No Dental Insurance, and Free Care Samples

Separate analyses are needed for the dental insurance and no dental insurance samples for two reasons:

First, the dental insurance group and no dental insurance group may not belong to the same population. As shown in Section IV, members of the insurance group have higher incomes and are more likely to be white than members of the no dental insurance group. Furthermore, a Chow test for the dental expenditures equations indicates that these two groups do not have the same linear relations between dependent and independent variables. Thus, separate analyses for these two groups are important.

Second, separating the dental insurance and no dental insurance groups eliminates the problem of endogeniety of the insurance variable encountered in the earlier model. In other words, the dental insurance variable no longer appears in either of these two equations. Thus, straightforward Tobit estimation is satisfactory and no bias exists. This separation estimation still provides a meaningful comparison of dental visits between insurance and no insurance groups.

Table 10 provides the results of the Tobit estimation of dental visits among the dental insurance group, no insurance group, and the free dental care group. Chi-squares show that the characteristics included in the estimation contribute significantly to the explanation of the utilization of dental visits.

Among the total sample, 9,946 individuals have no dental insurance, 811 have dental insurance, and 589 utilized dental services but paid nothing for them. The results for the no dental insurance sample are comparable to the results for the total sample shown in Table 7: males visited dentists less often; whites visited dentists more often than non-whites; income and education have positive effects on the demand for dental visits; children (except those under 5 years old) visited dentists more often than other age groups; and price and population per dentist have negative effects on the demand for dentists.

The patterns of significance for the dental insurance sample are less clear than for the no dental insurance sample. There are no statistically significant differences in dental visits between males and females or urban and rural samples. The effects of price and supply of dentists are not significant either. However, the equation does indicate that among individuals with dental insurance, whites visited dentists more frequently;

Table 10. Individual Demand for Dental Visits by Insurance Status, Tobit Results 1970

	Sample[a]		
	No Dental	Dental	Free
	Insurance	Insurance	Care
Variable	Sample	Sample	Sample
Constant	−7.23	−3.36	3.55
	(.71)	(1.50)	(1.02)
Male	−.80***	−.44	−.19
	(.15)	(.38)	(.29)
Urban	−.08	.58	.20
	(.20)	(.45)	(.49)
White	3.40***	1.18**	−.19
	(.20)	(.55)	(.31)
Family income	.000083***	.00012***	−.00000093
	(.000008)	(.00003)	(.00003764)
Education (none = 0)			
Education (1–7 years)	.22	−.60	.43
	(.46)	(.96)	(.61)
Education (8–12 years)	1.62***	−.08	−.036
	(.48)	(.90)	(.625)
Education (>12 years)	3.72***	.46***	−.22
	(.51)	(.01)	(.85)
Health (excellent = 0; good)			
Health (fair)	−.33	−.34	1.24***
	(.23)	(.65)	(.41)
Health (poor)	−1.25***	.02**	1.01
	(.40)	(.01)	(.64)
Age (<5)	−3.73***	−.05***	−2.21*
	(.66)	(.01)	(1.15)
Age (5–17)	2.78***	.01	−.75
	(.50)	(.91)	(.71)
Age (18–45)	1.40***	.02	−.19
	(.30)	(.56)	(.54)
Age (>45 = 0)			
Price	−.097***	.0089	
	(.040)	(.0885)	
Pop/dentist	−.00022***	−.00022	−.000098
	(.00007)	(.00020)	(.000156)
Fluoridation	.31*	−.80*	−.016
	(.16)	(.43)	(.316)

Table 10.   (Cont.)

Variable	No Dental Insurance Sample	Dental Insurance Sample	Free Care Sample
$\hat{\sigma}$	5.76	4.53	3.43
Sample size	9,946	811	589
Chi-square	121	128	156

Notes: [a] Values in parentheses are standard errors of coefficients.
   * Indicates the 10 percent level of significance (at two-tailed test).
  ** Indicates the 5 percent level of significance (at two-tailed test).
 *** Indicates the 1 percent level of significance (at two-tailed test).

higher income and more highly educated individuals visited dentists more frequently; individuals in poor health visited dentists less; and individuals who reside in fluoridated water areas visited dentists less frequently than those in unfluoridated water areas.

Since by definition free care individuals pay nothing out-of-pocket, the price variable is omitted from the demand equation. Only two variables are statistically significant: (1) individuals in fair health visited dentists more often than those of other health status, and (2) young children (under age 5) visited dentists less frequently than other age groups. Other than these two variables, no meaningful economic or policy interpretations can be drawn from this equation. This is partly due to relatively small sample size and to the complicated nature of free care (i.e., this category includes both poor individuals on Medicare and high-income individuals with industry fringe benefits).

To examine the possible different effects of income, price, and race on the demand for dental care among the dental insurance and no dental insurance samples, a similar estimation of price and income elasticities, probabilities, and expected number of dental visits were calculated. It is interesting to note that price is not a significant variable in the dental insurance sample. Presumably, once one has dental insurance, price is an unimportant factor in the demand for dental care. Since the price variable is not significant in the dental insurance sample and does not appear in the free care sample, only the no dental insurance sample provides the price elasticity at the sample mean value of $-.26$. The income elasticity for the no dental insurance sample is .18, and .33 for the dental insurance sample. Again, the income elasticity for free dental care is not statistically significant. Compared with the total sample estimates in Table 8, the no dental insurance estimates are in closer range than the estimated income elasticities for the dental insurance sample, although they are also quite inelastic.

Table 11 provides the estimated probabilities and expected number of dental visits for three separate sample groups: the no dental insurance sample, the dental insurance sample, and the free dental care sample. As expected, individuals with dental insurance have a higher probability of visiting a dentist than individuals with no dental insurance. Furthermore, individuals with free dental care service are twice as likely to visit a dentist than are the other two groups. In fact, among the free dental care sample, regardless of whether an individual is white or nonwhite, or has a low or average income, his expected number of dental visits is about three times higher than that of individuals with or without dental insurance. This finding implies that although nonwhite individuals with no dental insurance have a lower probability of visiting a dentist than do whites (.15 as compared to .34), the differences become narrower when both individuals have dental insurance (.37 for whites and .31 for nonwhites). When dental care is free, there are almost no differences among whites, nonwhites, males, females, children, and adults in their demand for dental visits, as shown in Table 11.

C. Subsamples of No Dental Insurance and Insured Groups

Previous analyses have attempted to compare the possible differences in demand for dental visits between individuals with and without dental insurance and have examined the factors affecting the demand for dental visits within these two groups. However, no attempt has been made to examine the demand for dental care within subgroups of the no dental insurance sample, such as white and nonwhite, male and female, child and adult, and high- and low-income individuals. This type of detailed separate analysis can eliminate the possible interactions among these sociodemographic variables. Furthermore, the demand function for dental visits may be different among each separate sociodemographic sample group. This type of detailed analysis requires large samples within each category that are available in the large total no insurance sample of 9,946 individuals.

Table 12 presents the Tobit results for the subsamples of the demand for dental visits among the no dental insurance sample. Among the above-poverty and below-poverty subsamples, the patterns of significance among these independent variables are very similar to those in the total sample as shown in Table 10. Among these variables, income has a positive and significant effect on the demand for dental visits. Males visited dentists less than did females; whites visited dentists more than did nonwhites; and the higher the education of the individual, the higher the number of dental visits. Urban above-poverty individuals visited

Table 11.   Estimated Probabilities and Expected Number of Dental Visits 1970 NORC Sample

	Estimated Probabilities $\left[F\left(\frac{\hat{I}}{\sigma}\right)\right]$			Expected Number of Dental Visits ($\hat{Y}$)		
Variable	No Dental Insurance Sample	Dental Insurance Sample	Free Care Sample	No Dental Insurance Sample	Dental Insurance Sample	Free Care Sample
High income[a]	.35	.40	N.A.[e]	1.30	1.66	N.A.[e]
Average income[a]	.34	.37	.80	1.23	1.59	3.29
Low income[a]	.31	.35	.81	1.14	1.57	3.30
White, male, age 18–45[a]	.34	.37	.80	1.23	1.59	3.29
Nonwhite[b]	.15	.31	.82	.50	.86	3.46
Female[c]	.39	.43	.82	1.54	1.70	3.46
Children (5–17 years old)[d]	.43	.39	.76	1.78	1.65	2.92

Notes: [a] Assuming one is a healthy white male between the ages of 18 and 45 who resides in an urban area, and given the mean value of dental fees and population–dentist ratio.
[b] Same assumption as in footnote a, except one is nonwhite.
[c] Same assumption as in footnote a, except one is female.
[d] Same assumption as in footnote a, except one is between 5 and 17 years old.
[e] N.A. indicates not applicable for the sample.

Sources: Data from Table 10.

Table 12.   Individual Demand for Dental Visits, Among No Dental Insurance Sample by Income Level and Race: Tobit Results

	Sample[a]			
Variable	Above Poverty	Below Poverty	White	Nonwhite
Constant	−6.11	−7.43	−3.31	−9.14
	(.87)	(1.11)	(.69)	(2.03)
Male	−.84***	−1.05***	−.83***	−.58
	(.18)	(.27)	(.16)	(.42)
Urban	.55**	−1.31***	.11	−1.83**
	(.26)	(.34)	(.19)	(.89)
White	3.13***	2.68***		
	(.26)	(.31)		
Family income	.000044***	.00028***	.000071***	.00027***
	(.000009)	(.00006)	(.000008)	(.00005)
Education (none = 0)				

Table 12. (Cont.)

Sample[a]

Variable	Above Poverty	Below Poverty	White	Nonwhite
Education (1–7 years)	−.078	.61	.12	.53
	(.62)	(.69)	(.50)	(1.22)
Education (8–12 years)	1.08*	2.08***	1.64***	1.96
	(.62)	(.71)	(.51)	(1.26)
Education (>12 years)	3.12***	3.88***	3.53***	4.53***
	(.65)	(.85)	(.54)	(1.38)
Health (excellent–good = 0)				
Health (fair)	−.13	−.43	−.33	−.26
	(.29)	(.37)	(.25)	(.59)
Health (poor)	−.010	−.79	−.95	−1.27
	(.58)	(.55)	(.42)	(1.11)
Age (<5)	−3.85***	−4.33***	−3.37***	−6.55***
	(.83)	(1.09)	(.69)	(1.88)
Age (5–17 years)	3.06***	1.90**	3.40***	−.26
	(.65)	(.75)	(.52)	(1.43)
Age (18–45 years)	1.20***	1.37***	1.52***	.45
	(.38)	(.50)	(.31)	(1.07)
Age (>45 = 0)				
Price	−.073*	−.097	−.13***	.046
	(.048)	(.074)	(.043)	(.113)
Pop/dentist	−.00025***	−.00016*	−.00024***	−.00018
	(.00009)	(.00010)	(.00007)	(.00024)
Fluoridation	.22	.071	.36**	−.097
	(.20)	(.29)	(.18)	(.44)
$\hat{\sigma}$	5.72	5.70	5.42	7.42
Sample size	5,639	4,307	6,758	3,188
Chi-square	864	338	978	225

Note: [a] Values in parentheses are standard errors of coefficients.
  * Indicates the 10 percent level of significance (at two-tailed test).
  ** Indicates the 5 percent level of significance (at two-tailed test).
  *** Indicates the 1 percent level of significance (at two-tailed test).

dentists more frequently than rural above-poverty individuals; the reverse was true for the below-poverty sample.

Again, the 5- to 17-year-old age group shows the highest number of dental visits, and children under 5 have the lowest number of dental visits.

The price variable has a negative sign in both the above-poverty and below-poverty samples, but only the above-poverty sample has a significant coefficient. Population per dentist has a negative sign in both groups and is statistically significant.

The significance pattern of the white subsample is very close to that for the above-poverty sample. The equation for the nonwhite subsample shows less significant statistical relations than the equation fitted for the white population. In spite of the less precise estimation, the nonwhite equation does reveal that income and education have positive effects on the demand for dental visits. Urban nonwhites have less demand for dental visits than do rural nonwhites. Among nonwhite subsamples, the price variable is not statistically significant.

Among the dental insurance subsamples, as shown in Table 13, the statistical relations between dental visits and independent variables are not as strong as those in equations for the no dental insurance subsamples. Two possible explanations come to mind. First, the dental insurance subsamples include only a small number of observations as compared to the no dental insurance sample. Second, dental insurance may affect the demand for dental visits among the dental insurance sample, so that other sociodemographic and economic variables become less significant.

Relative to the below-poverty and nonwhite dental insured subsamples, the dental insured above-poverty and white subsamples again reveal that income is a positive and statistically significant factor affecting the demand for dental visits whereas dental price is not a statistically significant variable. Children under 5 visited dentists less than other age groups did whereas individuals in the middle-age range (18–45) visited dentists more than older individuals did. Water fluoridation reduced the number of dental visits for white individuals but is not significant for above poverty individuals.

Among the below-poverty individuals, income is not a significant influence on dental visits, but price has a negative effect on the demand for dental care. Males visited dentists less than did females, and water fluoridation significantly reduced the number of dental visits. Residential location, race, education, age, and supply of dentists had no significant effect on the demand for dental visits.

Among nonwhite dentally insured individuals, neither income nor price had a significant effect on dental visits. The only significant variables were education (beyond high school), age (school-age children), and supply of dentists.

In order to compare the estimated probabilities of dental visits between no dental insurance individuals and dentally insured individuals, Table 14 provides comparisons of the estimated probabilities and expected number of dental visits among each subsample. It can be seen that the

Table 13.   Individual Demand for Dental Visits, Among Dental
Insurance Sample by Income Level and Race: Tobit Results

| | | | *Sample* | |
Variable	*Above Poverty*	*Below Poverty*	*White*	*Nonwhite*
Constant	−4.20 (1.54)	5.45 (7.30)	−1.05 (1.48)	−10.85 (6.12)
Male	−.085 (.381)	−3.17** (1.43)	−.40 (.38)	−.68 (1.54)
Urban	.57 (.45)	2.22 (1.97)	.61 (.41)	6.65 (6.71)
White	1.53*** (.59)	.33 (1.61)		
Family income	.00012*** (.00003)	.00032 (.00039)	.00012*** (.00003)	.000080 (.000142)
Education (none = 0)				
Education (1–7 years)	−.011 (1.02)	3.23 (2.63)	−1.16 (.96)	1.53 (4.22)
Education (8–12 years)	−.20 (.94)	1.71 (2.99)	−1.00 (.97)	3.62 (2.69)
Education (>12 years)	.45 (1.05)	1.71 (3.45)	−.64 (1.07)	6.25* (3.60)
Health (excellent– good = 0)				
Health (fair)	−.12 (.63)		−.30 (.67)	.093 (2.27)
Health (poor)	−2.10 (1.38)		−2.00 (1.38)	−19.19 (43.17)
Age (<5)	−4.00*** (1.37)	−15.32 (10.49)	−5.14*** (1.35)	−14.69 (14.95)
Age (5–17 years)	1.65* (.94)	1.42 (3.00)	.30 (.96)	5.87* (3.32)
Age (18–45 years)	1.45*** (.55)	2.42 (2.31)	1.45*** (.54)	1.74 (2.88)
Age (>45)				
Price	.040 (.085)	−1.01* (.61)	.0074 (.0900)	.13 (.54)
Pop/dentist	−.00022 (.00020)	.00019 (.00086)	−.00017 (.00019)	−.00038* (.00022)
Fluoridation	−.37 (.43)	−5.22*** (1.93)	−.94** (.45)	−.41 (1.57)

Table 13. (Cont.)

Variable	*Above Poverty*	*Below Poverty*	*White*	*Nonwhite*
			Sample	
$\hat{\sigma}$	4.23	5.67	4.13	6.73
Sample size	681	130	662	149
Chi-squares	109	171	108	19

Note: [a] Values in parentheses are standard errors of coefficients.
      * Indicates the 10 percent level of significance (at two-tailed test).
     ** Indicates the 5 percent level of significance (at two-tailed test).
    *** Indicates the 1 percent level of significance (at two-tailed test).

probability of visiting a dentist among dentally insured individuals is at least twice as high as that for no dental insurance individuals. The differences in terms of the expected number of dental visits in a given year (1970) were even greater. Dentally insured individuals have at least three times the expected number of visits (except for the below-poverty individuals within this group) than do their respective noninsured counterparts.

The differences in probabilities and expected number of dental visits between dentally insured and noninsured individuals as shown in Table

Table 14. Estimated Probabilities and Expected Number of Dental Visits, No Dental Insurance and Dental Insured Subsamples, 1970 NORC Data

Subsample	*Estimated Probabilities*[a] $\left[F\left(\dfrac{\hat{I}}{\sigma} \right) \right]$		*Expected Number of Dental Visits* $(\hat{Y})$	
	No Dental Insurance Sample	*Dental Insurance Sample*	*No Dental Insurance Sample*	*Dental Insurance Sample*
Above poverty	.37	.86	1.47	4.87
Below poverty	.35	.57	1.22	2.64
White	.36	.88	1.26	5.09
Nonwhite	.18	.46	.67	2.31

Note: [a] Assuming one is a healthy male between the ages of 18 and 45 who resides in an urban area with average income levels, and the mean value of dental fees and population/dentist ratio within each respective sample group.
Sources: Calculated from data in Tables 12 and 13.

14 are much greater than those shown in Table 9. In Table 9, the estimates assume that individuals with or without dental insurance come from the same population with similar sociodemographic and economic characteristics, except that one has dental insurance and the other has not. In Table 14, estimates are derived from each separate sample and take into account sociodemographic and economic differences. Therefore, each estimate in Table 14 reflects typical individual dental demand in each subsample. The sample statistics for dental insurance individuals indicate that this group has higher incomes, more whites, and more education, suggesting an upper-middle-income group. As dental insurance coverage expands to include other income groups in the future, it is likely that Table 9, not Table 14, will serve as a basis for predicting the impact of future dental insurance coverage on the demand for dental visits.

VI. EMPIRICAL ESTIMATION AND RESULTS: OUT-OF-POCKET DENTAL EXPENDITURES

One shortcoming of using the number of dental visits as the demand variable is that dental visits do not reflect a homogeneous service. Some visits are for cleaning or examination, whereas other visits entail extraction or orthodontic work, which results in the so called case-mix problem in the study of medical services since various dental services involve differing charges. To supplement the dental visit variable, out-of-pocket dental care expenditures provide an approximation of the case-mix as well as the extensiveness of dental care. It should be noted, however, that expenditure is a product of price and expenditure. Expenditure itself has its shortcomings as an approximation of the demand variable, since one cannot tell whether increases in expenditure are due to price or to quantity. The present study uses dental expenditures as a supplementary equation to enhance understanding of the demand for dental services.

The dependent variable is individual dental care expenditures. Independent variables fall into two categories: one relates to the characteristics of the individual, and the other to characteristics of the head of the household. The characteristics of the individual are race, sex, location, health status, and age. The reason for including the characteristics of the head of household, instead of characteristics of individuals, is that the number of dental visits among minors is determined by the head of household. The factors that affect the demand decision are the dental insurance status of the head of household, education level, family size, and family income.

A. Total Sample: Above-Poverty and Below-Poverty Samples

Table 15 provides regression results of out-of-pocket dental care expenditures for the total sample, above-poverty sample, and below-poverty sample. Most of the signs and statistical significance of the coefficients are consistent with each other between equations fitted by total and above-poverty samples, but they vary in magnitude. In the equation for below-poverty sample, however, the statistical relations between dependent and independent variables are less strong than in the other two equations. A comparison of these results reveals the following:

1. Family size has a significant negative effect on out-of-pocket dental care expenditures. As expected, the larger the family, the more competing expenditures as well as the more competition for dental care expenditures among individuals in the family, given the same budget constraints.

2. On the average, males spent less on dental care than females did by $3.00 to $4.50 among the total sample and above-poverty sample, respectively. However, there is no significant difference between males and females among the below-poverty sample. Urban individuals spend $6.70 to $11.00 more than rural individuals, among the total sample and above-poverty sample, respectively. Again, there is no significant difference among the below poverty sample.

3. Results among all three samples suggest that white individuals spent more than nonwhites on dental care. The differences are $10.74 for the total sample, $16.11 for the above-poverty sample, and $3.42 for the below-poverty sample.

4. The head of household with no education is the deleted dummy variable in the expenditure equation. Therefore, the coefficients of other education dummy variables reflect differences in dental care expenditures between the deleted variable and the included dummy variable. The results indicate that the higher the education level of the head of household, the greater the individual dental care expenditures. Again, the differences are much higher among the above-poverty sample than the below-poverty sample.

5. The health condition of an individual is not reflected in significant differences in dental care expenditures. The age differences indicate that young people between 5 and 17 spent more than other age groups in the total sample and above-poverty sample, whereas the age group between 18 and 45 spent more than other age groups in the below-poverty sample. Presumably, in the above-poverty group, more preventive dental work was done during the younger years than that done in the below-poverty group, who had more dental repair work done during the middle-age range than than above-poverty group.

6. Income has a positive and significant influence on dental care expenditures in all three equations. The estimated dental care expenditures elasticities with respect to income are .34 for the total sample, .24 for the above-poverty income sample, and .34 for the below-poverty sample (all evaluated at their respective sample means). These results are lower than those of previous studies. Furthermore, the expenditures elasticities are higher for the below-poverty sample than for the above-poverty sample. This finding is consistent with findings of price and income elasticities for dental visits in Table 8.

7. Dental insurance is a dummy variable in the expenditures equation. It is interesting to note that although the coefficient of dental insurance has negative signs, it is not significant for either the total sample or the above-poverty sample. Perhaps the insurance coverage is not extensive enough for individuals to significantly reduce their out-of-pocket dental expenditures. On the other hand, among the below-poverty sample, the

Table 15.   Out-of-Pocket Individual Dental Care Expenditures,
Total Sample and Subsample by Income, Classical
Least Squares (NORC 1970 Data)

	Sample[a]		
Variable	*Total Sample*	*Above Poverty*	*Below Poverty*
Constant	−2.51	−7.46	4.72
	(4.12)	(7.16)	(3.36)
Family size	−1.37***	−1.61***	−1.03***
	(.34)	(.62)	(.32)
Male	−3.06**	−4.77**	−1.69
	(1.36)	(2.13)	(1.22)
Urban	6.72***	11.15***	−.70
	(1.53)	(2.35)	(1.43)
White	10.74***	16.11***	3.42**
	(1.65)	(2.84)	(1.37)
Dental insurance	−.59	−3.14	7.44**
	(2.58)	(3.45)	(3.62)
Education (none = 0)			
Education (1–7 years)	7.23**	11.34*	4.02
	(3.37)	(6.00)	(2.63)
Education (8–12 years)	13.70***	18.63***	6.99***
	(3.33)	(5.78)	(2.69)
Education (>12 years)	26.80***	33.21***	10.26***
	(3.86)	(6.36)	(3.78)

Table 15. (Cont.)

Variable	Total Sample	Above Poverty	Below Poverty
		Sample[a]	
Health (excellent and good = 0)	.85 (2.03)	3.35 (3.33)	-1.29 (1.73)
Health (fair)			
Health (poor)	-4.46 (3.26)	-6.99 (6.32)	-.82 (2.45)
Age (<5 years)	-3.85 (4.16)	-5.15 (7.17)	-.93 (3.38)
Age (5–17 years)	6.55* (3.39)	12.93*** (5.75)	2.02 (2.83)
Age (18–45 years)	-1.85 (1.93)	-4.06 (2.87)	3.70* (1.93)
Age (>45 years = 0)			
Family income	.00075*** (.00009)	.00053*** (.00032)	.00073** (.00035)
$\bar{R}^2$	.035	.028	.019
F-ratio	29.27	14.09	7.12
Sample size	10,787	6,346	4,441

Note: [a] Values in parentheses are standard errors of coefficients.
* Indicates the 10 percent level of significance (at two-tailed test).
** Indicates the 5 percent level of significance (at two-tailed test).
*** Indicates the 1 percent level of significance (at two-tailed test).

insurance variable increases, not decreases, out-of-pocket dental care expenditures. There is no convincing argument to support this finding. It is possible that below-poverty individuals with dental insurance used more dental services (as shown in Section V), that dental insurance programs do not include enough coverage, or the amount deductible is such that individuals must pay additional fees for dental care.

B. No-Dental Insurance and Dentally Insured Samples

Dental expenditures analyses in Table 15 include the dental insurance variable in the equation. It may be argued that dental insurance is an endogenous variable or that dental care may differ between insured and noninsured individuals. Table 16 separates the total sample into dental insured and noninsured categories. Only 811 individuals have dental insurance as compared to 9,976 who do not.

The results presented in Table 16 indicate that the statistical relations between dental expenditures and independent variables are less strong among the insured sample than the noninsured sample. However, the basic patterns of relation between dependent variable and independent variables still exist. For instance, family size has a negative effect on individual dental care expenditures, males spent less than females, urban individuals spent more on dental care than rural individuals, and differences in health status have no significant effect on dental care expenditures. Although the income variable in both equations is highly positively significant, the magnitude of the coefficients is different. The dental care expenditures elasticities with respect to income, evaluated at the respective sample means, are .32 for the no dental insurance sample and .56 for the insured sample, respectively. The results indicate that dental insured individuals are more income responsive to dental care than the noninsured individuals.

Table 16. Out-of-Pocket Individual Dental Care Expenditures, No Dental Insurance and Insured Samples, Classical Least-Squares (NORC 1970 Data)

| | Sample[a] | |
Variable	No Insurance Sample	Insured Sample (Exclude Free Care)
Constant	−4.45	22.22
	(4.29)	(15.14)
Family size	−1.18***	−4.17***
	(.35)	(1.32)
Male	−2.41*	−9.87**
	(1.42)	(4.63)
Urban	6.54***	8.65*
	(1.60)	(5.10)
White	10.99***	6.16
	(1.71)	(6.36)
Dental insurance		
Education (none = 0)		
Education (1–7 years)	8.14**	−2.74
	(3.51)	(12.12)
Education (8–12 years)	14.36***	4.58
	(3.48)	(11.42)
Education (>12 years)	29.85***	−5.12
	(4.04)	(13.01)

Table 16. (Cont.)

Variable	Sample[a]	
	No Insurance Sample	*Insured Sample (Exclude Free Care)*
Health (excellent and good = 0)		
Health (fair)	1.21	− 3.47
	(2.10)	(7.85)
Health (poor)	− 3.69	− 20.11
	(3.34)	(15.45)
Age (<5 years)	− 2.84	− 17.77
	(4.34)	(14.38)
Age (5–17 years)	6.70*	4.06
	(3.54)	(11.76)
Age (18–45 years)	− 2.30	3.31
	(2.01)	(7.01)
Age (>45 years = 0)		
Family Income	.00073***	.0011**
	(.00009)	(.0004)
$\bar{R}^2$	.036	.032
F-ratio	29.89	3.04
Sample size	9,976	811

Notes: [a] Values in parentheses are standard errors of coefficients.
  * Indicates the 10 percent level of significance (at two-tailed test).
  ** Indicates the 5 percent level of significance (at two-tailed test).
  *** Indicates the 1 percent level of significance (at two-tailed test).

The no dental insurance sample indicates that the higher the level of education of the head of household, the higher the dental expenditures on young people between the ages of 5 and 17 years. However, the dental insured sample does not show any significant relations between dental expenditures and education or age variables.

VII. SUMMARY AND POLICY IMPLICATIONS

A. Summary

Utilization of dental care services has increased overall in recent years, but discrepancies still exist between low-income and high-income families in the use of dental services. To understand and predict the demand for dental care, it is necessary to analyze the factors affecting the magnitude of the demand for dental care services. Only when these factors are analyzed can the effects of type of financing of dental care services and the supply of dental manpower be meaningfully discussed. This study attempted to analyze the demand for dental care among different income classes by posing the following three questions at the beginning of the report:

1. What factors have affected the increase in demand for dental care services among low-income families during recent years? Is third-party dental coverage the only major factor?
2. Even though the number of dental visits among low-income families has risen rapidly, a large gap still exists in utilization of dental care services by high- and low-income families. Is income the most important explanatory variable here? What are the effects of other sociodemographic variables on dental services utilization?
3. To what extent have the supply of dentists and water fluoridation programs affected the utilization of dental services?

The empirical results of the present study are presented in response to these questions, followed by a discussion of the policy implications of the findings.

The empirical findings based on the 1970 NORC data indicate that income is the most important variable affecting the demand for dental care. Among the total sample of 10,787 individuals, price has significant negative effects on the demand for dental care, while dental insurance has a significant positive effect on the demand for dental care. This relation holds true for the below poverty level sample only; these two variables are not significant for the above poverty sample.

The ranges of price and income elasticities for dental visits among the various sample groups, i.e., above poverty, below poverty, dentally insured, and noninsured, are $-.10$ to $-.28$ and $.14$ to $.33$, respectively. The magnitudes of these estimated price and income elasticities are smaller than those cited in a number of previous studies. It may be that the inclusion of a dental insurance variable dampens the effect of price and income factors. In this study we found that below-poverty individuals are more price and income responsive to dental care than the above-poverty sample. Furthermore, individuals without dental insurance have higher price and income elasticities than insured individuals. The insurance variable in the low-income sample resulted in an estimated value of an average 1.54 visits for dentally insured individuals as compared to .81 visits for uninsured individuals. The differences are even more striking when the analyses are performed for separate dentally insured and uninsured samples: the expected number of dental visits among the insured group is more than double that of the uninsured group. This finding implies that increases in dental care coverage (in the form of either Medicaid for low-income individuals or fringe benefits for industry workers and their dependents) result in greater demand for dental care.

Among the other sociodemographic variables included, we found that females, whites, and highly educated individuals all visited dentists more frequently than males, nonwhites, and less educated persons. In terms of age, children between 5 and 17 have the highest number of dental visits.

It should also be noted that the supply of dentists (population per dentist) has a significant effect on the demand for dental visits. The higher the population per dentist, the fewer the dental visits made by individuals in the area. The effect of water fluoridation on the demand for dental care services, however, is unclear. The results are mixed and sometimes not significant.

Among the free dental care sample, the probability of visiting a dentist is about .80, with an expected number of dental visits of 3.0 to 3.5, regardless of sociodemographic and economic differences.

A separate analysis was made of dental care expenditures as a supplement to the analysis of demand for dental visits. The results are consistent with the dental visit equation. The estimated dental care expenditures elasticities with respect to income are .33 for the total sample, .23 for the above-poverty group, and .32 for the below-poverty group. Although they are inelastic, below-poverty households respond almost 10 percent higher to increased income than above-poverty households, thus supporting the finding on demand for dental visits that low-income individuals are more price and income elastic than high-income individuals.

B. Policy Implications

It is possible that within the next few years Congress will enact a national health insurance program. Several factors affect the type of health services that should be included under such a program. The following are high priorities: (1) health services that reduce mortality and mobidity, thus increasing benefits to the entire society; (2) health services that can place huge financial burdens on individuals; and (3) health services that are essential to individuals in spite of costs. Dental care services do not fall into any of the aforementioned categories, since dental care is usually considered cosmetic, hygienic, and preventive in nature. Therefore, it is likely that a future national health insurance program will not consider dental care services a top priority item when compared to hospital and physician services.

Government may intervene in a private market as a result of market imperfection, but it may also intervene for the purpose of income redistribution. For the latter reason, government may provide dental care services for a particular low-income subgroup of the population. An earlier study (see Feldstein, 1973, Table 2-12), showed that about 45 percent of low-income individuals visited dentists for extractions and dentures, while other income groups had more visits for cleaning, examinations, and fillings than for extractions. It is likely that if low-income individuals had access to preventive dental care they would have less nedd for serious dental treatments such as extractions and dentures. Furthermore, the empirical findings of this study indicate that low-income individuals visited dentists only about half as often as the above-poverty individuals. In view of the gap in utilization of dental care services between below-poverty and above-poverty individuals and the need for preventive dental care services for low-income individuals, removal of financial barriers may be warranted to encourage low-income individuals to seek preventive dental care.

National health insurance is still a few years away, and even if it is enacted it probably will not incorporate full dental coverage for the entire population. Currently, Medicaid programs in some, but not all, states cover dental care services for low-income families. Whether a national health insurance program includes dental coverage for low-income families or not, a more immediate step toward the improvement of dental care services for low-income families would be uniform dental care coverage under Medicaid programs in each state.

Low-income samples are disproportionately nonwhite, have fewer years of schooling, and have less accessibility to dentists. These are the same variables that this study found to have significantly negative effects on the utilization of dental care services. This study also found that low-income individuals are more price and income responsive than high-income individuals. In addition, low-income individuals with dental insurance are twice as likely to visit a dentist than those with no dental insurance. Thus, dental insurance coverage for low-income families appears to increase their demand for dental visits. This study also found that an increase in the number of dentists alone in a low-income area may increase the demand for dental visits. To fulfill the increased demand from low-income families will require additional dental manpower and financial resources to provide dental care services.

In order to prevent misuse of dental care insurance for low-income families, the type of dental coverage (check-up, cleaning, extraction, or orthodontic work) and the extent of financial coverage (the amount of deductibles or coinsurance rate) provided must be specified. If the emphasis is on preventive rather than on cosmetic dental work, then a fixed number of free check-ups and cleanings (say, once a year) is desirable. Other dental work, such as dentures and extractions, could entail coinsurance (such as 25 percent copayment). The problems of deductible insurance coverage are twofold: if it is too low, it defeats its purpose of preventing misuse; if it is too high, it defeats its purpose of removing financial barriers for low-income families. Therefore, a fixed number of free dental visits combined with a coinsurance rate seems a reasonable approach for financing dental care services among low-income families.

Another suggested priority for national dental insurance coverage is children's dental care. As shown in this study, children between 5 and 17 years old have the highest probability of dental visits. Dental care during this period is important for future dental hygiene. This study found that children from high-income families are twice as likely to visit a dentist than are children from low-income families. The need for dental care is much more urgent for children of low-income families than for children from high-income families. With limited financial resources, coverage for children of low-income families is a higher priority than coverage for all children.

It is beyond the scope of this study to design a particular type of dental care insurance for any particular sector of the population. To do this would require an analysis of costs and benefits of dental coverage as compared to other health services. For instance, according to U.S. Bureau of the Census estimates, in 1974 about 24.5 million people lived below the poverty level (*Current Population Report,* 1975, Series P-60). Under the proposed provision of one free visit per year for below-poverty individuals, the program would cost the government about $245 million a year (assuming $10 per visit). Given free care for the entire below-poverty population, at estimates of 3.3 visits per person (Table 11), the cost might be as high as $809 million. Would $245 million be too little or too much to spend to help low-income individuals to receive dental care? Is $809 million a worthwhile expenditure to ensure free dental care for low-income individuals, or would the money be better used for other preventive or emergency health care services? An increase of 24.5 million dental visits per year (assuming one free visit per person) would place a sudden burden on dental manpower, which in turn could raise the price of dental care for other income classes and increase waiting time for dental services. Further analysis of these and other issues is required.

C. Need for Further Research

This study is limited by the size of the sample of dental insured individuals. With the larger numbers of people being covered under dental insurance, future analyses of demand for dental care may have a larger sample base. A second limitation is that the definition of dental insurance in this study is very broad, and without knowing the type and degree of coverage it is difficult to provide meaningful policy recommendation. In terms of econometric estimation, it is desirable to consider dental insurance an endogenous variable. A technique recently developed by Heckman (1977) should prove to be a useful tool for reestimating the model specified in this study.

APPENDIX: EMPIRICAL ESTIMATIONS AND RESULTS—PROBABILITY OF INDIVIDUALS HAVING DENTAL INSURANCE

The NORC data contain information about whether a person has dental insurance coverage. However, the data do not reveal the extent of dental insurance coverage or the type of insurance carrier. For instance, some dental insurance covers only major orthodontal surgery, some requires substantial deductibles, some requires copayment, and some may offer 100 percent coverage. These variations in coverage may also relate to different types of carriers, such as Medicaid and Medicare sponsored by the government, or industry fringe benefits under Blue Shield or other commercial insurance. Due to the lack of detailed information, constraints are placed on the analysis of the probability of an individual having dental insurance and on the use of dental insurance as an explanatory variable, and these results should be interpreted with care.

The Probit analysis of the dental insurance model is specified in Section III. It is assumed that the probability of having voluntary dental insurance is a function of a set of sociodemographic and economic variables. Since most insurance policies are bought to cover the entire family, these sociodemographic and economic characteristics are represented by the head of the family. The explanatory variables are sex, location, race, education level, health status, occupation, age, and family income.

Table A.1 presents the Probit results for the total sample, above-poverty sample, and below-poverty sample. The results are not entirely consistent among the three equations. However, some variables do have a consistent sign and statistical significance. For instance, white individuals have a higher probability of having dental insurance, regardless of income level. Young (18–36) and middle-aged (36–45) households have a higher probability of having dental insurance than do older households, except for middle-aged individuals in below-poverty households, who have less chance of having dental insurance. Income has a positive effect on the probability of having dental insurance. There are no statistically significant differences between male or female heads of household in terms of having voluntary dental insurance.

Table A.1.   Probability of Individual Having Dental Insurance,
Tobit Results (1970 NORC Data)

Variable	Total Sample	Above Poverty	Below Poverty
		Sample[a]	
Constant	−5.07	−6.38	−6.30
	(0.64)	(2.33)	(−.83)
Male	0.02	0.03	t−0.17
	(0.06)	(0.06)	(0.17)
Urban	0.02	−0.04	1.04***
	(0.07)	(0.07)	(0.22)
White	0.52***	0.28**	0.85***
	(0.08)	(0.09)	(0.19)
Education (none = 0)			
Education (1–7 years)	1.12*	3.28	−0.13
	(0.63	(2.33)	(0.77)
Education (8–12 years)	1.57**	3.66	0.11
	(0.63)	(2.33)	(0.78)
Education (>12 years)	2.22***	4.23*	0.96
	(0.63)	(2.33)	(0.80)
Health (excellent and good = 0)			
Health (fair)	−0.21**	0.02	−0.53**
	(0.09)	(0.10)	(0.23)
Health (poor)	−0.18	0.52***	−1.76***
	(0.15)	(0.17)	(0.60)
Occupation (services = 0)			
Professional	−0.01	−0.23	0.41
	(0.14)	(0.15)	(0.43)
Managerial	0.12	−0.36***	−1.05***
	(0.11)	(0.13)	(0.41)
Kindred	0.59***	0.41***	0.20
	(0.09)	(0.12)	(0.20)
Farm	−0.30	−0.71***	0.46
	(0.19)	(0.27)	(0.34)
Age (18–30 years)	0.21**	0.19*	0.73***
	(0.09)	(0.10)	(0.22)
Age (31–45 years)	0.12*	0.23***	−0.53**
	(0.07)	(0.08)	(0.22)
Age (>45 years = 0)			
Family income	0.000018***	0.0000081**	0.00027***
	(0.000003)	(0.0000033)	(0.00004)
σ̂	1.81	1.70	2.00

Table A.1. (Cont.)

Variable	Total Sample	Above Poverty	Below Poverty
		Sample[a]	
Chi-square	707	561	121
Sample size	10,787	6,346	4,441

Note: [a] Values in parentheses are standard errors of coefficients.
   * Indicates the 10 percent level of significance (at two-tailed test).
   ** Indicates the 5 percent level of significance (at two-tailed test).
   *** Indicates the 1 percent level of significance (at two-tailed test).

Some variables do not show a consistent pattern among the total sample, above-poverty sample, and below-poverty sample. Higher educational attainment is linked with the likelihood of having dental insurance among the total sample and above-poverty sample but not in the below-poverty sample. For the entire sample, there are no differences between urban and rural populations, but for the below-poverty population the urban poor have a higher probability of having dental insurance than the rural poor. Presumably the urban poor are more aware of and likely to use Medicaid programs.

Excellent or good health status is the omitted dummy variable. For the total sample and the below-poverty sample, less healthy individuals are less likely to have dental insurance than those in good health, but among the above-poverty sample, a person in poor health has a higher probability of having dental insurance.

Table A.2. Estimated Probabilities of an Individual Having Dental Insurance (1970 NORC Data)

Variable	Total Sample	Above-Poverty Sample	Below-Poverty Sample
		Sample	
White[a]	.08	.11	.02
Nonwhite[a]	.04	.08	.01
Services Occupation[b]	.08	.11	.02
Kindred Occupation[b]	.13	.16	.03

Notes: [a] Assuming one is male, resides in an urban area, has 8–12 years of education, good health, is between the ages of 31–45, in a service occupation, and with mean income of respective sample groups.
   [b] Assuming one is a white male residing in urban area with 8–12 years of education, good health, and with mean income of respective sample groups.

Sources: Estimated from Table A.1.

Among the different occupational dummy variables, service occupation is the omitted variable. Except for kindred occupations, other types of occupation show no significant difference between the service occupations for the whole sample and above-poverty sample. This finding may reflect an association between labor unions, such as those that are represented among kindred occupations, and higher probability of having dental insurance. However, the 1970 data showed that those in managerial occupations or farm occupations have less probability of having dental insurance than individuals in service occupations in the above-poverty sample. The same conclusion holds for managerial occupations among the below-poverty sample.

Taking into account the similarities and differences among these three equations, a summary of the differences in the probabilities of an individual having dental insurance can be estimated. Since some of the sociodemographic variables are not significant in these equations, only significant characteristics are used for comparison. Thus, Table A.2 provides the estimated probabilities of having dental insurance by race and two occupations, assuming other sociodemographic characteristics of individuals are the same and using the mean income of each sample group. The results indicate that on the average a white individual (urban, middle-aged, and high-school educated; see footnotes in Table A.2) has about an 8 percent probability of having dental insurance as compared to 4 percent for nonwhites. A person in a kindred occupation has a 13 percent probability as compared to 8 percent for one in a service occupation.

There is a big difference in the probability of having dental insurance between the above-poverty and below-poverty sample. An above-poverty white individual has an 11 percent probability of having dental insurance as compared to only 2 percent for below-poverty white individuals. A nonwhite individual has an 8 percent probability of having dental insurance among the above-poverty sample and only 1 percent among the below-poverty sample. It can be seen that income plays an important role in determining the probability of having dental insurance. Again, this is a preliminary analysis; more detailed data collection is required for a full investigation of dental insurance coverage.

ACKNOWLEDGMENTS

Many people contributed their time and knowledge to this project. Kwok-wing Shum performed all of the computer work for the study. Staff members at the National Opinion Research Center at the University of Chicago provided data information. Dr. Lien-fu Huang provided the computer program and advice on methodology. A preliminary version of this study was presented at the Western

Economic Association meetings at Anaheim, California, June 1977, where Alex Maurizi and Rachel Boaz made a number of useful suggestions. Needless to say, while these persons made many improvements in the study, the responsibility for any errors or omissions lies with the authors. The analyses and views expressed are those of the authors alone and do not reflect the position of any other individual, agency, or institution.

A report supported by the National Center for Health Services Research, HRA Grant No. 3 R01 HS 02273-01S1.

NOTE

1. Congressional Budget Office, *Health Differentials Between White and Nonwhite Americans,* Congress of the U.S., U.S. Government Printing Office, Washington, D.C., September 1977.

REFERENCES

Acton, Jan Paul (1975), "Nonmonetary Factors in the Demand for Medical Services: Some Empirical Evidence," *Journal of Political Economy 83,* 595–614.

American Dental Association (1956, 1971, 1976), *Survey of Dental Practice.* Chicago, Illinois.

Andersen, Ronald, and Benham, Lee (1970), "Factors Affecting the Relationship Between Family Income and Medical Care Consumption," in *Empirical Studies in Health Economics* (Herbert E. Klarman, ed.). Baltimore: Johns Hopkins Press.

Andersen, Ronald, Kravits, Joanna, Anderson, Odin, and Daley, Joan (1972), *Health Service Use: National Trends and Variations, 1953–1971.* U.S. Dept. of Health, Education, and Welfare Publ. No. (HSM) 73-3004.

Andersen, Ronald, Kravits, Joanna, Anderson, Odin, and Daley, Joan (1973), *Expenditures for Personal Health Services.* U.S. Dept. of Health, Education, and Welfare Publ. No. (HRA) 75-3105.

Andersen, O. W., and Newman, John F. (1972), *Patterns of Dental Service Utilization in the United States: A Nationwide Social Survey.* University of Chicago Center for Health Administration Studies, Research Ser. XX30.

Ast, David, et al. (1970), "Time and Cost Factors to Provide Regular, Periodic Dental Care for Children in a Fluoridated and Non-Fluoridated Area: Final Report," *Journal of the American Dental Association* April.

Becker, G. S. (1965), "A Theory of the Allocation of Time," *Economic Journal 75,* pp. 493–517.

Fein, R. (1970), "An Economic Analysis of Variations in Medical Expenses and Work-Loss Rates: Comment," in *Empirical Studies in Health Economics* (H. Klarman, ed.). Baltimore: Johns Hopkins Press.

Feldstein, Paul (1973), *Financing Dental Care: An Economic Analysis.* Lexington, Mass.: Heath.

Gibson, Robert, and Mueller, Marjorie (1977), "National Health Expenditure, Fiscal Year 1976," *Social Security Bulletin* April, pp. 3–22.

Heckman, James J. (1977), "Dummy Endogenous Variables in a Simultaneous Equation System," Center Rept. No. 7726, Center for Mathematical Studies in Business and Economics, University of Chicago.

Holtmann, A. G., and Olsen, E. Odgers (1976), "The Demand for Dental Care Production:

A Study of Consumption and Household Production," *Journal of Human Resources* pp. 546–560.

Maurizi, Alex (1975), *Public Policy and the Dental Care Market*. Washington, D.C.: American Enterprise Inst.

Manning, Willard, and Phelps, Charles (1977), *The Demand for Dental Care: Putting Your Mouth Where Your Money Is*. The Rand Corporation, R-2157-HEW (1977).

McClure, F. J. , ed. (1962), *Fluoridated Drinking Water*. Bethesda, Md.: U.S. Dept. of Health, Education and Welfare.

Meyer, Mitchell (1976), *Dental Insurance Plans*. New York: The Conference Board.

National Institutes of Health (1969), *Fluoridation Census*. Bethesda, Md.: U.S. Dept. of Health, Education, and Welfare.

Phelps, Charles E., and Newhouse, Joseph P. (1974), *Coinsurance and the Demand for Medical Services*. The Rand Corporation, R-964-1-OEO (Oct.).

Silver, Morris (1970), "An Economic Analysis of Variations in Medical Expenses and Work-loss Rates," in *Empirical Studies in Health Economics* (Herbert E. Klarman, ed.). Baltimore, Md.: Johns Hopkins Press.

Upton, Charles, and Silverman, William (1972), "The Demand for Dental Services," *The Journal of Human Resources* Spring, pp. 250–261.

U.S. Congressional Budget Office, (1977), *Health Differentials Between White and Non-white Americans*. Washington, D.C.: U.S. Government Printing Office (Sept.).

PHYSICIAN PRICING, COSTS, AND INCOME

Michael Redisch, Jon Gabel and Martha Blaxall

I. INTRODUCTION

From a national survey of 1,014 office-based physicians this paper presents findings on physician fees, income, practice costs, and productivity during 1975. Based on descriptive statistics and reduced form equations we suggest that in the market for physician services the price mechanism is not performing an equilibrating function. We conclude that continued increases in physician supply under current institutional arrangements will exacerbate, not alleviate, the existing inflation in the health care sector.

Since the expiration wage and price controls in April 1974, inflation in the health care sector in general and in the physician component in particular has outpaced the overall rate for the economy. The physician

Advances in Health Economics and Health Services Research, Vol. 2, pgs. 197–228.
(Volume 1 published as Research in Health Economics)

component of the consumer price index (CPI) has risen at an annual rate of 11.7 percent since controls expired, compared with an overall CPI annual rate of increase of 7.6 percent. If inflation is examined in terms of expenditure increases, the situation is more ominous. Expenditures for physician services increased by 15.5 percent per annum between April 1974 and July 1976 (Gibson, 1977), with the rate of increase even higher in the public programs. During that same period, physician outlays in Medicare grew by 23.7 percent per year and in Medicaid by 16.2 percent per year (Gibson, 1977).

The inflation in the physician sector during 1974–1976, the most rapid escalation of prices of the post-Medicare period, coincided with a 7 percent increase in the number of physicians per capita (American Medical Association, 1976). This fact drew the attention of Eric Severeid, who stated in the CBS news on April 27, 1977:

> The barbaric costs of staying alive in America deny the basic criteria of a civilized society, and once again, the economic laws of supply and demand do not work. We have a surplus of hospital beds, but their cost does not go down. We have more and more doctors per capita, but their fees do not go down.

Other observers and many research findings in the economics literature have concluded that the market for physician services may not function as an ordinary competitive market. The evidence is often ambiguous. Most physician inputs, i.e., nurses, equipment, and rent are lumpy, suggesting potential economies of scale; yet the majority of physicians remain in solo practice (American Medical Association, 1976). The steady rise in physician incomes has been accompanied by a decline in physician hours worked per week (American Medical Association, 1976). The Institute of Medicine (1976) reported that the highest Medicare fees in the country are to be found in Manhattan, where the physician-population ratio is six times the national average.

Throughout this paper the assumption is made that individual physician decisions on pricing, hours worked, productivity, practice costs, and income are highly interdependent and ofter determined simultaneously. To observe the effect of an individual variable requires the disentangling of the relevant supply-and-demand factors. In Section II we briefly review the literature in the area and propose a model that is intended to disentangle these supply-and-demand factors. In Section III we report selected descriptive findings from the survey results. In Section IV we show results from reduced form equations. Finally, we conclude with a discussion of the relevance of our research for policy development in the area of physician reimbursement.

II. DEVELOPING A MODEL OF PHYSICIAN PRICING, PRODUCTIVITY, AND INCOME DETERMINATION: FOOD FOR THOUGHT

This paper should be viewed as an empirical exploration of a particularly rich microdata base containing information on individual physician's pricing and production decisions under a variety of market settings. Since our unit of observation is the individual physician's office practice, the variables we will be most interested in "explaining" (i.e., our set of endogenous variables) include the price of the physician's services, the number of hours the physician chooses to work in a typical workweek, the quantity of services produced and sold by the physician in an hour and in a week, the level of the physician's practice costs, and the level of net income per hour and per year generated by the physician from his or her practice.

It is clear that we have set ambitious goals for ourselves, and the empirical section of this paper will amply demonstrate that we have barely begun to interpret our data base. This current section is intended to provide the reader with a grasp of the "mindset" with which we choose to analyze the market for physicians' services and to tie certain of our ideas and findings to previous work in this area.

The term *mindset* is used to imply that the empirical model we are attempting to estimate is loosely based on a heuristic (or intuitive) model of the ways in which physicians and their patients behave; we have not yet agreed upon a precise, formal, mathematical statement describing our view of their market behavior. In part, this reflects the general proclivities of the authors. We adhere to the extended utility maximization school of physician behavior (the distinction between this school and the views of adherents to the simple utility maximization school or to the profit maximization school are discussed later in this paper in some detail). The only combination of utility function maximands and production function constraints resulting in structural and reduced form equations appropriate for estimation are quite restrictive (and often pathological). Instead of assuming in an ad hoc way a set of these restrictive forms we shall assume in an equally ad hoc fashion an empirical model relating our variables of interest to one another and to a set of exogenous variables.

At this point it should prove useful to discuss some of the controversy surrounding the ways by which the market for physicians' services operates at the level of the individual office practice and to set forth some of our views. There are three interrelated questions that we discuss in turn: (1) Does the individual office practice operate within a competitive or a monopolistic market framework? (2) Do supply parameters enter into the "demand" function for physicians' services, i.e., can physicians induce utilization? (3) Do office practices maximize physician profit or utility, and—if the latter—what are the principal components in the utility function?

A. Competitive or Monopolistic Market Framework

When economists refer to a competitive market framework they are really thinking of a set of characteristics an economic market must exhibit in order to be included within this market category. These characteristics include conditions such as homogeneous products, free information concerning both price and product, unimpeded entry and exit of individual firms, and the apparent absence of collusive pricing agreements. Many of these factors appear to be missing from the market for physicians' services. Since our unit of observation is the individual office practice, we shall address these issues as they relate to the local level. We omit for the present a discussion of how the overall level of physicians' incomes could be at a monopolistic level due to the past success of physician trade organizations at limiting (until recently) aggregate entry levels into medical schools, utilizing occupational licensure laws to severely impair competition from related fields, and stifling growth of new organizational arrangements (e.g., prepaid group practice) that directly compete with fee-for-service office practice. While these restraints could create monopoly rents for the medical profession, it would still be theoretically possible for individual physicians to operate within a relatively competitive environment. However, we do not believe that this is the case. Our view of the physician is not as a "price taker" but as a "price setter" facing a downward sloping and possibly "unstable" demand curve. We are persuaded of this through a line of informal reasoning and by a growing body of data. A discussion of the concept of an "unstable" demand curve (i.e., the possibility of an extreme case of monopoly power through which the physician may be able to induce shifts in the demand schedule he or she faces) will be withheld until the next section. For now, we limit our remarks to the more traditional concepts related to monopoly and competition.

The classic article concerning the extent of monopoly power in the market for physicians' services was that of Kessel (1958). He argued that physicians operated as price-discriminating monopolists, charging different prices to different classes of patients to eliminate as best as they could any semblance of consumer surplus from the market. The control exhibited by county medical societies over hospital staff privileges was used as an effective barrier to keep potential price-cutting physicians from entering local markets. Sloan, Cromwell, and Mitchell (1978) suggest that price discrimination at the level of the individual physician is now relatively unimportant. However, what still may be going on unnoticed is a movement away from the type of price discrimination where two patients (with different levels of demand) are billed at separate rates for the same procedure. Instead, the level of patient demand may now be related to the number and types of billed services for what might otherwise be expected to be identical visits. For example, American Health Systems (1977) has shown that the mix of billings per visit within a set of fee-for-service group practices is strongly related to whether or not a patient has insurance coverage.

Further evidence of possible monopoly power at the local market level comes from measurement of fee dispersion in local areas. Newhouse and Sloan (1972) reported a coefficient of variation of about 0.2 to 0.3 in New York City and Chicago for specialty-specific fees for appendectomies and for initial and follow-up office visits. Sloan and Feldman (1977) reported that Mathematica, Inc. will soon make public similar findings. Data from our 1975 physician survey indicated that in New York City the coefficient of variation for a routine follow-up hospital visit for internists was 0.2 and for obstetricians–gynecologists, 0.9. These results are much higher than the coefficients of variation exhibited by prices of most competitive products in local markets.

Stigler (1961) noted that "price dispersion is a manifestation—and, indeed, it is the measure—of ignorance in the market." It is this ignorance that allows individual firms to enjoy a degree of monopoly power. However, certain caveats must be kept in mind before the Stigler prescription is applied full force to the market for physicians' services. Much of the fee dispersion may be related to product differentiation. This can be due to higher "quality" care (as perceived by the patient), by more "amenities" (plusher carpets, air-conditioned offices, etc.), or by lower time prices of care (e.g., shorter waiting times). The as yet unmeasured part of fee dispersion that is best related to physician monopoly power is the part that is due to the high search costs of patients for low-cost physicians and to the inability of patients to effectively judge product quality, often even after the product is consumed. Both of these market imperfections had been greatly exacerbated by the ability of physician associations to ban advertising relating to fees, physician credentials (e.g., board certification, medical school, and place in class, etc.), and product quality (e.g., procedure-specific surgical mortality rates). In fairness to physicians, it must be said that analysis of fee dispersion can only go so far. If the coefficient of variation is "too small," economists can talk of price

collusion within the local market area. If it is "too large," then economists can suggest monopoly power being concentrated at the level of
the individual office practice.

Other types of control mechanisms could also be utilized at the local
level to provide some degree of monopoly power for small groups of
physicians. The courts eroded many of the flagrant abuses of physician
associations documented by Kessel (1958) in determining eligibility for
hospital staff privileges. (For example, you no longer have to be a member in good standing of the local county medical society to be considered
for staff privileges at the local hospital.) However, medical staff members
of hospitals still retain a certain amount of control over the decision to
grant staff privileges to physicians considering entrance into a local market area. Under the guise of "quality of care" a group of physicians with
staff privileges at a local hospital can often suggest that a potential
competitor is qualified to practice medicine anywhere in the state as long
as he or she does not admit patients into their hospital. In areas with
few hospitals, physicians with practices that depend heavily on hospital
care for their patients may thus be able to construct effective barriers
to be used against physicians seeking to enter that market area to set
up a similar (i.e., competing) practice.

B. Do Supply Parameters Enter into the Demand Function?

In an insightful piece, Evans (1976) suggests a novel nomenclature that
may be used to divide into two distinct groups that set of economists
with a professional interest in the market for medical services. The first
group is labeled N (for narrow). Economic practitioners assigned here
are traditionalists who believe that, given production constraints (i.e.,
supply curves), the primary motivating force behind the allocation of
medical goods and services is expressed consumer preferences.

The second group is labeled B (for broad). A standard belief among
its members is that the provider (typically personified by the physician),
rather than the patient as consumer, is the dominant force in determining
medical care utilization patterns. Evans, himself a B, is aware that B
economists have a fine grasp of anecdote but so far have failed to express
their views within the context of a complete and rigorous analytic model.

Evans notes almost parenthetically that, within the context of the
Perlman (1974) book of conference papers he is reviewing, the N group
is composed in its entirety of Americans while the B group reflects the
rest of the world plus a few American defectors. This should not be too
surprising since most countries other than the United States have adopted
some form of universal and comprehensive national health insurance.
With money price no longer allowed to play its traditional role of allocator

of resources within markets for medical care services, foreign economists have been forced to look elsewhere to make sense out of utilization patterns. A dominant physician has often fulfilled this need. It is easy to find an informal rationale to justify this perspective. The physician appears to have the ability to effectively alter both the patient's perception of his or her individual needs and the capacity of modern medical technology to satisfy them. To the foreign economists, supply-and-demand schedules were often confusing in medical markets where the supplier (typically an authoritative physician) tells the "demander" (often a medically unsophisticated patient) what the latter needs and wants in terms of medical resources.

American economists have been slow in following this lead. Even in the hospital sector, where over 92 percent of revenues are currently generated by third-party payment, most economists have clung to the belief that utilization within our fee-for-service system is determined primarily by patient preference. Yet, as noted in Redisch (1978), it is the physician who recommends admission, takes responsibility for ordering diagnostic procedures and therapeutic measures, and determines when the patient is fit to leave the hospital. In addition, it is the physician who typically engages in a lobbying effort with hopes of committing the administrator and trustees to invest in additional bed space, in personnel to help the physician provide more and better care, and in new and expensive technology; all of these will be used by the physician to affect the level of future "demand" for care. (In our empirical work we hope to measure the dependency of office-based physicians on hospital resources, the physician's "rent-free workshop", by inserting a variable representing hospital intensity—hospital beds per 100,000 population—in our regression equations.)

In the office practices that underlie our data base, the market situation is somewhat different than it is for care completely within the hospital. Patients not requiring hospitalization are typically suffering from a less acute and/or less fear-inspiring illness. Furthermore, patients also have a greater relative financial stake in physician (as opposed to hospital) resources that are consumed. Vohavich and Aherne (1973) note that in 1970 fee-for-service physicians obtained 52 percent of their gross revenues from private and government insurance. However, this percentage varies greatly by specialty and is related to the proportion of patients seen in a hospital setting. For example, pediatricians and general surgeons, two specialties represented within our sample, received 20 percent and 68 percent of revenues from third-party sources, respectively.

On the other hand, even for office-based physician practices with patients facing positive money prices, there is a broad and growing base of empirical evidence in support of the B group philosophy. Much of this evidence is anecdotal, such as the *Washington Post* story by Myers (1977) that told of an internist who admitted to supplementing his income during a slack year by initiating among his patients the concept of an annual physical examination.

More involved empirical analyses of this issue are concerned with attempts to measure the ability of new suppliers of medical services in a market area to fulfill Say's Law of inducing or outwardly shifting patient "demand." Note that the concept we are discussing is distinct from the traditional view of an economic market whereby new supplies (i.e., a rightward shift in the supply schedule) are absorbed by consumers at a lower price as a movement down a stable demand schedule occurs. Instead, B economists talk of the ability of medical care supply parameters to enter directly as positive shift parameters into a "demand" function. We have chosen to put quotation marks around the term "demand" since, if this scenario holds, the concept of patient "demand" begins to lose much of its traditional meaning. We, therefore, prefer the term "supply-induced utilization" to "supply-induced demand," but will still find ourselves using both interchangeably throughout the rest of this paper.

Most of the evidence cited in favor of the "physician dominance" hypothesis in the market for physicians' services relates to the impact of the local physician–population ratio on physician fees and workload. In particular, evidence can be cited to show that physician workloads appear to be relatively insensitive to the local intensity of physicians (as reflected by the physician–population ratio) whereas physician fees are related in a positive, not negative, manner to this local intensity.

This conflicts with a more traditional model of the market for physicians' services in which the local levels of per capita income, insurance coverage, and the physician–population ratio all act as simple shift parameters to the patient demand curve faced by an individual office practice. Under this scenario, a decrease in per capita income would be expected, ceteris paribus, to decrease patient demand (i.e., to shift the demand curve downward and to the left), assuming physicians' services are a normal good. Much of the same effect would be expected from a decrease in insurance coverage (a rotation of demand downward to the left with the strong possibility of a rise in demand elasticity). Finally, a similar effect would be expected from a rise in the local physician-population ratio. Each office practice would be forced to share the potential area patient load with a larger number of physicians. Not only would fewer patients be available to each practice at any specific price level, but individual practices would also be expected to find their patient load more price sensitive (i.e., an increased elasticity of demand) as more competitors enter the market area.

Under each of these circumstances (fall in per capita income, fall in insurance coverage, rise in physician-population ratio) the traditional model would predict that on average (i.e., except for unusual rotations of the demand schedules or for changes in side conditions) prices of physicians services and practice workload would both fall.

Yet much empirical evidence exists to show that this is not the case as the physician-population ratio varies over a cross-sectional sample. For example, Evans (1974) shows that in British Columbia physician workload is barely related to physician density in a system where patients face zero money prices. Fuchs and Kramer (1972) estimate that, *ceteris paribus*, an increase in the level of physicians in a state by one percent would decrease physician workload by only six-tenths of one percent. May (1975) used household survey data to show that, *ceteris paribus*, the increased availability of health resources leads to higher family utilization rates. Fuchs et al. (1972) demonstrate that the level of surgical activity in an area is related more to the availability of surgeons than to apparent technical necessity.

Further evidence of the ability of physicians to control demand is presented in Table 1, which contains American Medical Association (AMA) data abstracted from Cantwell (1976). As area population increases from the 10,000–25,000 range to over 5 million the population per physician ratio decreases by over 75 percent (from 2,092 to 518). Yet the mean hours practiced per physician falls only 10 percent (from 52.6 to 47.0) while the mean initial office visit fee, unadjusted for cost of living or specialty mix, actually rises substantially (from $12.22 to $25.16).

Table 1. Evidence of the Ability of Physicians to Control Demand

Population of the Area	Population–Physician Ratio	Physician Income	Mean Hour Practiced	Mean Initial Office Visit Fee
Entire population	812	$48,562	49.9	$19.56
10,000–25,000	2,092	47,186	52.6	12.22
25,000–50,000	1,412	48,037	52.1	12.92
50,000–500,000 SMSA	822	52,081	51.0	18.75
500,000–1,000,000 SMSA	724	49,267	51.1	20.03
1,000,000–5,000,000 SMSA	605	47,704	49.3	21.10
Over 5,000,000 SMSA	518	47,107	47.0	25.16

Source: James R. Cantwell, "A Cross-Section Econometric Analysis for Physician Location and Pricing," paper presented at the Medical Economics Session, Midwest Economics Association Meeting, Apr. 3, 1976.

There is additional evidence that a rise in the physician–population ratio leads to a rise, not a fall, in the price of physicians' services. Huang and Korapecky (1973) obtain this result. Steinwald and Sloan (1974) and Sloan (1976) get mixed results using AMA survey data. Different impacts of physician density on fees are estimated for different specialties. New-house and Phelps (1976) estimate an elasticity of price with respect to the physician-population ratio equal to 0.40 (t = 4.5). They find this one of the more striking findings of their study and warn that "this casts doubt upon the notion that an increase in the number of physicians will mitigate physician price increases."

While these studies hint at the ability of physicians to induce utilization, they are not conclusive. For example, Sloan and Feldman (1977) suggest that quality of care, amenities, and patient waiting time vary systematically with the physician–population ratio and that this explains much of the apparent induced demand.

In a slightly different context, Feldstein (1970) concludes that the market for physicians' services exists in a constant state of excess demand. Price is allowed to remain below a market clearing price to enable physicians to choose a more "interesting" patient load. Note that cross-sectional studies (such as the ones we have previously referenced) would have trouble empirically differentiating between one situation in which there was permanent excess demand whose level was correlated with the physician–population ratio and an alternative situation in which the market was in equilibrium (i.e., there was no excess demand) but physicians had to induce utilization. In the context of a Feldstein-type model, it is the shelter provided by permanent excess demand that gives physicians the discretionary power to vary both their prices and their services supplied.

Where demand inducement completely dominates the physicians' services market, there is an implication that the price variable no longer plays its traditional market-clearing role. Instead, market clearance would come about through an informal rationing system. The physician, acting as patient agent, would play the central role.

If demand inducement is present but not completely dominant (i.e., traditional demand variables still matter), then demand models are still misspecified unless they include explicit consideration of physician behavior. However, under these circumstances, it becomes particularly difficult to empirically disentangle supply-and-demand effects. To the extent that utilization is supply determined, what has often passed as demand equations would in fact represent supply equations. This mixing of demand and supply forces arises directly from the incomplete "agency" relationship of physician and patient. Due to consumer ignorance of the health production process, the physician is designated as the patient's surrogate and is given freedom to choose a bundle of medical resources that the patient is to consume. If this agency relationship were complete (i.e., if the bundle of resources chosen by the physician on behalf of the patient were identical to the bundle that would have been chosen directly by the patient if he or she had full knowledge) then the traditional concept of demand would still be a viable one. However, the physician who is made the patient's agent is also often the fee-for-service provider of one of the medical resources that is being chosen. It is this distortion that creates an incomplete agency relationship and allows supply parameters to enter into demand functions. Society has attempted to minimize the distortion created by this case of market failure. This has taken the form of repeated indoctrination of physicians, outside a market context, with a set of ethical standards.

C. Profit vs. Utility Models of Physicians Behavior

In addition to a concern with empirical verification of the extent of an individual physician's monopoly power, economists have also been interested in what maximand (objective function) would prove most useful in conjunction with a fee-for-service office practice. Arrow (1963) noted that the demand for physicians' services was widely held to be price inelastic and that this was not compatible with profit-maximizing behavior (since a physician facing such an inelastic demand curve could presumably increase revenues and decrease output, costs, and hours worked simply by increasing price). However, the inelastic demand curve that is referred to by Arrow appears to be an industry (or market area) demand curve. This could still be compatible with profit-maximizing behavior as long as individual office practices faced elastic demand schedules. Studies by Newhouse and Phelps (1976) and by Steinwald and Sloan (1974) do estimate less than unitary price elasticities of demand for physicians' services, but neither performs what we would consider the conclusive test of observing the impact on utilization of a group of office practices that have raised their fees relative to other office practices in their respective market areas.

There are less formal reasons for expecting a low demand elasticity. As insurance for physicians' services has grown, the time price of care has assumed a greater and greater share of total patient costs. A large proportional reduction in money prices may, therefore, only represent a small decrease in total costs faced by the patient. In addition, Grossman (1976) points out that the patient's demand is for health, not for specific medical service inputs. Since the demand for physicians' services is considered within this context to be a derived demand for an input with few close substitutes, we would expect a low price elasticity.

A more telling argument against the profit maximization hypothesis is initiated by considering the office practice as a simple, owner-operated firm. This situation was discussed many years ago by Scitovsky (1943), who postulated that firms might choose to maximize a function of profits and of owners' or managerial leisure. It was this type of simple utility maximization model that was used by Sloan (1975) and by Vahovich (1973) to explain the physician's choice of hours worked per week and weeks worked per year. The traditional labor vs. leisure choice within the theory of the household was revised somewhat, since the physician faces an endogenous price for his own labor. It would appear that there exists a declining marginal product of physician time in an office-practice setting. [Reinhardt (1972) estimates the marginal impact of physician hours on practice patient-billings peak at 24 hours per week and steadily declines until it turns negative at the hypothetical level of 120 hours per week.] Yet it is difficult to estimate the impact of hours worked on the marginal hourly wage. This is confounded by the fact that a portion of a physician's net practice income is not a direct return to labor services but a return on his or her ownership of physical capital (x-ray equipment, etc.). For now we plan to estimate reduced form physician hourly wage equations.

So far we have been discussing a "simple utility maximization" model of physician behavior. However, a two-argument function, with a positive marginal product for income and a negative marginal product for hours worked, may not be appropriate. This function would still imply that, for a given level of hours worked, physicians maximize net practice incomes. It would also imply that, for a given level of income, physicians minimize hours worked.

We would like a model of physician behavior that incorporates the possibility of physician-induced utilization. Yet the preliminary evidence presented earlier of demand shifts caused by supply variables implies that inducement takes place under some sets of circumstances but not under others. (If physicians induced all the demand they possibly could at all times, then the demand schedule would be invariant with respect to supply parameters and would always be pushed out as far to the right as possible.) To surmount this hurdle we borrow from Evans (1974) and define a new variable that appears as a third argument in the physician's utility function. The new variable is called D, and represents physician discretionary power to induce demand. Ceteris paribus, increases in D decrease a physician's utility due to the ethical standards a physician has been indoctrinated to uphold. However, increases in D can also raise a physician's income, leading to an increase in utility. Only at relatively low levels of income does the trade-off appear to be in favor of increasing D. Thus this "extended utility maximization model" is compatible with a situation in which physician income is not maximized for every level of hours of work.

Our model can be generalized still further. Reinhardt (1972) estimates that physicians in office practice could profitably double the employment of aides. He suggests that this example of non-profit-maximizing behavior is due to psychic costs that the physician feels are attached to the employment and management of aides. This may not be a complete explanation. Aides appear to be utilized most effectively in physician-scarce areas. As the physician–population ratio rises, physicians see fewer patients and employ far fewer aides. Since actual physician hours appear to hold fairly steady or decline slightly (see the AMA data in Cantwell, 1976), the physician input assumes a greater and greater share of total practice input costs. Note that if you do not impute a shadow cost to physician time, then office practices such as these where the physician performs a disproportionate amount of work appear to be comparatively efficient (in terms of nonphysician practice costs per phycian) when just the opposite may be the case.

If practices in physician-dense areas do in fact reject the option of maintaining net income by employing more aides and decreasing the physician input, than this may be a case wherein physicians receive positive utility from practicing medicine some minimal number of hours a week. On the other hand, it may simply be a case of increasing physician intensity of practice caused by a fall in the marginal physician shadow hourly wage (since physicians earn less in high physician density areas) relative to the cost of aides (whose wages are positively correlated to physician density caused by a joint association with cost of living).

III. SUMMARY OF DESCRIPTIVE STATISTICS OBTAINED FROM THE 1975 PHYSICIAN SURVEY

A number of cross-tabulations were prepared with the data obtained from the national survey of 1,014 physicians to examine the relationship, by specialty, between physicians' incomes, fees, productivity and practice costs, and certain exogenous variables such as physician density and the cost of living in an area relative to the national average. Although the precise nature of these relationships cannot be quantified with these cross-tabulations, they do permit certain inferences to be drawn which can be tested more rigorously using regression analyses.

For example, as shown in Table 2, for all physicians there does not seem to be a decline in the mean net income level as physician density increases from the physician scarce areas to areas where the physician population ratio exceeds 150 per 100,000 population. For general practitioners, general surgeons, and pediatricians, the trend is mixed for a

Table 2. Mean Net Incomes of Physicians in 1975 by Specialty
and Physician Density

Physicians per 100,000 Population	General Practitioners	General Surgeons	Pediatricians	Obstetricians– Gynecologists	Internists	All Physicians
0–50	$43,461	$69,545	$65,000	$52,000	$48,333	$51,765
	(26)	(11)	(3)	(5)	(6)	(51)
51–100	49,848	42,667	46,875	63,571	48,182	49,850
	(33)	(15)	(16)	(14)	(22)	(100)
101–150	43,919	59,194	46,094	63,910	51,557	52,000
	(111)	(62)	(32)	(56)	(61)	(322)
151–200	47,619	67,286	58,750	62,529	56,772	56,872
	(105)	(56)	(40)	(51)	(79)	(337)
200+	37,143	60,710	44,615	71,143	55,404	53,008
	(42)	(31)	(39)	(35)	(57)	(204)
Total	44,826	61,286	50,077	64,563	53,947	53,614
	(317)	(175)	(130)	(167)	(225)	(1014)

Note: ª Numbers in parentheses indicate number of doctors reporting.
Source: 1975 Physician Survey, Abt Associates—National Opinion Research Center.

variety of reasons. General practitioners are more likely to be located in rural areas and may be the only doctor available, thereby generating higher incomes through higher volume. Pediatricians and general surgeons, like general practitioners, have much higher workloads in rural areas than in physician dense areas without major differentials in the mean fee levels (Tables 3, 4, and 5) and thereby generate the high incomes in physician-scarce areas through the larger workloads. Internists generate incomes in the areas with relatively more physicians by charging relatively higher fees and maintaining roughly comparable workloads to their colleagues in more physician-scarce areas.

The data on obstetricians are less useful since a significant portion of their revenue is probably generated through global fees for the total costs of providing prenatal, delivery, and postpartum services. Data for these charges are not available from the survey. The much higher income levels of obstetricians/gynecologists in the physician-dense areas may reflect the fact that abortion services tend to be concentrated in metropolitan areas and may constitute a considerable volume of obstetricians/gynecologists services in those areas.

What is most interesting, as discussed elsewhere in the paper, is the fact that fee levels seem to be positively related to physician density. Unadjusted fee levels are highest in areas where physician density is

Table 3. Mean Usual Fee for Hospital Follow-Up Visit by Specialty and Physician Density

Physicians per 100,000 Population	General Practitioners	General Surgeons	Pediatricians	Obstetricians– Gynecologists	Internists	All Physicians
0–50	$11.29 (21)	$12.26 (11)	$14.49 (3)	$9.02 (5)	$15.68 (5)	$11.93 (45)
51–100	11.97 (32)	11.33 (14)	13.11 (16)	8.22 (11)	14.06 (22)	12.22 (95)
101–150	11.92 (92)	12.91 (53)	13.34 (31)	11.55 (42)	14.32 (59)	12.72 (277)
151–200	13.91 (100)	12.26 (54)	15.11 (38)	11.82 (47)	17.35 (77)	14.30 (316)
200+	12.59 (35)	14.69 (28)	14.28 (39)	9.07 (29)	14.79 (57)	13.36 (188)
All regions	12.67 (280)	12.82 (160)	14.13 (127)	10.74 (134)	15.51 (220)	13.30 (921)

Note: [a] Numbers in parentheses indicate number of reporting physicians in each cell.
Source: 1975 Physician Survey, Abt Associates—National Opinion Research Center.

Table 4. Mean Usual Fee for Office Follow-Up Visit by Specialty and Physician Density

Physicians per 100,000 Population	General Practitioners	General Surgeons	Pediatricians	Obstetricians– Gynecologists	Internists	All Physicians
0–50	$8.22 (25)	$9.89 (11)	$9.03 (3)	$10.57 (5)	$11.34 (5)	$9.20 (49)
51–100	9.93 (33)	10.06 (14)	9.54 (16)	12.09 (12)	11.66 (22)	10.54 (97)
101–150	9.65 (109)	11.01 (60)	10.03 (32)	12.77 (50)	13.07 (60)	11.11 (311)
151–200	10.58 (103)	11.25 (54)	11.05 (40)	14.16 (56)	14.52 (79)	12.29 (322)
200+	10.19 (40)	10.52 (29)	11.03 (39)	12.77 (35)	14.14 (57)	11.98 (200)
Total	9.95 (310)	10.85 (168)	10.36 (130)	13.14 (158)	13.69 (223)	11.53 (989)

Note: [a] Numbers in parentheses indicate number of doctors reporting.
Source: 1975 Physician Survey, Abt Associates—National Opinion Research Center.

Table 5.   Average Number of Encounters (Unweighted Visits) per
Week, by Specialty and Physician Density

Physicians per 100,000 Population	General Practitioners	General Surgeons	Pediatricians	Obstetricians– Gynecologists	Internists	All Physicians
0–50	243.3	253.7	321.1	244.8	150.8	239.4
	(26)	(11)	(3)	(5)	(6)	(51)
50–100	217.0	146.9	192.4	217.4	178.2	194.1
	(33)	(15)	(16)	(14)	(22)	(100)
101–150	192.5	147.1	197.1	174.3	137.0	170.5
	(111)	(62)	(32)	(56)	(61)	(322)
151–200	177.2	129.7	195.1	158.1	147.9	161.3
	(105)	(56)	(40)	(57)	(79)	(337)
200+	138.8	165.8	164.6	137.0	135.0	146.5
	(42)	(31)	(39)	(35)	(57)	(204)
Total	187.0	151.5	189.0	166.7	144.7	168.4
	(317)	(175)	(130)	(167)	(225)	(1014)

Note: [a] Numbers in parentheses indicate number of doctors reporting.
Source: 1975 Physician Survey, Abt Associates—National Opinion Research Center.

between 151 and 200 physicians per 100,000 population and, for office
follow-up visits, are consistently higher in the most physician-dense regions than in those where the physician to population ratio is less than
100.

As discussed earlier, it can be seen that cost-of-living indices are not
a good prediction of physicians' practice costs (Table 6). Physicians in
lower-cost regions seem to have higher practice expenses in total but
on an adjusted visit basis (Table 7) are shown to be less costly. This
latter finding may be more related to the use of physicians' assistants
and their types of aides in rural practices than in metropolitan areas (i.e.,
more efficient production functions for medical care) than to real differences in the level of factor prices.

IV.   ANALYTIC FINDINGS

This section will present empirical findings from reduced-form equations
in which all variables endogenous to our system have been regressed on
a simple linear function of our exogenous variables. We have made use
of the stepwise ordinary least squares (OLS) regression routine that is
part of the SPSS software package. Our discussion will concentrate on
parameter estimates of two variables: (1) number of physicians per capita,

Table 6. Mean Physician Practice Costs by Specialty and Cost of Living Level

Cost-of-Living Index (100 = National Urban Average)	General Practitioners	General Surgeons	Pediatricians	Obstetricians–Gynecologists	Internists	All Physicians
70–89	36,140.59 (63)	48,015.15 (33)	42,158.14 (27)	58,548.14 (35)	56,410.09 (37)	46,851.20 (195)
90–100	41,980.58 (109)	39,958.16 (61)	42,087.29 (40)	36,825.63 (55)	43,933.81 (77)	41,243.09 (342)
100+	28,025.92 (134)	31,005.33 (72)	32,626.70 (61)	45,455.97 (72)	43,620.18 (99)	35,541.45 (438)
All regions	34,667.36 (306)	37,676.70 (166)	37,593.67 (128)	45,341.14 (162)	45,955.28 (213)	39,803.36 (975)

Note: [a] Numbers in parentheses indicate number of physicians reporting.
Source: 1975 Physician Survey, Abt Associates—National Opinion Research Center.

213

Table 7. Mean Practice Costs Per Visit Unit,[a] by Specialty and Cost-of-Living Level[b]

Cost-of-Living Index (100 = National Urban Average)	General Practitioners	General Surgery	Pediatricians	Obstetricians– Gynecologists	Internists	All Physicians
70–89	3.35 (64)	4.25 (35)	3.67 (27)	4.17 (38)	6.60 (39)	4.33 (203)
90–100	4.16 (112)	4.97 (66)	4.70 (40)	4.16 (57)	7.16 (81)	5.05 (356)
100+	3.53 (141)	4.38 (74)	3.96 (63)	6.22 (72)	6.74 (105)	4.90 (455)
All regions	3.72 (317)	4.58 (175)	4.13 (130)	5.05 (167)	6.87 (225)	4.84 (1014)

Notes: [a] One Visit Unit equals the number of minutes reported to conduct an office visit. All procedures were converted into Visit Units by dividing the number of minutes reported as necessary to perform a procedure by the number of minutes in one Visit Unit. Total practice costs were then divided by the total number of visit units reported per year to determine mean practice costs per visit unit for each physician.

[b] Numbers in parentheses indicate number of doctors reporting.

Source: 1975 Physician Survey, Abt Associates—National Opinion Research Center.

214

and (2) hospital beds per capita. These variables were selected because the impact of physician concentration within a locality on our endogenous variables can shed light on the ability of physicians to induce utilization of their services. Also, parameter estimates of hospital beds per capita should indicate the extent to which hospital resources constitute free, complementary inputs of office-based physicians.

For regression analysis, the national sample of 1,014 physicians was subdivided into two groups: primary care physicians (317 general practitioners, 130 pediatricians, and 225 internists) and surgical specialists (175 general surgeons and 167 obstetricians–gynecologists).

Table 8 lists the variables, their definitions, and the variable means and standard deviations for the dependent variables used in the primary care reduced-form equations. Table 9 displays the identical information that was used in the reduced-form equations for the surgical specialists.

For purposes of discussion, the independent variables have been classified into three groups: (1) economic; (2) physician characteristics; and (3) practice characteristics. All independent variables in our reduced-form equations are considered exogenous because they are determined prior to the pricing, output, hours, etc. decisions of the individual office practice. Thus, while physician-pricing decisions may substantially determine the long-run question of area physicians, to the individual physician the number of practicing area physicians is predetermined prior to making this year's price decision. For purposes of discussion endogenous variables have been classified into four categories: (1) productivity; (2) costs; (3) prices; and (4) income. They are determined by this year's pricing and output decisions.

With the exception of the number of physicians and hospital beds per capita, data used in the regressions are from the physician survey. Many of the variables are estimated from the physician's personal estimate from the last full week of practice. This method may be a source of additional noise, reducing the predictive power of the equations.

As noted in the preceding section, comparisons with other studies suggest that in the survey physicians tended to overestimate their productivity, especially in terms of the number of hours worked and the number of patients served. Prior analysis of the physician response bias found that physicians' ideological positions were in some cases correlated with their productivity: physicians who were vehemently opposed to government intervention tended to work longer hours and treat more patients. To correct for this possible response bias, we have included the independent binary variable coni, with a value of 1 assigned to anti-interventionist physicians.

Regression results for the primary care physicians are displayed in Table 10 and for surgical specialists in Table 11. Regressions were run

Table 8. Definitions of Variables Used in Primary Care Specialists Reduced Form Equations

Variable	Definition	Mean	S.D.
Dependent Variables			
Sum visit	Total patient encounters, unweighted	176.42	91.48
Hours	Total weekly patient care hours	50.05	15.58
VISPHR	Patient encounters per hour	3.61	1.81
TCPER$_2$	Total practice costs	36,133	33,414
COSTPENCE	Cost per encounter (unweighted)	5.33	4.72
NCOSTVIS	Cost per weighted visit	4.97	4.53
OFF FEE	Usual office visit follow-up fee	11.34	3.77
GIPENC	Gross income per encounter	12.18	10.08
GI	Gross income	85,481	49,445
NETINC	Net Income	49,348	24,188
Independent Variables			
Economic Variables			
PRIMDEN	Primary care physicians per 100,000 population	NA for independent variables	
HOSBPOP	Hospital beds per 100,000 population		
NI	Percent of physicians patients that are noninsured		
PCTHINC	Percent of physicians that are high income		
PCTBLACK	Percent of physicians patients that are black		
Physician Characteristics			
Age	Age of physician		
Sex	Sex of physician (1 = female; 0 = male)		
CONI	Politics of physician (1 = vehemently antigovernment)		
HI	Health status of physician (1 = bad health)		
Board	1 = Specialty board certification		
Mother	1 = Mother of child under 18		
Father	1 = Father of child under 18		
Outside	1 = Nonmedical income $10,000		
APPT	1 = Medical school faculty appointment		
PED	1 = Pediatrician		
INTMED	1 = Internal medicine		
TWFMG	1 = Third-world foreign medical graduate		
Practice Characteristics			
EXS	1 = Group practice, expense sharing; 0 = other		
EQSH	1 = Group practice, income shared equally; 0 = other		
UNEQ	1 = Group practice, income shared equally, 0 = other		

in a stepwise manner, with each independent variable entered into the equation in the order of the size of the F statistic of its partial correlation coefficient. The displayed equation is the equation in which the R^2 was at a maximum. Therefore, for equations that omit an individual independent variable, we may assume that the T statistic for that omitted coefficient is less than 1 and is thus insignificant. For those variables that are displayed, the top number represents the ordinary least squares (OLS) parameter estimate, with the significance level in parentheses below.

The regression results are generally supportive of the model hypothesized in Section II. Two aspects of the model distinguish it from earlier studies: (1) the relationship between the physician and the hospital, where the hospital is viewed as the physicians' rent-free workshop; and (2) a labor–leisure tradeoff curve where the utility of work may be valued positively up to a rather high threshold level. The possibility of a positive marginal utility of work may be helpful in explaining much of the seemingly nonorthodox behavior of physicians.

In general, the regressions indicated that increased physician density tended to lower physician productivity in terms of the number of visits per week and visits per hour. (See Table 12 for partial elasticities.) The effect of increased physician density on hours was less clear; there was no statistically significant effect on surgeons' weekly hours and a negative effect on primary-care physicians. It is interesting to note that the "hours" equations had the lowest explanatory power of the 10 equations for both surgeons and primary-care physicians.

The number of patients served decreased with increasing physician density and total nonphysician practice costs tended to fall, although unit nonphysician costs tended to rise. This could be explained by the fact that fewer patients per hour require fewer aides, leading to lower total practice costs. However, with fewer patients over which these costs can be spread, unit costs rise. These generalizations were never statistically significant for both specialty groups *simultaneously*. Primary-care physicians' total costs fell significantly, but not their unit costs. Surgeons' unit costs rose significantly (partial elasticities were .71 for COSTPENC and .77 for NCOSTVIS), but their total practice costs did not fall significantly.

Both specialties exhibited pricing behavior that was compatible with an extended utility maximization model and in conflict with a neoclassical profit-maximizing one. We viewed the price variables as a pure price measure, and the gross revenue per visit as a combined measure of price and overall complexity of service mix. We would expect that physicians' efforts to maintain income target levels in the face of increased physician–population ratios could be achieved by increasing the volume of

Table 9. Definitions of Variables Used in Surgical Specialists
Reduced Form Equations

Variable	Definition	Mean	S.D.
Dependent Variables			
Sumvisit	Total patient encounters, unweighted	162.77	85.87
HOURS	Total weekly patient care hours	56.33	20.45
VISPHR	Patient encounters per hour	2.93	1.29
TCPER$_2$	Total nonphysician practice costs	41,677	47,787
COSTPENCE	Cost per encounter (unweighted)	6.21	5.57
NCOSTVIS	Cost per weighted visit	4.80	4.61
HOS FEE	Usual hospital visit follow-up fee	12.14	5.20
GIPENC	Gross income per encounter	16.97	13.39
GI	Gross income	105,473	66,113
NETINC	Net income	63,796	38,693
Independent Variables			
Economic Variables			
SURGDEN	Surgeons per 100,000 population	Not available for independent variables	
HOSBPOP	Hospital beds per 100,000 population		
NI	Percent of physicians patients that are non insured		
PCTHINC	Percent of physicians patients that are high income		
PCTBLACK	Percent of physicians patients that are black		
Physician Characteristics			
Age	Age of physician		
Sex	Sex of physician (1 = female; 0 = male)		
CONI	Politics of physician (1 = vehemently antigovernment)		
HI	Health status of physician (1 = bad health)		
Board	1 = Specialty board certification		
Mother	1 = Mother of child under 18		
Father	1 = Father of child under 18		
Outside	1 = Nonmedical income $10,000		
Appt	1 = Medical school faculty appointment		
O.B.	1 = Obstetrics–gynecology; 0 = General surgery		
TWFMG	1 = Third-world foreign medical graduate		

Table 9 (Cont.)

Variable	Definition	Mean	S.D.
Practice Characteristics			
EXS	1 = Group practice, expense sharing; 0 = other		
EQSH	1 = Group practice, income shared equally; 0 = other		
UNEQ	1 = Group practice, income shared unequally; 0 = other		

ancillary services as well as the complexity and cost of office visits (brief visits become extended visits), etc. These efforts would be reflected in the gross revenue per visit statistics. Three of the four price measures were statistically significant at the 0 alpha level—a 1 percent increase in surgeons per capita is associated with a .69 percent increase in gross income per encounter. For primary-care physicians, the gross income per encounter figure increased by .33 percent related to a 1 percent rise in primary-care physicians per capita, while their fees measured by routine follow-up office visits increased by .25 percent. We suspect the statistically insignificant relationship between surgeons per capita and the routine hospital charge can be traced to the inadequacy of the hospital visit as a representative price for surgeons services (for some surgeons the follow-up charge is included in the fee for the surgical procedure itself).

Physician density exhibited no statistically significant relationship to net or gross income for either surgeons or primary-care physicians. This may imply that by charging higher prices and by offering a more expensive basket of goods, physicians in counties with high physician–population ratios were able to achieve income levels similar to those in counties with low ratios. This occured in spite of the fact that the physicians from the physician-rich counties processed almost 50 percent fewer patients.

In Section II, we examined the hypothesis that physicians use the hospital as a rent-free workshop for physicians. To begin to test this relationship we used as a measure of local hospital capacity the number of hospital beds per 100,000 population. This is admittedly a crude measure, which may not capture some of the necessary refinements. For example, surgical suites are complementary inputs for surgeons, but outpatient clinics staffed by residents may be substitutes for primary physicians' office practices.

For the surgical specialists, the hospital beds variable exhibited a strong statistical relationship with productivity, cost-and price-dependent variables, and a weaker relationship with income. No statistically sig-

Table 10. Estimated Coefficients in Primary Care Reduced-Form Equations[a]

		Productivity		Cost			Fees		Income	
	SUMVISIT	HOURS	VISPHR	TCPER 2	COSTPENC	NCOSTVIS	OFFFEE	GIPENC	GI	NETINC
Independent Variables	$\bar{R}^2=.14$	$\bar{R}^2=.04$	$\bar{R}^2=.10$	$\bar{R}^2=.11$	$\bar{R}^2=.14$	$\bar{R}^2=.19$	$\bar{R}^2=.31$	$\bar{R}^2=.11$	$\bar{R}^2=.11$	$\bar{R}^2=.10$
Economic Variables										
PriMDEN	−.886	−.105		−138.45	.014	.013	.0523	.0760	−75.7	−64.5
	(0)	(.003)		(.066)	(.178)	(.185)	(0)	(0)	(.39)	(.243)
HOSBPOP	.026	.0037		9.820	.001	.001	8.378			10.16
	(.233)	(.312)		(.199)	(.182)	(.166)	(.231)			(.078)
NI				−1103.3	−.06	−.06	−.05		−1350	
				(.0)	(.18)	(.14)	(.12)		(.01)	
PCTHINC	−.529		−.01		.01	.01	.02	.042		77.7
	(.01)		(.01)		(.28)	(.28)	(0)	(.05)		(.14)
PCTBLACK	.411		.12		−.2	−.1	.01		140	100
	(.08)		(.01)		(.22)	(.28)	(.29)		(.27)	(.13)
Physician Characteristics										
Age	−.324	−.051	−.01	236.8	.03	.03		.06	.97	
	(.243)	(.31)	(.20)	(.02)	(.02)	(.02)		(.04)	(.19)	
Sex	−42.9	−6.4	−1.1	−10903			−.5		−26618	15920
	(.013)	(.17)	(.03)	(.09)			(.42)		(.01)	(.0)
CONI		1.7		5430	.7	.6	.39	1.44	9050	3213
		(.18)		(.04)	(.06)	(.11)	(.14)	(.08)	(.02)	(.10)
H.L.			−.16				−.76		−5399	3480
			(.45)				(.05)		(.33)	(.22)

220

	1	2	3	4	5	6	7	8	9	10
Board			-.12 (.51)		.6 (.25)	.5 (.30)		1.3 (.19)		3940 (.07)
Mother		5.9 (.30)	.6 (.37)					2.7 (.28)		
Father	29.72 (0)	4.4 (.01)	.4 (.03)	4708 (.11)		.7 (.13)		1.1 (.21)	7549 (.09)	2971 (.16)
Outside					.78 (.09)		.41 (.22)	2.61 (.02)	7029 (.16)	5184 (.04)
APPT				14621 (0)	1.3 (.03)	1.4 (.02)	1.3 (0)	1.5 (.26)	17332 (.01)	
PED	-8.3 (.355)		.32 (.17)	-4635 (.24)	-1.8 (0)	-1.3 (.02)		2.5 (.05)		
INTMED	-35.6 (0)		-.67 (0)	6467 (.04)	1.6 (0)	2.4 (0)	3.1 (0)	3.1 (.0)	13295 (.01)	14230 (.05)
TWFMG			-.42 (.15)						-8226 (.29)	-7304 (.15)
Practice Characteristics										
EXS				-15179 (.01)	-.9 (.17)	-1.0 (.11)		-2.7 (.07)	12201 (.09)	
EQSH		1.4 (.41)		6117 (.10)	1.4 (.01)	1.4 (.01)	-.24 (.49)		11295 (.04)	4792 (.08)
UNEQ	19.8 (.121)			11581 (.02)	2.4 (0)	2.4 (0)			21625 (.01)	10280 (.01)

Note: [a] *Alpha levels appear in parenthesis.*

221

222

Table 11. Estimated Coefficients in Surgical Specialists Reduced-Form Equations[a]

Dependent Variables (n = 260)

Independent Variables	Productivity			Costs			Price		Income	
	SUMVISIT $\bar{R}^2=.16$	HOURS $\bar{R}^2=.05$	VISPHR $\bar{R}^2=.13$	TCPER 2 $\bar{R}^2=.05$	COSTPENC $\bar{R}^2=.19$	NCOSTVIS $\bar{R}^2=.21$	HOSFEE $\bar{R}^2=.06$	GIPENC $\bar{R}^2=.12$	GI $\bar{R}^2=.08$	NETINC $\bar{R}^2=.09$
Economic variables										
SurgDEN	-209.4 (0)	-6.71 (.344)	-2.63 (0)	-34.48 (.015)	10.885 (0)	9.09 (0)	2.353 (.196)	28.76 (0)		
HOSBPOP	.118 (.003)		.0015 (.013)		-.01 (0)	-.008 (0)		-.024 (0)	35.48 (07)	
NI	1.56 (.21)			-1128 (.12)	-.18 (.02)	-.11 (.08)	.07 (.40)	-3.35 (.08)	1358 (.16)	
PCTHINC	.27 (.39)	.08 (.20)		190.2 (.29)	.03 (0)	.08 (0)		.14 (.01)	139 (.57)	
PCTBLACK	.5 (.08)		.01 (.02)		-.08 (.09)	-.06 (.24)		-.09 (.06)		
Physician Characteristics										
Age	1.0 (.10)		.01 (.09)	30815 (.28)	.31 (0)	.15 (0)				
Sex			-.8 (.07)							
CONI										
H.L.	-43.3 (.01)	-7.4 (.09)	.42 (.13)	-14041 (.17)	1.7 (.13)	2.41 (.01)			-38790 (.01)	-23785 (.01)

	C1	C2	C3	C4	C5	C6	C7	C8	C9	C10
Board				10615 (.11)				2.6 (.17)	16327 (.09)	5749 (.30)
Mother		6.2 (.02)					3.1 (.31)			
Father	12.6 (.32)				-2.1 (.01)	-2.2 (.01)	-1.6 (.02)	-3.4 (.05)	9678 (.27)	
Outside					2.0 (.02)	1.4 (.04)		2.7 (.19)	13713 (.71)	8876 (.13)
APPT	24.1 (.07)		.48 (.02)					-3.1 (.13)		
O.B.	18.6 (.07)		.35 (.03)					-2.9 (.07)	8933 (.28)	
TWFMG	-26 (.12)		-.31 (.23)				-1.3 (.35)		-13888 (.31)	-10897 (.16)
Practice Characteristics										
EXS	43.9 (.03)	4.9 (.32)	.46 (.13)		-3.44 (.01)	-2.95 (.01)	1.5 (.24)		19956 (.21)	
EQSH	34.2 (.01)	4.9 (.09)	.42 (.02)	-19866 (.09)	-.85 (.22)	-.67	1.4 (.07)	-6.7 (.01)	16597 (.07)	20504 (0)
UNEQ		-7.1 (.15)	.51 (.01)				1.9 (.13)			

Note: [a] Alpha levels appear in parenthesis.

Table 12.   Estimated Partial Elasticities for Physician Density
Variables and Hospital Beds Per Capita Variable[a]

| | Partial Elasticities | | | |
| | Surgical Specialties | | Primary Care Specialties | |
Dependent Variable	Surgeons per Population	Beds per Population	Primary Physicians per Population	Beds per Population
SUMVISIT	− .52	+ .30	− .27	+ .07
HOURS	− .05		− .11	+ .03
VISPHR	− .36	+ .27	− .15	
TCPER 2		− .44	− .20	+ .14
COSTPENC	+ .71	− .90	.14	.14
NCOSTVIS	+ .77	− .87	.14	.14
HOSFEE	+ .07		NA	NA
GIPENC	+ .69	− .76	+ .33	
GI		− .18	− .05	
NETINC			− .07	+ .10
OFFFEE	NA	NA	+ .25	− .10

Notes: [a] These elasticities were calculated at the means. If T static was less than 1, variable was not
included in the equation and, therefore, elasticity does not appear.
[b] NA = not applicable.

nificant relationship was found for the primary-care physicians in any equation. We will confine the remainder of the discussion to the surgical specialists.

Hospital beds served as a complementary input with regard to productivity and cost measures; with the exception of the hours equation, the parameter estimates were always significant at an alpha of .01. A 1 percent increase in beds per capita was found to be associated with a .30 percent increase in weekly encounters and a .27 percent increase in visits per hour. The elasticities for the cost measures emphasize the free nature of hospital services to the surgeon and the substitutability of these services for those provided in the physicians' office at the physician's expense. A 1 percent increase in beds per capita was associated with a .44 percent decline in total costs, a .90 percent decline in costs per encounter, and an .87 percent decline in costs per weighted visit.

HOSBPOP parameter estimates from the fee equations are more difficult to interpret (Table 11). No significant statistical relationship was found to exist between beds per capita and the follow-up hospital visit fee. We noted previously that the follow-up visit fee for surgeons may be a poor example to represent the price of surgeons' services, and in the future we plan to substitute a surgical procedure or an index of surgical fees.

Increasing beds per capita was associated with decreasing gross revenue per encounter. One would expect greater hospital bed capacity to result in an increased volume of surgery and thus increased revenue per encounter. It does appear that physicians are sensitive to unit costs, shifting them forward to their patients.

Beds per capita had an insignificant relationship to net income and a significant one to gross income (alpha = .07). A 1 percent increase in beds per capita was associated with an .18 percent increase in gross income.

In this paper, we have not emphasized the issues of economies of scale associated with group practices. Further work is needed to disentangle the sometimes countervailing effects of practice size and practice arrangements, income sharing, expense sharing, etc. In our reduced-form equations, we attempted to control for group practice economies and group incentive effects through the use of three binary variables: (1) EXS—group practices that share expenses but not income; under this arrangement, marginal costs to the individual physician are less than marginal costs of the practice, and we would hypothesize that this should lead to inefficiencies and higher practice costs. (2) EQSH—groups that share expenses and income equally; (3) UNEQ—groups that share expenses and income unequally. We would hypothesize that the third method provides the greatest incentives for efficiency and productivity for the marginal costs and revenues of the individual physician and group would be roughly equivalent. Solo practices receive a value of zero for all three variables. Thus, the parameter estimates for the three variables are in relation to solo practice.

A cursory glance at the regression results indicates that many a priori assumptions were not realized. EXS was associated with significantly lower unit costs, total costs, prices, and gross revenues for primary care physicians. Surgical expense sharing tended to have higher weekly and hourly visits relative to solo practitioners: UNEQ and EQSH were associated with higher costs, higher productivity, higher fees, higher revenue per visit, and higher incomes.

V. CONCLUSION

This paper has presented preliminary findings from a national survey of 1,014 office-based physicians. The authors have designated themselves as members of the B (broad) school whose standard belief is that the physician, rather than the patient, is the dominant force in determining medical care utilization patterns. Two modifications were proposed to B school dogma. The first was a labor–leisure utility function, in which work may have positive marginal utility up to some critical level. The second modification is that physician pricing, productivity, costs, and incomes can be better understood by the relationship between the physician and their rent-free workshop, the hospital. Reversing a previous work by Feldstein (1970), the analysis looked at the effect of the hospital as a complementary input for the physician's office practice.

Empirical findings are based on cross tabulations and reduced form equations. The results are generally supportive of our modifications. Weekly physician hours proved to be the most difficult endogenous variable to explain. Surgical specialists' weekly hours were unaffected by varying levels of physician density, in spite of significantly falling workloads. Primary care physicians' weekly hours were found to decrease as the area physician per capita ratio rose.

Surgical specialists' productivity and costs were found to be sensitive to the availability of hospital resources, as measured by beds per capita. Our findings did not reject the hypothesis that the hospital is used as a free "workshop" by the physician. The average elasticity for the beds per capita variable in the unit cost equations was $-.89$; this same variable averaged .28 in the patient flow equations. At no time was a statistically significant relationship uncovered between beds per capita and the 10 endogenous variables in the primary-care equations.

Parameter estimates of the physicians per capita variable were usually supportive of "B" school doctrine. Increased local physician per capita ratios (measured as primary-care physicians per 100,000 or surgical specialists per 100,000) were associated with falling patient flow (visits per hour or per week), generally falling total, nonphysician costs, and rising unit nonphysician costs. Yet, gross and net incomes did not fall. By charging higher fees and offering a more complex overall service mix (the elasticities in the gross revenue per visit equations were .69 for surgeons and .33 for primary physicians), practitioners in physician-rich counties were able to achieve income levels comparable with their peers in physician-scarce counties.

When a stable gross income per physician statistic is multiplied by an increasing physicians per capita figure, the product is increased physician expenditures per capita. And the effect of increased physican supply on the hospital sector may be even greater.

Today, medical school enrollments are double those of 15 years ago, and they are projected to increase further. If cost containment is a priority goal in health policy, two alternatives are apparent. The first is to curtail the number of physicians entering the market. The second is to drastically restructure the present fee-for-service system that we think leads to induced utilization and renders increases in supply inflationary in terms of both unit prices and total expenditures.

ACKNOWLEDGMENT

An earlier draft of the paper was delivered at the Western Economic Association Meetings, Anaheim, California June 20, 1977.

Michael Redisch is an economist with the Interstate Commerce Commission. Jon Gabel is an economist with the National Center for Health Services Research. Martha Blaxall is a Department of Commerce economist. At the time this article was written, the authors were employed by the Health Care Financing Administration.

REFERENCES

American Health Systems (1977), *An Examination of the Impact of Methods of Reimbursement on Physicians' Income.* Paper presented at SSA Physician Reimbursement Methodology Conference, Mar. 10–11, 1977.

American Medical Association (1975), *Profile of Medical Practice.* Chicago: AMA Center for Health Services Research and Development.

American Medical Association (1976), *Journal of the American Medical Association* Dec.

Arrow, Kenneth J. (1963), "Uncertainty and the Welfare Economics of Medical Care," *The American Economic Review 53*(5), 941–973.

Cantwell, James R. (1976), *A Cross-Section Econometric Analysis of Physician Location and Pricing.* Paper presented at Midwest Economics Association Meetings, Apr. 3.

Ernst, Richard (1976), "Ancillary Production and the Size of Physicians' Practices." *Inquiry, 13*(4).

Evans, Robert G. (1974), "Supplier-Induced Demand: Some Empirical Evidence and Implications." In *The Economics of Health and Medical Care.* (Mark Perlman, ed.). London: Macmillan, pp. 162–173.

————(1976), "Review of *The Economics of Health and Medical Care,* M. Perlman, ed., " *Canadian Journal of Economics 9*(5), 532–537.

Feldstein, Martin, (1970), "The Rising Price of Physicians' Services," *The Review of Economics and Statistics 52*(2), 121–133.

Fuchs, Victor R., and Kramer, Marcia J. (1972), *Determinants of Expenditures for Physicians' Services in the United States 1948–68.* Washington: National Center of Health Services Research and Development.

Gibson, R. (1977), "National Health Expenditures, Fiscal Year 1976," *Social Security Bulletin* Apr. pp. 40–41.

Grossman, Michael (1976), *The Demand for Health.* New York: National Bureau of Economic Research.

Huang, L. F., and Koropecky, O. (1973), *The Effects of the Medicare Method of Reimbursement on Physicians' Fees and on Beneficiaries' Utilization.* Washington, D.C.: Nathan Associates.

Hughes, E. F. X., Fuchs, V., Jacoby, J., and Lewit, E. M. (1972), "Surgical Work Loads in Community Practice," *Surgery 71*(3), 315–327.

Institute of Medicine (1976), *Medicare Medicaid Reimbursement Policies,* Chap. 10. (Mar.).

Kessel, Reuben A. (1958), "Pricing Discrimination in Medicine," *Journal of Law and Economics. 1,* 20–53.

May, J. Joel (1975), "Utilization of Health Services and the Availability of Resources," in *Equity in Health Services* (R. Andersen, J. Kravits, and O. Anderson, eds.). Cambridge, Mass.: Ballinger, pp. 131–150.

Myers, Lawrence (1977), "Report of an Interview with an Internist," *Washington Post,* June 12.

Newhouse, Joseph, and Phelps, Charles E. (1976) "New Estimates of Price and Income Elasticities of Medical Care Services," in *The Role of Health Insurance in the Health Services Sector* (R. Rosett, ed.). New York: National Bureau of Economic Research, pp. 261–320.

Newhouse, Joseph, and Sloan, Frank (1972), "Physician Pricing: Monopolistic or Competitive: Reply," *Southern Economic Journal 38,* 577–580.

Perlman, Mark, ed. (1974), *The Economics of Health and Medical Care.* New York: Macmillan.

Redisch, Michael (1978), "Cost Containment and Physician Involvement in Hospital Decision-Making" in *Hospital Cost Containment: Selected Notes for Future Policy* (Michael Zubnoff and Ira Raskin, ed.). Milbank Memorial Fund.

Reinhardt, Uwe E. (1972), "A Production Function for Physicians," *The Review of Economics and Statistics 54*(1).

————(1975), *Physician Productivity and the Demand for Health Manpower.* Cambridge, Mass.: Ballinger.

Scitovsky, Tibor (1943), "A Note on Profit Maximisation and Its Implications," *The Review of Economic Studies 11.*

Sevareid, Eric (1977), Transcript of April 27 Commentary, CBS Nightly News.

Sloan, Frank, and Feldman, Roger (1977), *Monopolistic Elements in the Market for Physicians' Services.* Paper presented at a conference on Competition in the Health Care Sector, Washington, D.C., June 1–2.

Sloan, Frank (1975), "Physician Supply Behavior in the Short Run," *Industrial and Labor Relations Review 28*(4), 549–569.

————(1976), "Physician Fee Inflation: Evidence from the Late 1960's," in *The Role of Health Insurance in the Health Services Sector* (R. Rosett, ed). New York: National Bureau of Economic Research, pp. 321–354.

Sloan, Frank, Cromwell, Jerry, and Mitchell, Janet (1978), *Private Physicians and Public Programs.* Lexington, Mass: D.C. Health and Co.

Steinwald, Bruce, and Sloan, Frank (1974), "Determinants of Physicians' Fees," *Journal of Business 47*(4), 493–511.

Stigler, George J. (1961), "The Economics of Information," *The Journal of Political Economy 49,* 213–225.

Vahovich, S. G., and Aherne, P. (1973) *Profile of Medical Practice.* Chicago: American Medical Association.

INCENTIVES AND ORGANIZATIONAL STRUCTURE IN HEALTH MAINTENANCE ORGANIZATIONS

David Whipple

I. INTRODUCTION

The level and significance of the rapidly rising health care costs in the United States has been sufficiently documented and will not be belabored here. Although it could be asserted that the growth of spending in a major sector of the economy indicates a positive contribution to a healthy fiscal environment, most would also agree that this phenomenon in the health care sector is cause for concern. Berry (1977) speaks for this group when he points out that our concern is motivated by the perception that the health care "market" is significantly imperfect. These imperfections, which will be analyzed below, cause us to doubt that the level

Advances in Health Economics and Health Services Research, Vol. 2, pgs. 229–267.
(Volume 1 published as Research in Health Economics)
ISBN: 0-89232-100-8

of health care produced is even in the neighborhood of that associated with the equation of marginal social benefit and marginal social cost, and thus cause us to be concerned with the magnitude of the resulting social opportunity cost.

The emphasis these days is therefore on "cost containment" and ways to realize its benefits in the health care sector. After years of almost unfettered operation, the cost-plus type reimbursement mechanisms erected to facilitate financial lubrication of the various cogs of the health care delivery system (HCDS) are not only under close scrutiny but have been the object of significant endogenous and exogenous attempts at modification. The historical, descriptive, and generally passive analytical/regulatory approach has given way to numerous attempts to understand and develop methodologies which will foster more directly less costly ways to provide for the health care needs and demands of "consumers," professional as well as patient. Economists have motivated a portion of these efforts by providing estimates of the present and projected opportunity costs of the present HCDS.

However, the macro emphasis of these studies has begun to give way to micro efforts as the probable marginal gains from further aggregate projects have fallen. That has meant more research into the determinants of costs, productivity, operational structure, and management of the specific entities which together make up the HCDS. For example, past concern with ensuring sufficient physicians to care for a growing population whose demand for services was further facilitated by increases in the use of third-party payers led to policies designed to foster an increase in the rate of growth of the stock of physicians. However, although the stock has grown much faster than in the past, we find that we are not getting the *type* of physicians we most needed (primary care) and that the new doctors are not locating in the rural and inner city areas where their presence is most needed. Rather, physicians continue to open practices in seemingly well-supplied areas and somehow find patients who "need" their services. Thus, subsequent studies attempted to answer the following kinds of questions: *Why* was the observed behavior in response to the policy measure not as desired? *What* kinds of revised policies might yield results closer to those which originally motivated the attempts to increase physician supply? *How* were physicians able to profitably locate in areas with seemingly sufficient stocks of providers?

More specific to the content of the present paper, consider the case of the HCDS financial intermediaries which for years had designed coverage packages for their insurance and prepayment plans to minimize (they thought) overutilization and hence costs. To this end they utilized retrospective reviews of claims from institutions in order to ensure that the requested payments were appropriate. However, with the acceleration of these costs, research efforts increasingly began to be devoted to understanding the behavior of those institutions and providers to whom the payments were made. This necessitated analysis of the incentives extant in the system and the influence of the operational structure and its management on the observed costs. The result was an increase in attempts to prospectively determine reimbursement. Although not necessarily a totally accurate measure of the applicability of the results of these efforts, the continuing proposal at the federal executive level for an aggregate blanket percentage lid on cost growth in nongovernment hospitals would seem to indicate that as yet there exists no widely accepted effective prospective reimbursement methodology.

A major source of the problem is that the organization of the HCDS is generally fragmented. The private sector portion of the HCDS has been allowed to operate under a set of rules and structures resembling free enterprise. This has led to the evolution of a variety of financial and direct care structures governing the delivery of health care. Therefore, the analyst is faced with the need to address these specific structures when dealing with such basic economic questions as efficiency, equity, and incentives. While in a competitive market sector the interaction of supply and demand forces tend to result in a natural incentive to control production costs, this incentive has been found lacking in the traditional health care market (Falk, 1973). This stems in part from the combination of the professional providers' control over both aspects of supply and demand and the ability of the providers to pass along increased costs to third-party payers. Since the consumer neither controls the amount of the resources to be consumed during an illness episode nor has a direct interest in the total cost of those resources, assuming some form of coverage which reduces out-of-pocket costs, a perverse incentive situation exists. Therefore, due in part to this imperfect market system, there are insufficient inherent incentives to produce health care outputs efficiently. Moreover, in many production processes the specification and measurement of output units can be relatively easily accomplished. But due in part to the multiproduct nature of health care services and the limits of medical technology, the identification and measurement of its outputs is an extremely difficult task. To date, no adequate methodology for measuring health care output has been developed. This lack of a natural incentive for seeking efficient production of health care, compounded by the inability to adequately measure health care output, results in insufficient management control over costs within the HCDS.

Many analysts, myself included, have posited that the growing prepaid group practice, health maintenance organization (PPGP/HMO) sector could well provide not only the prototype of a more efficient systemic component than the solo practice, fee-for-service (FFS) mode of delivery but also significant competition for the existing components of the HCDS which embody the aforementioned imperfections and collectively constitute the "market" of which we are therefore suspect. The hope has been that deviations from "appropriate" market operations would therefore be minimized without a more direct form of regulatory intervention. However, for the reasons to be detailed in this paper, it is not clear that PPGP/HMOs as presently structured will fulfill these hopes to any significant degree. Fortunately, a more holistic and basic look at the genesis of the barriers to this fulfillment indicates that there may well be a feasible strategy for the HCDS in which restructured PPGP/HMOs have a critical part to play. The former assertion stems from my research conclusion that *insufficient attention has been paid to date to the need for incentive structures within PPGP/HMOs to correct the rational—but undesirable—economic behavior of providers and patients that leads to the social inefficiencies with which we are concerned.* Recognition of the roots of this problem holds the promise of its solution in the form of modified incentive and organizational structures, for PPGP/HMOs as well as the fee-for-service sector. The major questions are these: What authority and responsibility structures must exist? What must be the rewards and penalties for the managers and providers? Moreover, how can efficiency be identified, measured, and reported so that these rewards and penalties can be meted out objectively and corrective actions taken when portions of the system are not as efficient as possible? In other words, what general form must the PPGP/HMO management control system take?

The remainder of this paper analyzes and attempts to answer these and related questions on the basis of research undertaken as a part of a project attempting to assess the potential efficacy of the adoption of capitation budgeting (CB) in the military HCDS. Section II discusses the problem of PPGP/HMO structure and incentive relationships in greater detail, while Section III draws lessons and examples from both the literature and the management interviews which were a part of the CB research project. Section IV then uses the military HCDS as a vehicle to illustrate more specifically the problem as well as to suggest possible solutions. Section V sketches the outline of a proposed solution strategy which may provide useful to private sector PPGP/HMOs as well.

II.   THE PROBLEM: GOALS AND INCENTIVES

Not until absolute health care costs and their proportion of gross national product (GNP) began to rise at rates significantly higher than those in other sectors was the structure of the health care market questioned. The situation has deteriorated to the point where private third-party payers and Blue Cross have been forced by increasingly binding budget constraints (tightened in many cases by governmental rate review bodies) to begin to switch from their historically perceived role as fiscal supporters of physicians and hospitals to "honest adversaries." The federal government has shifted to a position of such active resistance to health care cost increases that the spector of heavy government resulation hangs over the health care market. When the Deputy Assistant Attorney General of the U.S. Dept. of Justice's Antitrust Division publishes an article entitled "The Need For Regulatory Reform in the Health Care Industry" (Sims, 1978), the members of that industry must see all sorts of handwriting on the wall.

The suggestions for reform and regulation of the procedures of health care in the United States are myriad. They range from the effective nationalization of all health care resources to Band-Aids covering the body of the existing HCDS. It is far beyond the scope of this paper to detail these proposals; however it is within its purview to note that one type of regulatory proposal attempts to restore some competitive aspects to the health care market and therefore rely on a more decentralized approach to regulation than that associated with strategies traditionally employed in other markets. [The latest proposal in this vein is that by Enthoven (1977) for a voucher-based Consumer-Choice Health Plan (CCHP).] Such plans envision increased competition, at least partially motivated by the more prominent existence of PPGP/HMOs. However, the problem of choosing the most nearly correct cost containment regulatory strategy is compounded by our lack of sufficient knowledge of the causes of the symptoms about which we are concerned. As Berry (1977, p. 589) puts it, "the real constraint on cost containment policy may be the sheer magnitude of the gap between what is known about the structure of the hospital industry and especially the behavioral patterns within the industry." It appears that analysts have too long been preoccupied with the symptoms themselves and their quantification rather than with the environmental parameters, spanning many disciplines, which combine to generate the problem. One might say that we know almost precisely the magnitude, duration, and incidence rates of the country's health care "headaches" but have little idea of how to prevent them because the cause is so complex.

The increasing recognition by economists, systems analysts, and organizational behaviorists of the special nature of the health care market may well change this. For example, although the agency relationship in various markets has been the subject of significant generic investigation, such research specific to the health care market, and physicians in particular, has been relatively sparse (Whipple, 1975). It has been conjectured that there exists such a unique type and degree of agency here that a careful exploration of this portion of the health care market operations may well yield valuable insights facilitating cost containment.

Even more specific to the provider's role in containing costs in PPGP/HMOs is recognition that the basic problem is to identify appropriate incentive and managerial structures to ensure consistency between the likely differing goals of those who allocate resources or cause them to be allocated. It is well-known that goal congruence is not automatic and that the specific environment will, in large part, determine the appropriate response in terms of management strategies and incentive structures. The goals of the various individuals at the different levels need not be identical, for then it would be sufficient merely to provide correct information to the various levels and personnel. Rather, goal congruence means that, even if the specific goals of the individuals and/or portions of the organization are different, the *impact* of each pursuing its own goal may still be, or may be caused to be, consistent with the other element's optimization process, i.e., that effects of the pursuit of the individual goals may still be consistent with those of the organization. Thus, if an insurance company wants to maximize income, and its salesmen want to maximize income, the latter purpose is consistent with the organization achieving its objectives. Such goal congruence does not appear to be present to a sufficient degree in PPGP/HMOs.

To further illustrate the problems inherent in managing such an organization, consider next the relationship between, on the one hand, the hospital and health plan administrators and, on the other hand, the provider community which makes the daily decisions affecting the resource utilization and output determinations associated with direct patient care. Whereas the administrators may have the aggregate potential patient population as their target group, the providers deal with the individual members of that group who actually come in contact with the HCDS. To establish the probable noncongruence of goals between these providers and the administrators, consider two polar types of providers: The first we term the *total altruist*. He/she wants to do his/her best for the patient and thus will tend to prescribe care (inpatient or ambulatory) up to the point where its absolute marginal benefit to the patient reaches zero. The second is the *effort minimizer* who realizes that he/she is "on salary" and therefore has no personal financial gain to be realized from "excess" patient care. Thus, an effort minimizer will tend to see only as many patients as necessary and will provide care which just satisfies the constraints associated with one's professional ethics. It should be clear that the effects of the actions of the total altruist are most probably inconsistent with the goals of the administrator faced with limited resources relative to projected patient demands.

One might suppose at first glance that the actions of the effort minimizer may be more consistent with the goals of the administrator in that it would seem resource utilization would be minimized as compared with the more altruistic provider. However, this is almost certainly not the case. First, effort minimization is defined on the individual provider who practices it, *not* on the patient. Thus one may observe excessive referrals from such a practitioner. Second, the tendency to minimize effort at one encounter level may allow disease to go undiagnosed or insufficiently treated and thus cause follow-up encounters which require even heavier resource use than had the case been treated by the total altruist initially (e.g., hospitalization when adequate medication initially prescribed would have effected the cure). Third, the perceptions of the patients must be taken into account. To the extent that they feel shunted about or insufficiently cared for, their utilization may actually increase in terms of costs. That is, they may return for more of what has been termed "worried well" type care than they might had they felt the care originally provided was adequate.

The conjecture might next be that neither polar example of provider motivation is accurate and therefore that some combination midway between the two poles may in fact provide goal congruence. However, we point out that such an occurrence would only be coincidental, even for a single provider, and the likelihood of its collective existence is small. The problem of "bounded rationality" and associated "satisficing" is even *more* likely at this level of the organization and the strong professional identification makes such decisions more acceptable. That is, the provider faced with the complexities and uncertainties surrounding the operation of the organization can substitute professional standing for organizational approval. Providers, especially physicians, are generally "winners" in the organizational structure by virtue of their knowledge and expertise. Thus they are likely to be resistant to managerial exhortations to change accepted methods of practice in the name of organizational efficiency and goal enhancement. They may well view innovation as a threat to their traditional status and power which does not offer sufficient potential resources because of institutional rigidities or the immeasurability of the "product" of their labors.

In the situations just sketched managerial recognition is needed, at all levels, of the requirement for an effective and equitable "social contract" between the organization and its members. That is, there must be a balance between the desired contributions of the members to the goals of the organization and the inducements which are offered to them in return. The "Path/Goal" theory of leadership indicates that the inducements must be tied to the desired behavior or contributions. It also makes clear the difference between "compensation" and "inducements." A straight salary may easily be viewed as compensation for minimum expectations and not as an inducement for periodic innovation or even acceptance of innovations in the pursuit of efficiency.

The process of innovation is generally problem induced. Thus, as opposed to the providers, who are generally "winners" as we said, the managers may be "losing" the most in that they must face the systemic problems which motivate the need for organizational change, and thus they may be more willing to innovate. However, the implementation of innovations in many cases lies outside of their area of control and involves direct patient care. Thus they must have at their disposal the means to both educate the provider community (or the hospital administrators if we are speaking of the Health Plan managers) and to provide inducements for the desired changes where the direct benefits are not clear or where there is in fact a real or potential individual loss.

For example, if the Health Plan administrators desire the facility administrators to optimize rather than satisfice and to give up or reduce the rational tendency to build up "organizational slack" (asking for larger budgets, building workload to justify it, etc.), to help deal with uncertainty, they must be willing to provide the opportunity for the manager to benefit from acceptance of the risk associated with such a change in behavior. This may mean that the organization is willing to finance some level of organizational slack outright from which innovation "search costs" may be financed and inducements to the provider community may be offered.

Consider next the problem of local controllability of costs. First, the hospital manager may be given an annual operating budget which includes both controllable and noncontrollable (to him) costs. Although he is charged with the responsibility for seeking efficiency and reducing the cost of operations, the rewards generated from such behavior may not be strong enough to elicit that behavior. Rather such a manager may seek to control cost only insofar as an overspending of the fixed, present year budget does not occur. In addition, such managers may view certain personnel resources as free because of central funding. Thus, in determining overall personnel needs, centralized (i.e., plan) management may program for the total system as well as budget for the specific facility or responsibility center. In doing so, the central manager in large part determines the quality and quantity of the personnel mix. These personnel costs may be perceived as being non-controllable by the local manager, especially in the short run. Therefore, since central management both determines allowable costs for a portion of personnel and authorizes these costs, local managers may view them as "noncontrollable" and therefore not a true cost to their operation. This suggests that a perverse incentive may exist due to the degree of centralized decision making, since the local manager may perceive his role as one mainly consisting of custodial duties. Thus his emphasis may be merely to supervise operations to ensure that they continue to provide for—and sustain—the system during current operations under the constraints given him rather than to pursue greater efficiency.

We posit that the foregoing is a reasonable description of the state of the "internal market" of the average PPGP/HMO and that it is therefore unrealistic to expect them, individually or collectively, to exert any significant influence on cost containment.

III. HEALTH MAINTENANCE ORGANIZATIONS AND COST CONTAINMENT

A. Organizational Overview

Luft (1975) summarizes the key features of HMOs as follows:

1. The HMO assumes a contractual responsibility to provide or assure the delivery of a stated range of health services. This includes at least ambulatory care and inpatient services.
2. The HMO serves a defined population that is enrolled.
3. There is a fixed annual or monthly payment by the consumer that is independent of use of services. (There may be small charges that are related to utilization but these are relatively insignificant.)
4. There is voluntary enrollment of subscribers.
5. The HMO assumes at least part of the financial risk and/or gain in the provision of services.

Luft specifically does not list group practice or capitation reimbursement of physicians as integral parts of HMOs since medical foundations and independent practice associations are HMOs which are not group practices and whose physicians are compensated on a fee-for-service basis. An examination of a sample of well-known PPGP health plans (see "Professional Performances," 1976) reflects the general organizational response to these key features:

1. The enrolled population
2. The health plan or administrative division
3. The physician/provider group
4. The hospitals/physical facilities

The exact relationship between the separate parts is certainly not uniform over all plans. For example, some own their hospitals (Kaiser), while others contract for inpatient care (HIP). Some directly employ physicians while others contract for their services, etc.

The literature is replete with studies which examine the relative cost effectiveness of HMOs in providing health care (Donabedian, 1969; American Public Health Assoc., 1971; Roemer and Shonick, 1973; Luft, 1978). The basic conclusion has been that this form of health care delivery has cut the costs of providing comprehensive care to large enrolled populations, mainly by controlling the inpatient care where feasible and reducing some types of elective surgery. These elements, along with the existence of peer review for utilization control as well as quality control are posited by many to contribute to the kinds of cost controls that lead, for example, to the lower rates of cost increases for PPGP/HMOs as compared to fee-for-service insurance plans cited by Strumpf (1976) and Luft (1978).

On the other hand, although generally accepted as the most (relative) cost effective mode of care for their enrollees, PPGP/HMOs have operational elements about which questions have been raised. For example, McNamara and Todd (1970), Bailey (1968), and Luft (1975, p. 45), among many, have questioned the efficiency of group practice per se in effectively reducing costs of delivering care. The uncertainty in the literature over the existence and range of economies of scale with respect to hospital size raises questions about the need for hospital-based HMOs. The existence of reimbursement experiments, such as those at HIP (Densen et al., 1971; Jones et al., 1974), indicate that merely "capitating" physician group services may not generate optimal utilization patterns or minimize associated costs. A recent study by Gaus et al. (1976) led to the conclusion that while group practice HMOs had significantly lower hospital utilization than fee-for-service groups, foundation HMOs did not. The study concluded: "This seems to indicate that capitation payment to an HMO alone is not significant enough to produce major changes in utilization and that the organized multi-specialty group practice arrangement with largely salaried physicians may be more significant." Finally, there is the question of HMO management. William McLeod, director of HEW's office of HMO Qualification and Compliance, has said, "A successful HMO requires hard-nosed management, rigorous financial planning and a good understanding of the health insurance and employee benefits industry" (Group Health Association of America, 1976). George Strumpf, Deputy Director of HEW's Division of HMO points out that "Authors of studies of unsuccessful medical group practices have concluded that failure to observe basic principles of organization and management was the cause . . ." (1976, p. 7), while Mc-

Namara and Todd (1970, p. 1310) note that "Groups with prepayment seem to show no unique organizational characteristics when compared with all groups". Strumpf (1976, pp. 4,8) further notes that his studies have shown lack of management capability to be one of the major causes of HMOs having their funding terminated under PL 93–222. This conclusion has been borne out in another study (Penchansky and Berki, 1976).

Strumpf (1976, p. 7) has noted that HMO "failure can result from organizational objectives which lead to organizational policies in conflict with the professional role or from failure to define or support organizational objectives as a central theme around which the organization is operated." Thus, goal consistency (or congruence) and managerial effectiveness must be actively fostered. Great care must be exercised in formulating operational strategies and structuring incentives. In terms of questions we have raised above, whether or not scale economies exist in present group practices may not be as important as whether they *can* exist or whether they can be extended in an internally restructured and appropriately managed system. As Pauly (1970, p. 123) has pointed out, the past events condition to a large extent the possibility of significant increases in efficiency in the short run, no matter how hard administrators may seemingly try. Thus, although agreeing with Dunlop's (1965) statement that "It is changes in the way we practice our medicine that are likely to affect most significantly the constraints on costs and financial stringency over the next decade," we would only caution that we must be willing to realistically examine our capability to reap the benefits of whatever changes are made. In particular, we cannot assume that we have a congruent set of incentives and internal management controls, and so we must ensure that the system is structured in such a way that it will have the inherent tendency to mitigate future costs.

B. *Physician Incentives*

Since it is clear that the physician, as the predominant health care provider, exerts majority influence on the resources used in the HCDS, it is important that we examine his likely response to incentives within the HMO, in particular under various HMO organizational structures.

Dr. Cecil Cutting of Kaiser has said, "There is no doubt that the multi-specialty group organization represents a step toward more efficient coalescence of medical specialists, more efficient utilization of equipment and facilities, ease of consultation, and support to quality" (see Somers, 1971). Thus, Kaiser has made group practice one of the six major principles forming their organizational "Genetic Code." On the other hand, Newhouse (1973) and others (Pauly, 1970; Sloan, 1974) have pressed the probability that the dilution of the individual physician provider's incentive to control costs in a group practice situation will tend to cause unit costs to rise, ceteris paribus.

Consider, for example, the research by Rosett (1974) on the clustering of proprietary hospitals at relatively small bed sizes. He conjectures and establishes the reasonableness of the hypothesis that as size increases the individual physician owners of such facilities tend to lose their incentives to be efficient (since increased bed size means more doctors sharing the costs of using the facility). Thus, physicians tend to use the hospital staff as an adjunct and substitute input for their own effort, driving up the ancillary services' costs and lowering the profits of the facility as an organization. Thus, larger facilities tend to be not-for-profit.

Newhouse found that the overhead costs of private physicians in solo (or small) single-specialty group practice were below those of large, multispecialty groups practicing in outpatient clinics and that whatever economies of scale might exist were exhausted at relatively low total patient visit levels. He concludes that "the findings should give pause to those who believe that large clinics and large groups can give more efficient care than physicians working alone or in small groups . . ." (Newhouse, 1973, p. 38). He goes on to point out that although "some groups attempt to take account of the individual's effort to generate additional revenue by making his share dependent upon gross revenues generated . . . almost none . . . appears to recognize extra effort to control cost" (p. 39). He posits that solo practitioners have a competitive incentive (even though the cross elasticity of demand is low between physicians) to keep costs down whereas in clinic situations this tends to be mitigated because of the pass-through aspect of costs to third-party payers and the existence of philanthropic and government subsidies. The empirical work presented supports his contentions, showing multispecialty clinic overhead costs to be greater than those of single specialty groups or solo practitioners by a factor of 3, i.e., $14.24 to $4.54. His explanation of the source of this disparity is a simple matter of overstaffing: "Given the traditional low salaries in hospitals and their ability to pass along costs, it is quite plausible that hospitals have not adjusted very quickly to a change in the factor prices which they face" (p. 43).

On the basis of his own research, Sloan (1974) agrees and points out that "If decision making within groups primarily takes place at the individual group member level, then practice output, price, and input purchase decisions will reflect individual member marginal costs and returns rather than those of the group. . . . The principal reason for policy concern is . . . that incentives inherent in groups may reduce productivity; they may result in lower output at a higher resource cost per unit."

Newhouse points out that in larger groups it may (does) behoove the group to hire a business manager to combat the tendency toward wastefulness (X inefficiency) fostered by diluted individual incentives. We return to this aspect later. Although his analysis points to the probable existence of economies of scale (in terms of group size), they cease at the relatively low level of 860 visits per month. Newhouse finds that "a solo practitioner with 400 visits per month has lower estimated average salary costs than a group which shares costs regardless of the number of visits" (1973, p. 45; see also Scheffler, 1975).

Let us now look more closely at the theory and reality of the contribution of prepayment to the cost effectiveness of the PPGP model of health care delivery. Newhouse (1973, pp. 51–52) is not alone in differentiating the contribution of prepayment from that of group practice. For example, Reinhardt, in his comprehensive summary paper (1973) notes "The important thing to keep in mind . . . is that it is the prepayment feature and not necessarily the group practice setting that yields the desired efficiency gains in prepaid group practices. . . ." However, he cautions that the theoretically attractive notion of prepayment may not work in the expected manner in practice.

The complicating factor is that in large PPGPs there usually exists a *combination* of incentives which may not capture the posited totality of the prepaid environment. For example, although the medical group may be reimbursed on a capitation basis, its individual members are salaried. In addition, there is the problem that the physician group has little say over the size of their overall panel, so that capitation is weakened. That is, the group can't say, "That's it; we don't want any more members (physicians) or enrollees."

As Montgomery (1974) has rightly pointed out, individual salaries with bonuses and fringes for providers and capitated payments to the group and institutions are necessary to allay the "maximum loss" fears of physicians under total vertical capitation (because of random or adverse selection, etc.). However, Pauly (1970) cautions: "The incentive effects of salaried practice obviously depend upon the way in which salaries are determined. To take the extreme case, if salaries were based only on number of years of practice, the physician would have an incentive to minimize the amount of labor he performs, as under a capitation scheme, but with no offsetting incentive to seek additional enrollees by giving good service." We must, however, point out the assertion of Pineault (1976), which tends to counteract this undesirable feature, namely, that in a PPGP setting less extreme than the one cited above physicians are more dependent upon a colleague's reviews and evaluations for promotion, advancement, and recognition than is the case in solo, fee-for-service practice. This peer review then tends to offset the lack of incentive to care about costs, etc., even given strict (i.e., no bonus) salaried practice. In fact, Pineault (1976, p. 121) concludes that "These results . . . provide supportive evidence for the widely held notion that prepaid group practice, through changing the nature of the incentives to physicians and introducing professional regulations, leads to a more efficient way of providing medical care by reducing the use of costly resources". (See also Glaser, 1970.)

Although physicians coupled with other types of providers may be more effective/efficient in groups associated with prepaid health plans than their colleagues in fee-for-service, solo practice, the fact remains that we have witnessed many experiments and proposals over the past few years which had as their avowed purpose the increased effectiveness and efficiency of these PPGP providers. Bauer and Densen (1974) reported on a study which, although dealing largely with incentive reimbursement experiments in the fee-for-service sector, includes some PPGP plans and concludes that they too may gain from a further investigation of incentives faced by providers. For example, in the plans these authors reviewed, although it is clear that one "should offer rewards or penalties to those people who are in positions to bring about the kinds of changes in performance that the system wants to encourage, . . . almost without exception [they] are directed to *institutions,* not to the individual decision makers within them" (Bauer and Densen, 1974, pp. 83–84). Thus it is not surprising that a PPGP health plan like HIP, concerned with rising costs, attempted to motivate further cost containment by providing additional provider incentives, even though the organization already possessed the maximum incentive under prepayment. That is, the managers of the Health Plan recognized areas wherein the system or organizational incentives did not seem to be effective at the most appropriate level and attempted to "extend" the incentives and thus foster additional cost containment.

C. Innovations for Cost Containment

Having suggested the likely existence of X inefficiencies in PPGP/ HMOs and the need for systematic and systemic management efforts to counter them, we must now delve more deeply into the problem setting and discuss those elements which are essentially barriers to both static and dynamic improvement in the HMO's resource allocation and input determination processes, as well as to the elimination of these X inefficiencies. Specifically, we must ask how cost containment might be realized and identify the classes of costs most likely to be amenable to reduction. Next we must ascertain the (generic) means probabilistically associated with the motivation of discovery and implementation of changes that will lead to cost containment.

Luft (1978) recently reconfirmed and quantified the widely held belief that the majority of HMO cost savings vis-à-vis the FFS sector are attributable to lower overall occupied bed days (OBDs) per member. He further finds that this is due almost entirely to lower admission rates; that average length of stay shows little difference; and that there is no real evidence of reduction in discretionary or "unnecessary" admissions by HMOs. These facts, coupled with the theoretical and empirical foundation we have laid in the foregoing discussion, lead to the conjecture that the most probable and productive sources of cost reduction in PPGP/ HMOs lie in the discovery and use of more innovative modes of care and "patient management." We further posit that, aside from a cautious attitude toward adoption of costly new technology, the most fertile areas for such innovative behavior lie in the ambulatory clinic settings. However it is doubtful that there are sufficient endogenous incentives in presently structured HMOs to ensure such activity. For example, one would posit that the PPGP/HMO has an inherent *organizational* incentive to educate its enrolled population with respect to the most appropriate and efficacious use of the plan's health care resources and to discover the most efficient mix of these resources to care for the resulting level of appropriate client demand. The question remains how one obtains the cooperation of the providers and midlevel managers in achieving these organizational goals. As an example, consider the efforts of Kaiser/Northern California to deal with the utilization of their ambulatory resources by the "worried well." Because of the lack of a monetary rationing mechanism, they have been concerned for years about the number of asymptomatic patients using the facilities. However, because a portion of this population in fact turns out to be sick, and because it was not possible to reduce the residual demand administratively, a pilot program was proposed and implemented by the research group in cooperation with the medical group provider staff. Introduced was the use of paramedical personnel to screen out those who really did not need to see a physician (Garfield et al., 1976). This "reduced total resources used throughout the year by $32,550 per 1000 entrants, and proved very satisfactory to patients, and generally so to staff." Thus, the organization perceived an area where costs might be reduced through a modified system structure and use of more nonphysician providers. The administration was able to obtain the cooperation of the physicians in large part because of the provider's lack of a monetary incentive to see each individual patient. However, it was not a physician-motivated study. In addition to the assertion of the author, Sidney Garfield, clearly a man who should know, that "adaptation to new methods in traditional medicine is often a difficult and strongly resisted process" (1976, p. 430), we must also cite as a probable cause the provider's tendency toward organizational myopia discussed earlier. Again as Garfield puts it, "Preoccupied with their traditional methods, they care for their own groups of patients and may not see the need for new methods to fill the gap between the sick-care needs of the relatively few and the total health-care needs of the many in the population that they have contracted to serve''.

This same sort of conclusion has been expressed by Yankauer (1970), who states that "there are serious interpersonal obstacles to institutional and social change of the sort which must be overcome before such change can occur on any significant scale." He continues: "These obstacles may be more difficult to work through in large medical groups than in smaller practice settings faced with mounting demands for care." Specifically, there may be less direct positive (monetary) incentives to innovate or to respond to innovation in such settings.

The illustrative innovation discussed here is the increased use of non-physician providers, which have consistently been shown to be cost-effective in many areas in large PPGP/HMO settings (Golladay et al., 1976; Freidson, 1964). The obvious point is that the adoption of the most efficient provider combination is not automatic even in a PPGP/HMO setting. As Reinhardt (1973) has noted: "In the final analysis, the effective constraints on any factor substitutions in the hospital sector may, of course, be found not to be *technical* at all, but instead to result from certain institutional factors characteristic of that sector. Foremost among the latter is . . . the increasing professionalization of health-manpower in the hospital. This process has produced a rather rigid occupational hierarchy with fairly impenetrable barriers between occupations, and with specific tasks associated with each rung on the hierarchial ladder." For example, Steinwachs et al. (1976) noted that a portion of the managerial structure of the Columbia Medical Program thought it desirable that more nonphysician providers be utilized to care for their catchment population. When they saw that this was not being accomplished, they initiated a training program which resulted in the desired increase. However, since the number of physicians was not reduced the relative factor substitution was facilitated through Plan membership growth and *managerial* catalyst.

D. Illustrations from Management Interviews

The previous sections have attempted to substantiate the assertion that there is sufficient reason to believe that HMOs, and even PPGP/HMOs, must look to an internal restructuring of incentives and organization if they are to achieve their potential as truly cost-effective elements in the HCDS. While it is not clear what exact form such modified internal markets should take, it seems clear that some type of relative performance measurement will necessarily have to be developed and integrated into the PPGP/HMO resource allocation process. This will be discussed in a later section.

To further illustrate the problem facing us in deriving an effective performance measure with appropriate incentives for cost containment, I will briefly discuss the ways in which three necessarily anonymous PPGP/HMOs allocated resources internally during 1976. These methodologies seem to be fairly representative of existing practices. The three important questions are as follows:

1. How is the PPGP/HMO premium determined?
2. How is the capitation rate paid to the physician group calculated?
3. How is the budget of the individual hospital/health plan facility set?

Plan A. In the first plan, the capitation rate paid to the physician group is indirectly derived:

Let
- c = physician capitation payment (per enrollee)
- M = total dollars paid to the medical group
- E = total enrollees in the budget year
- E_o = total enrollees in the previous year
- r = enrollees per physician target ratio (historically given)
- α_i = percentage of total physicians in specialty i
- s_i = salary of providers in category i
- p_i = number of providers in category i
- e = expected growth rate of enrollees
- P = total number of physicians for the budget year

Then the capitation payment, c, is derived as follows:

Step 1. $\dfrac{(1+e)E_o}{r} = \dfrac{E}{r} = P$

Step 2. $\alpha_i p = p_i,$ for all i.

Step 3. $\Sigma_i s_i p_i = M.$

Step 4. $\dfrac{M}{E} = c.$

Here $s = (s_1, s_2, \ldots, s_1, \ldots)$ is negotiated each year under a constraint called the "equal lifetime earnings" concept. Under this concept the salary $s_i = (s_i^{t}, s_i^{t^2}, \ldots, s_i^{t^n})\forall_i$, are set such that a physician in specialty i who came to the plan directly after finishing training (residency, postdocs, etc.) would make the same total amount as a physician of specialty j (for all j) if they both worked until retirement at the Plan. Thus *relative* salaries (i.e., between specialties) are constrained with only few exceptions. Across-the-board salary increases are the subject of the annual negotiations.

Also, α_i can be negotiated to provide for expanded use of nurse practitioners (NPs), physician assistants (PAs), MEDEXs, etc. In general all nonphysician providers except nurses are included in the medical group budget and ratio calculations [e.g., NPs = 1/3 M.D. position while PAs = 1/2].

Thus the heart of the yearly derivation of the capitation rate c is the estimate of e, the agreement on r and α_i ($\forall_i$), and the negotiation of the salary schedule. These then determine c after the fact, rather than using c to foster the choice of r, α_i, etc. Further, in this Plan the overall monthly premium rate is set by estimating total costs for the Plan and the number of enrollee months for the coming year and dividing the former by the latter. In addition to the total physician costs, M, discussed above, there are the hospital, lab, nursing, administration, etc., costs to be figured. To derive these costs they have a budget cycle in which the *central administration* estimates the various expected workloads of the facilities and then asks the facilities to "cost them out." When the facilities submit these budget figures, the central administration checks the projected costs on the basis of selected output measures to determine whether they are acceptable. This appears to be in violation of the spirit and supposed efficiency of capitation budgeting since the capitation rates are, in each case, determined by many calculations which should be minimized in this system.

Plan B. In the second group, the basic medical group capitation rate is determined as follows: There exists an established rate which is adjusted (upward) each year (it is not clear where the first one came from). It is *negotiated* with the Medical Group Council (the consortium spokesman for the various medical groups), and the amount is limited by the local area marketability of the premium given the rate and is based in part on inflation, hiring salary needs of the groups, and changes in workload. These data (on utilization) are collected and used to mitigate—or at least argue against—the size of the rate increases. Utilization rates are "fairly stable" according to the Plan spokesperson. Further, there were no real physician/enrollee ratios followed by the Plan. This is due mainly to the fact that, of the 1,100–1,200 members, only 400 are full-time physicians and provide about 60% of the enrollee services. Thus, its ratio would be a vague measure of requirements at best. It is essentially up to the physicians to ensure that they have enough personnel. Any non-M.D. providers (NPs, PAs, etc.) used by the groups are hired and controlled by them, with some cost sharing by the Central Plan.

There are no hospital PAs, etc., since 75% of the enrollees admitted are in non-Plan hospitals. There was a pending proposal to use PAs, NPs, etc., in the one hospital-based group practice.

Plan C. Representatives from another major PPGP/HMO interviewed presented a general outline of the cost and revenue calculations made each year. These figures form the basis of their prospective subscription rate setting, or, as they call it, "the community rate increase forecast." Their two major expense categories are the medical group and hospital (or facility) costs. First, the basic contractual payment (BCP) for the physician group as a whole is calculated. This involves the physicians' estimate of the number of doctors (themselves) that will be required to care for the forecast member population. This is done generally using the aggregate rule of 1 M.D. per 1,000 members. Then they decide, on the basis of their subjective judgement (i.e., there is no hard internal formula) the distribution of the physicians by specialty. They also decide on the average percentage increase in salary compensation they want to realize in the coming year and then combine these two elements to come up with the requested, or estimated, BCP (e.g., $4.32 per member per month that year). The next category of expenses includes Health Plan administrative and capital costs as well as the negotiated Medical Group Bonus amount. Thus their simplified cost estimation would appear:

M.D. BCP	$^x1
Medical Group Bonus	$^x2
Other Health Plan costs	$^x3
Total costs	$\Sigma^x i$

The revenue projections are straightforward, although certainly stochastic:

Member dues	y_1
Other revenue	y_2
Total revenue	Σy_i

where y_1 = the product of *expected* membership enrollment and premium costs;

y_2 = the sum of expected fee-for-service revenues from non-members, Medicare reimbursement, etc.

Then $\Sigma y_i - \Sigma x_i$ yields the expected shortfall and $-(\Sigma y_i - \Sigma x_i)/y_i$ yields the proposed community rate increase. The expense projections for the health plan and hospital elements are based upon membership projections communicated to the various elements and coupled with historical utilization rates. Each department, or budget entity, takes these projected workloads and makes cost and staffing projections, and estimates the nonpayroll budget as well. This is analogous to the incremental budgeting, or "wish list," approach and these budget submissions are trimmed by the constraints on the marketability of the indicated or associated community rate increase projections. These trimmings involve negotiations between the Regional Director, Medical Director, etc., on down the line. They continue until the necessary associated rate increase is "acceptable."

On the basis of this sample of our indicative research, and that previously discussed, the following conclusions are offered:

- The existing incentive structure for providers in PPGP/HMOs appears too weak to motivate any significant new cost containment measures, either in implementation or development.
- The management and organizational structures are too traditionally designed to counteract the basic economic and psychological forces which cause an insufficient level of goal congruence. This contributes to the same sort of behavior *within* PPGP/HMOs as that in the overall FFS-dominated HCDS which has led to the existence of an imperfect health care market.
- Further analytical and empirical research is necessary to specify the parameters of the problems and to begin to measure the potential for improvement through innovative internal structural change in PPGP/HMO organizations.
- The required research seems clearly to encompass a wider set of disciplines than previously embodied in such research. These include economics, systems analysis, organization psychology, and sociology. The research projects should integrate these considerations as their effects do not appear to be separable.
- It appears some of the most fruitful classes of restructuring are the following: (a) fixed capitation subbudgets used at clinic or department levels analogous to those conceptually used between the health plan and the medical groups as a whole; (b) productivity and innovation bonuses tied to provider-subset performance, and a sharing of the costs saved when realized; (c) performance-related incentive pay for managers at all levels; (d) use of trained personnel to "facilitate" the significant changes in organizational structure in the recognition that direct, solely monetary rewards may not be sufficient to overcome individual and organizational inertia; (e) joint management- and provider-supported patient education programs aimed at knowing when it is really necessary to contact the HCDS and how unnecessary visits may be avoided through a combination of telephone consultations and self-care.

The goal of these efforts is to first recognize and then design effective incentives to partially counteract the forces which have traditionally led to the health care market imperfections. By providing sets of *locally* effective incentives in PPGP/HMOs, one would hope that a macro program of "decentralized regulation," such as embodied in CCHP, will be successful in containing health care costs in the long run. As things stand, although greater reliance on PPGO/HMOs in a large-scale enfranchisement scheme such as NHI would seem to help mitigate the cost spiral in the health care sector, their actual contribution will probably be much less than that hoped for.

In the following section we use the Military HCDS and its present quest for cost containment as a vehicle for further elaboration and analysis.

IV. THE MILITARY HCDS AS AN HMO

A. Introduction and Background

The recently issued report of the MHCS (Military Health Care Study, 1975) includes a recommendation for the use of capitation budgeting (CB) as a replacement for the historical workload budgeting (WB) on an incremental basis which has characterized the various components of the Military Health Services System (MHSS) to the present. The motivation for this recommendation was to provide additional endogenous cost containment incentives to further enhance the MHCS determination of the comparative cost effectiveness of the MHSS in delivering health care to the population presently eligible to use it. The CB recommendation actually stems from its universal use in prepaid health plans which have been able to cut the costs of delivering comprehensive health care benefits to their enrolled beneficiaries as compared with fee-for-service type plans such as we have discussed earlier.

Since the more than 9 million beneficiaries of the MHSS are, from their point of view, members of a prepaid plan and since military providers are paid on a salary rather than a fee-for-service basis, it seems a reasonable conjecture that CB rather than WB is an appropriate managerial step from a systemic point of view. In CB, the organizational entity (health plan, physician group, etc.) generally receives a per capita payment—usually on a monthly enrollment basis—for each person for whom it accepts treatment responsibility. Thus the number of enrollee-months times the capitation payment yields its yearly budget, theoretically eliminating the need for the cumbersome and costly WB process.

(However, as noted in the previous subsection, WB tends to be the basis for facility budgets.) The hope was that coupling a more logical budgeting system with a HCDS which on the surface closely resembles private-sector prepaid health plans that successfully use CB would lead to cost containment in its almost $4 billion budget. However, it remains generally true that there are no easy answers to complex questions. It was and is our conjecture that the mere superposition of CB on the existing operational and managerial structure of the MHSS might in fact cause costs to rise faster rather than to fall. Consider only the following example of the source of our skepticism.

A major concern of the MHCS was the existence of generally higher utilization rates within the MHSS as compared with those in PPGP/HMO plans such as Kaiser. Although in many important ways the MHSS does approximate an extremely large PPGP/HMO plan, the utilization comparison belies this point. Thus, since the recommendations for the MHSS to adopt capitation budgeting stem in large part from analyses which assume MHSS characteristic elements to parallel a PPGP/HMO, we must ask why such discrepancies in utilization exist. Our assessment of the problem, of which this is but one manifestation, is that a consistent and sufficient set of management and operational incentives are lacking in the MHSS, as it exists, making it unlikely that the inherent efficiencies of prepayment will be fully realized. Thus, to expect cost containment to result from the singular adoption of capitation budgeting in this system is naive and potentially damaging in the sense of limiting the probability of necessary systemic structural changes in the future.

The U.S. Department of Defense (DOD) decision makers face the problem of maintaining an adequate HCDS to meet the contingency needs associated with caring for casualties in a military operation and to ensure a fit fighting and support force. In addition, they desire to provide a quality fringe benefit to the active-duty force in order to motivate enlistments and retention in the All Volunteer Force sufficient to maintain force readiness. However, they face the resource allocation problem of trying to expend the minimum number of dollars to operate the MHSS at a level which will produce their desired results. Thus the managers of the MHSS must compete for resource dollars with the other program elements in the DOD budget. The MHCS was, of course, an attempt on the part of the DOD to determine if there was a more cost-effective way to accomplish their goals. The recommendation for use of capitation budgeting, which motivated the research upon which this paper is based, was in turn an attempt to influence the MHSS to become even more cost-effective, an attempt of extra-MHSS DOD managers to change the incentive structure of the MHSS organization and its managers in order to induce behavior more consistent with their own more centralized goals and needs.

The MHSS is actually composed of three essentially independent direct care elements corresponding to the three major branches of the service—Army, Navy, Air Force—with independent administrative (or "Health Plan") offices. In addition, there is an umbrella fiscal office (CHAMPUS) at the DOD level that funds utilization by eligible beneficiaries of private-sector direct care facilities and provides ("out of plan" utilization). The Navy's Health Plan office, the Bureau of Medicine and Surgery (BUMED), will serve as our focus of discussion.

BUMED receives resources from DOD, which has received them in appropriations from Congress. BUMED then must distribute these resources among its "member facilities" throughout the United States and abroad. Some of these facilities, in turn, have responsibility for smaller facilities in their geographic area. In each case, providers are uniquely identified with a specific facility and are under the authority of that facility's commanding officer. Further details of the structure and operation of the MHSS, BUMED, and the direct care facilities it controls will emerge during our analysis and discussion.

We posit that BUMED wants to use its budgeted dollars received from DOD's central decision makers to fulfill its obligations to care for an aggregate population of eligible "clients" of the MHSS–Navy. It needs (because of its legitimate desire to remain in existence) to demonstrate to "the fleet" that its operational health care needs are met, while simultaneously providing an appropriate quantity and quality of care to the various dependent and retired eligibles. Thus it distributes its limited resources among the field activities in such magnitudes as to maximize its organizational subjective probability of being able to accomplish these goals.

On the other hand, it seems reasonable to posit that each "member facility" in turn wants to be as prepared as possible to respond to the health care needs of that subset of the aggregate population for which it is responsible. Since there tend to be an infinite number of possible demands which such a catchment population can make on a facility, the more dollars it can convince BUMED to allocate to itself, the better it will be able to respond. Thus a reasonable response by a Regional Medical Center Commanding Officer/Manager is to attempt to maximize the budget allocation of BUMED to his facility. This would yield the greatest flexibility in dealing with the health care needs of his eligible client population. This does not imply greed or undue selfishness. It simply reflects the decisions of a rational manager dealing with uncertainty and a nebulous product against the output of which his managerial proficiency will be measured. Thus, even though he may be aware of the overall goals and constraints facing BUMED, most are outside of his direct control and he therefore must manage and optimize that for which he is responsible and controls—his specific facility.

This sort of situation often leads to a "means/ends inversion" in which the manager attempts to protect that position (facility) for which he is responsible, rather than positively reacting to the broader organizational goals. Such instances of "bounded rationality" caused by complex and information-scarce relationships between the parts of the organization and its central managers cause "satisficing" rather than optimization strategies to be adopted. We posit that the MHSS facility manager has in the past been a cost-based revenue maximizer, a role which is hardly consistent with the goals of the system at large.

Montgomery (1974) has previously dealt with some of the basic incentive similarities with PPGP/HMOs and discussed difficulties and ramifications for their implementation in the MHSS. We build upon some of the basic principles he abstracted from the literature, as well as the potential problems he identified, to discuss the general problem of CB in the MHSS. In particular, while Montgomery concentrated his efforts on outlining the broad categories of differences in the provider incentives of fee-for-service vs. prepaid medicine and the effects on utilization of consumer participation in payment, we are looking more deeply within the system to identify specific classes of incentives, *given* the system structure, and to analyze what impact these may have on the possibility for cost containment in the MHSS. For example, Montgomery (1974, p. 29) concludes: "In terms of provider reimbursement . . . there is one system which theoretically approaches the ideal. This is capitation payment of providers. It constitutes the only situation in which incentives for cost-consciousness and quality are, at least theoretically, simultaneously present". It is exactly the perceived disparity between the theoretical vs. the operationally capturable efficiencies of prepayment and CB with which we are here concerned.

Montgomery concludes that "Capitation payments to military providers to cover the costs of care are not feasible under present conditions" (1974, p. 36). The elements of the vector of "present conditions" which he cites include the need for true enrollment, service package definition, and more effective restriction of "out-of-plan" utilization under CHAMPUS. We believe that the conditions he sets forth are, in fact, necessary for the viability of an effective cost-containment program through CB. However, we do not believe that they alone are sufficient to ensure this desired goal.

The work by Penchansky and Berki (1976) deals with analogous problems faced by the Health Networks they studied. They specifically recognize the role of goal congruence in contributing to the probability of success of these new organizational structures built on existing foundations.

The question then appears to be this: Can we design positive incentives for the MHSS which will enhance the probability of cost containment by providers even though we have no medical or physician group with whom we contract? Further, can these systemic incentives encompass the motivation for innovations in general which might assist in cost containment? For example, will the incentive exist for hospital and clinic managers to attempt patient education measures/experiments to cut unnecessary utilization?

B. The Normative Role of the Manager

Two items regarding management structure emerged and steadily grew in importance as our research progressed: one was the emphasis that successful private-sector plans placed on the "management input" of operational personnel; the other was the general failure of MHSS central administrative personnel to perceive the relationship between the successful use of CB and such input.

Consider the latter point first. Capitation budgeting is logically based on the recognition that it is either not possible or undesirable for central decision makers to control *effectively* the total operations of the system. That is, the use of CB is an attempt to transfer at least a portion of the risk faced by the "Health Plan" with respect to potential utilization (and hence resource costs) to elements of the HCDS closer to the point of service decision—namely, to the providers. This stems from the implicit recognition of the probable existence of goal incongruence between, on the one hand, the central administration and provider levels of the system and, on the other, the desire to overcome its harmful (costly) effects by interposing the opportunity to profit by matching one's behavior to the organization's goals (or the chance of loss if the systemic goals are ignored). The salient point which must be emphasized is that CB is therefore unambiguously associated with a decentralization of decision-making authority and responsibility. It seems impossible for CB to yield any significant benefits in terms of cost containment if those who are receiving the now capitated budget are constrained from making cost-saving decisions (and taking the responsibility for them) which may yield the cost savings hoped for.

If BUMED knew, for the given population, exactly what its average utilization was going to be in the coming year, and also the optimal treatment mode and input combination for each, then CB would be superfluous. The "production" of this average utilization could then be costed out and the total budget sum derived for that facility. Although managers at the facility level would be necessary to provide the associated support services of local administrators and to guard against obvious inefficiency, they would not be required to make decisions significantly affecting resource use and hence costs. In fact, in our view, this has been the mistaken impression (in general) of the central MHSS managers, and has resulted in the past use of especially inappropriate forms of WB. While the persistence of significant cost increases and the high absolute dollar size of the MHSS composite budget has forced a rethinking of the operational characteristics of the MHSS and led to the recommendation to switch to the use of CB, the necessary modifications to the organizational structure and decision-making responsibilities as well as the budgetary proceduresmay not yet be clear. This will require an active and effective management in place of the somewhat passive role played and allowed in many instances under the present system.

The role of management varied among the private-sector plan managers whom we interviewed. However, there was a number of these private-sector representatives who stressed that, without the existence of facility managers who had both the responsibility for cost containment and quality assurance and the authority to make changes in pursuit of these goals, CB would be a useless exercise in the MHSS. However, they perceived the role of the manager to be much narrower than one might have thought. For example, although it was pointed out that the economics of group practice do have drawbacks in terms of diluted incentives for cost containment among providers, the representative's view was that the role of management is to constantly keep the topic of costs before the providers. This requires an appropriate information system to report the most pertinent data and the feedback from the management level to the providers to make them aware of the organizational opportunity cost of their actions. However, as we indicated at the end of Section III.D, above, they fail to go far enough. On the basis of the increasing number of studies which recognize and examine the role of the manager in the efficient and effective provision of health care (Golladay et al., 1976; Shortell and Brown, 1976; Strumpf, 1976), as well as from our analysis of the aforementioned research management interviews, we posit that more benefits may be attainable if more careful thought and application of generally accepted organizational principles are brought to bear on the MHSS.

C. Summary of Project Recommendations

In the pages which follow, we discuss the recommendations resulting from our research effort that are applicable to the topic of this paper. Suffice it to say it appears likely that CB will be implemented in some form in the MHSS in the near future and that our goal was to provide a set of recommendations that would maximize the probability that CB would accomplish its major desired end—cost containment. To this end we specified the dimensions of the problem as we saw it and examined a broad spectrum of the relevant published and unpublished literature. In addition, we interviewed a significant number of managers and researchers from private-sector plans familiar with CB and a sample of the same personnel types from the MHSS. From these interviews we abstracted what we considered to be the applicable lessons to be learned for our purposes in the MHSS. These, in conjunction with the analyses of the related literature, form the basis of our recommendations, which we believe are suggestive of guidelines applicable to the private-sector PPGP/HMO community.

The recommendations that follow are presented as elements of four specific categories. There are clearly many dimensions to each and more than one recommendation in some categories. However, we believe that the following taxonomy, which will be discussed at greater length in the next section, captures the full scope and import of the normative results of the present research effort. The ordering of the recommendations has no necessary intended relationship to eitherimportance or implementation, since we have taken a holistic view of the problem and thus perceive the proposed course toward its solution in the same light.

1. *Total regional systems costs must be included in the capitation budget and allocated to the various facilities in that region by a regional authority.* Although there are many facets to this proposal, the majorimport is that, to be effective, the budget authorizations from DOD should be to triservice, regional authorities and should include the CHAMPUS cost allowance for the catchment population as well as the military personnel costs for those assigned to elements of the MHSS in that area, which are presently separately budgeted.

2. *There must be effective direct and indirect monetary incentives provided at the hospital and clinic levels.* To foster cost containment we must be willing to share the fruits of these efforts with those most responsible for their realization. This means the implementation of innovative and effective fringe benefits for the managers and providers who have daily responsibility for the decisions which determine resource utilization.

3. *Managers and decision makers at the field level must be given substantially increased authority to pursue cost-effectiveness.* One cannot tie the hands of those who have been given a mandate to cut costs. We must be willing to grant them broad new power to affect the day-to-day management decisions and innovations which will lead to cost containment.

4. *The capitation rate setting methodology developed must reward efficiency and motivate cost containment. Thus, an objective set of performance indicators must be developed and integrated into the budget decisions.* The budget process under CB must be understandable to the field-level participants. This requires that it provide, as well as require, information upon which they may base future decisions concerning internal resource allocation and their search for areas which may yield cost savings. In addition, the rate-setting methodology must be such that the facility and regional managers are assured that their performance on behalf of their facilities will be objectively incorporated into the rate-setting process. This requires that there exist a well-defined set of performance indicators which are directly tied to the *relative* rate-setting process (i.e., among facilities) to ensure that arbitrary budget allocation decisions are at an absolute minimum.

In the following subsection, we speak to each of the recommendations in turn in more depth, explaining the basis for each and relating them to the research which has preceded them.

D.   Discussion and Amplification of Recommendations

1.   The rationale underlying the "Total Systems Cost" recommendation is simple: if one wants to accurately reflect the cost of operation, one mustn't segregate portions of those costs and make them "uncontrollable." The more constraints and the greater the number of "pockets" out of which these resource costs come, the less likely that the optimal choices of provider mix, mode of patient care delivery, etc., will be made. The duplication of facilities' capabilities and use of CHAMPUS as "no cost safety valves" when otherwise constrained reosurces get "tight" at the military hospitals are but examples of the results of isolating the various kinds of budgets as is presently done.

We must include CHAMPUS costs in the capitated budget for the region in order to motivate coordinated (among services) and effective (within facilities) efforts to be cost effective. If the area has x people eligible to use the MHSS, then the total regional budget (simplified) for the period should be $c \cdot x = \$R$. Out of this budget should come *all* the costs of providing health care to that given population. Thus, if $F are aggregate (essentially) fixed costs of operating all the direct care facilities in the region, then $(R - F)$ represents the funds left to cover the internal variable costs (i.e., those which depend upon to what extent the direct care system is used by dependents) *and* the CHAMPUS costs associated with those who do not use the direct care system. Thus, if these CHAMPUS costs are high relative to $(R - F)$, the ability of the regional facilities to respond to the demands on its resources is going to be significantly diminished. Thus, all the managers of the various services in the region will tend to be more cooperative in order to be able to meet such constraints. If the CHAMPUS dollars are not included, as in the past, then there will tend to be the shifting of some care to CHAMPUS, either by design on the part of the institutions' managers and providers or indirectly by providing less acceptable care to the clients who then decide for themselves to use CHAMPUS. The private sector prepaid plans know full well that such uncontrolled out-of-plan utilization can be extremely costly.

In addition, if the budget given to a region is triservice and based on the total eligible population, then it does the individual service facilities in the region no good in their budget negotiations with Washington to fight over who's responsible for what portion of the population. The attempts to double count the eligibles (i.e., two or more facilities claiming they are responsible for the same people) may still exist within the region, but the incentive is to be more realistic and more receptive to the elimination of the duplication of facilities. This occurs since they are no longer competing with all the other military facilities for their specific budget based on their calculations of catchment population, but rather only with the other facilities in their region for the fixed total dollars available there.

Next, it is essential that the capitated budget include the cost of military health care providers and staff. One of the largest potential sources of cost containment in HCDS is in the substitution of less expensive providers and in the development of labor-saving innovations such as patient education and utilization control. If, however, the cost of military personnel is not under the control of the field level managers, having been excluded from the budget and only weakly associated with the facility's cost of operation, then the incentive to discover and implement these labor cost–saving innovations is almost nonexistent. The point (again) is that if we want to save money, then we should provide the largest possible visible target for these savings and eliminate any incentives to disregard significant portions of the costs such as CHAMPUS and military personnel.

2. We spent a great deal of time in our review of the literature examining the possibility that cost containment might result solely from the implementation of capitation budgeting. I believe that any objective review of these writings supports the conclusion that there is little reason to expect cost containment as an automatic consequence of using CB. Rather, the more reasonable conjecture is that the close correlation between the relatively cost-effective care provided by PPGP/HMOs as compared with fee-for-service plans has to do with the removal of the perverse incentive to hospitalize patients and the provision of a positive,

although weak, incentive to substitute ambulatory for inpatient care via the physician bonus. The fact that any comparison of inpatient utilization rates between the MHSS and the PPGP/HMO private sector is not favorable to the MHSS, coupled with the fact that the organizational structure of the MHSS precludes even the relatively weak direct monetary incentives for physicians (and other providers) possible in the private-sector plans, implies that extreme skepticism should confront those who would adopt CB in the MHSS without significant accompanying changes in its incentive and organizational structure. The results of our interviews of private-sector personnel support this conclusion. However, we propose to go even further than have our private-sector colleagues in distributing the incentives throughout the organization.

In particular we propose that, with some reservations for start-up funds, etc., any savings from the estimated and allocated capitated budgets for the regions, facilities, and internal departments be shared realistically with those managerial and provider personnel responsible for the related operational elements. Thus, if out of the total regional budget there are documented savings (i.e., monies which were not needed because of cost-containment efforts) of x, the region collectively should get to keep $\$\alpha x$ $(0 < \alpha < 1)$. Some of these savings may obtain as a result of the regional authority's managerial effort, e.g., if they had instituted specific innovative programs to reduce CHAMPUS enrollment so as to more appropriately utilize the direct care system. These savings would stay totally (in terms of discretion) at the regional level. However, we conjecture that the majority of savings would accrue as the result of facility-specific managerial or provider actions. Thus, the region would have an internal sharing formula with each of its accountability centers, e.g., the Naval Regional Medical Center (NRMC). Thus, given that out of every dollar saved, α of it would stay in the region, the regional authority would allow some percentage, β $(0 < \beta < 1)$ to stay at the facility which generated the saving. Thus, if $\$y$ total were generated by the facility, $\beta \cdot \alpha \cdot \$y$ would be available for the facility and/or its providers to use.

Further, the facility level managers would also have an internal sharing formula. That is, if the Family Practice Clinic was able to document savings of $\$y_f$, since the facility as a whole would get to keep $\beta \cdot \alpha \cdot \$y_f$, the command managers must be willing to allow γ of the net savings to stay with the group of providers and staff which were responsible for its generation. Thus, out of each dollar saved by any organizational element, $\gamma \cdot \beta \cdot \alpha \cdot \$y_f$ would be available for that entity's (department, say) use.

Consider the following illustration: Suppose $40 million is allocated to the region by BUMED or some other central budget entity. A portion of this budget, say, $20 million, is allocated to the NRMC. Suppose in turn that the NRMC allocated $.5 million to the operation of its Family Practice Clinic (FPC), which has 5,000 people for whom it is responsible. We have proposed that a significant percentage of each dollar the FPC saves through the efforts (productivity) of its managers, providers, and staff be kept by the FPC for its use either by the organization or by the individual members which will enhance the motivation toward cost containment. Likewise, a portion of the savings should accrue to the overall command level at the facility for reasons we shall discuss below. Thus, given our proposal above, suppose:

α = .6 (60% of savings stay in the region);
β = .9 (90% of net regional savings stay at the facility);
γ = .8 (80% of net facility savings stay in the responsible department).

Then suppose that the FPC "saves" $20,000 in the period. They get to keep $\gamma \cdot \beta \cdot \alpha$ of it, or (.432)$20,000 = $8,640. The command, in turn gets to keep $(1 - \gamma) \cdot \beta \cdot \alpha$ of it, or (.108)$20,000 = $2,160. Likewise, the regional authority gets to collect $(1 - \beta) \cdot \alpha$ of it, or (.06)$20,000 = $1,200, while the central authority gets $(1 - \alpha)$ of it, or .4(20,000) = $8,000. Although the percentages used are illustrative, they conform to the *relative* incentive structure we want to construct. For example, the largest absolute share goes to those most ostensibly responsible— the members of the FPC—while a large share also goes to the DOD level to reduce overall MHSS costs. In this case, since local managers will tend to be more responsible for facilitating cost containment at the department or clinical service level, they receive a significant share. The regional managers who probably have little to do with this type of cost containment receive only a small sum so as to be able to build up a fund to facilitate other improvements. Both theory and reality as surveyed indicate clearly to us that it is naive to expect significant (in terms of effects), continuing cost containment efforts without the provision of endogenous, visible, and reasonable incentives.

It is true that we in a real sense are recommending going "further" in terms of incentive provision and sharing than has been the general case in private-sector plans. We do this for at least two reasons. First, the special structure of the MHSS and the relationship between its providers and the organization precludes some of the direct sharing possibilities, e.g., no productivity salary bonus is possible as it stands at present. Second, some of the private sector plans have recognized that the present incentive/sharing relationship, as represented by the Physician's Group bonus, is too weak to provide the level of effort toward cost containment necessary in the present environment in which health care dollars are no longer sacrosanct and, because of their size, must now face competition from non–health care demands.

3. It should be abundantly clear that we are convinced that no significant cost containment measures will result from the implementation of CB unless the intermediate and field-level managers are given the authority to make the decisions which will lead to cost containment. We have emphasized throughout this study that CB is a measure designed to decentralize decision-making. It is impossible for such a measure to be productive if CB is all form with no content. For example, it is unreasonable to believe that a chief of some clinical service is going to invest the time and energy to figure out a more cost-effective mix of providers to serve his patients if he knows from the beginning that he does not have the authority to change the provider mix in his own department. Decision-making authority must be vested at the lowest level consistent with the required level of organizational control, information costs and availability, and competence.

4. The use of CB requires that a methodology be developed which will generate an "average price" for which a representative member of an identified or target population may be provided health care in the specified period. Clearly, we want this capitation rate to be a necessary, or minimum possible, price. In discussing the various methodologies used by the private-sector plans during our interviews, one fact became increasingly clear: It would be both difficult and generally undesirable to attempt to adapt their overall rate-setting methods for our purposes in the MHSS. In general, private-sector PPGP/HMO rate setting depends much more on historical workload data than we believe is advisable.

One alternative is to attempt to define some benchmark production unit(s), cost them out, and then extrapolate to get at least a first approximation to a viable budgetary methodology. "Optimal panel-sizing" and the like should also be carefully considered in conjunction with some baseline data on average cost per beneficiary by facility and region. This, then, must be adjusted by both the demographic characteristics of the catchment population and the facility-specific parameters (such as renal dialysis capability). However, note that the existence of endogenous incentives to discover cost-saving innovations will, in contrast to existing PPGP/HMO budgetary processes, tend to make the year-to-year baseline data more believable.

We should recognize the "two-way" feature of this rate-setting methodology. It is part of a budgetary process and, given the costly and uncertain nature of the commodity "health care," we can expect that, even with the best intentions, not all of the budget submissions will be able to be met, just as under WB. Thus, an objective, equitable, and efficient adjustment mechanism must exist in conjunction with the basic rate-setting methodology to allocate the always insufficient total or central budget among the competing regions (facilities). Suppose that the total amount requested from all the regions is greater than the amount allocated by Congress. The question is how to "spread" this shortfall over the facilities. A proportional cut implies that all the regions or facilities are equally efficient and/or needy. As we have pointed out, the large, multi-institution private-sector plans have realized that this is both naive and costly.

An answer to this dilemma is the construction of a set of facility/region Performance Indicators using the CB rate-setting methodology. Thus, in the simplest case, if one efficient region/facility had an index number of 2 and another less efficient facility had an index number of 1, then the former's share of the revenue cut would be one-half of the latter's. Thus, efficiency would be objectively regarded in the budgeting process rather than penalized as is the case when inefficient facilities with large budget requests end up getting relatively more than do efficient ones with smaller and/or more reasonable requested amounts.

V. A PROPOSED SOLUTION STRATEGY

In this section we sketch some rudimentary guidelines for the construction of an integrated, goal-congruent resource allocation methodology and performance measure for use in the PPGP/HMO sector. The concepts and their deviation from other PR attempts are actually quite simple. Our approach is to recognize the advantage a closed, essentially prepaid system (of whatever size) has in motivating efficient behavior in the production of necessary health care services over the fee-for-service sector. This enables the methodology to be *based on catchment population directly,* rather than on the intermediate outputs used in other prospective reimbursement (PR) attempts, in order to motivate the provision of the appropriate level of health care at minimum cost.

There are two major parts to reaching an overall optimum minimum cost level: the first is deriving the correct or necessary level of output, and the second is motivating (informing) the hospital and its providers to move toward it at the lowest possible cost. In the work-load-based-fee-for-service sector, a facility does not have a specific catchment population. Rather, it "services" a group of providers who prescribe use of its facilities as independent contractors with their patients. We argue that the very best such a facility can be expected to do is to produce the associated level of care at the cheapest price, that is, to operate "on" its short-run average cost curve. As we have discussed earlier, participation in PR programs with no upper limits on total revenues/costs may in fact cause suboptimal levels of care to be produced.

Even in the PPGP/HMO sector where the hospital administrator has even less direct control over admission/discharge policy, our previous research indicates that insufficient attention has been given to the incentives necessary to drive HMO facilities to operate *on* their short-run average cost curves. Thus, for example, suppose that the capitated budget used between medical group and the health plan/administration of a PPGP/HMO sufficiently defines the optimal (necessary) level of output for a facility in terms of OBDs and admissions. There exists significant doubt that there are sufficient positive incentives for the hospital management to ensure they minimize costs for that level of output. Uncertainty, organizational slack, and perceived difficulty in implementing innovative staffing and delivery patterns all combine to make probable operation somewhat less than otpimal. Of course, these same sorts of obstacles exist for the medical group in terms of the likelihood that the optimal level of output will be determined by them.

The first step is to outline the change in organizational structure necessary to support the resource allocation and performance measure methodologies with an incentive structure consistent with the internal goal congruence we have extensively discussed and analyzed earlier. We shall use the term *Health Plan* to designate the administrative component of the overall "system" under scrutiny. In the case of Kaiser of Southern California this would denote the central administration component which has aggregate responsibility for the operation of the several major medical centers and separate outpatient facilities. The term *Medical Group* will denote the aggregation of all providers with whom the Health Plan traditionally negotiates. *Hospital Administrator* identifies the person or group of decision makers officially responsible for the day-to-day operation of a single specific health care delivery facility. A *unit* is an identifiable subset of the hospital/facility health care system, e.g., the pediatrics clinic or emergency room/walk-in clinic.

We may summarize our proposed guidelines for restructuring as follows:

1. The Health Plan estimates the aggregate expected costs and revenues of the Plan for the coming year. This is based upon adjusted historical costs and projections of the future enrolled population and its major subsets. This sets the upper bound on the total revenue accruing to the system as a whole.

2. These expected revenues are allocated to the various major medical facilities on the basis of their catchment populations and necessarily unique delivery capabilities.

3. Although the Medical Group will remain intact as a formal subset of the overall system, the negotiations to determine provider base salaries will be influenced by the facility to which the provider is "assigned."

Thus differential salaries for "identical" providers (e.g., pediatricians with 5 years of seniority) *may* be established dependent upon which catchment population subset the provider is associated with.

4. Bonuses and productivity differential sharing with providers will be totally based on the fiscal performance of the facility/catchment population with which the provider works or is "affiliated".

5. Each facility (or group of facilities under the aegis of the major (or "responsible") facility will determine unit subbudgets for its organizational components. These will be based on the demographics and prior utilization of the catchment population.

6. Units may choose to further disaggregate the budget process through the use of "Team budgets" within the unit.

7. Sharing formulas for distribution of the excess revenues attributable to the lowest level of disaggregated budget entities—Facilities, Units, Teams—shall be established through negotiation.

8. "Managers" at each of the various levels shall have the authority and responsibility to see to it that their group operates at less than or equal to its prospectively set budget. Thus they shall be able to determine the mix of providers and staff necessary to fulfill the health care needs of the catchment population.

9. Each of these managers will be judged and rewarded or penalized on the basis of his or her ability to contain costs under his/her control while at the same time seeing to it that sufficient quality/access standards are met. These will be determined through a combination of peer review, patient satisfaction monitoring, and turnover rates among *their* population.

10. The basis for succeeding years' calculations of steps 1 through 9, above, will then be based on the outcome of the cost containment efforts motivated by this system. This will tend to mitigate the rate of cost/premium increase and substitute the resulting cost experience for the overall market premium upper bounds presently used.

In steps 1 and 2, above, a measure of the average (and group-specific marginal) costs of caring for subsets of the catchment population is estimated. This is a variation of the "average cost per beneficiary" approach, but one which attempts to recognize region/facility-specific vagaries analogous to the case-mix adjustment methodologies. It is designed to help develop "regional" and facility-specific budgets by providing the associated "efficiency" comparisons of these entities in terms of their catchment populations. Thus, we suggest the regression of the regional/facility total health care costs on the numbers of members of the various subsets of the catchment population defined by beneficiary category and demographic profile. The feasibility of estimating a cost function dependent upon "output" in terms of beneficiaries is dependent upon the existence of sufficient variation in the mix of this catchment population across regions/facilities. However, presuming the presence of this variation, estimates of the marginal costs of providing health care (really being *responsible* for providing the care) to additional members of these specific groups can be calculated.

Of course, a number of potential "nuisance" parameters must also be estimated. For example, the presence of the capacity to perform some types of specialized procedures within a region may involve significant fixed personnel and support costs not directly related to the population to be served. However, we believe that, correctly structured, such a plan will contain significant incentives to minimize duplication of costly tertiary services. Hence, a facility cost function estimated with this full complement of variables will take account of variations which are peculiar to the facility as well as differences in the catchment population. The model, when fully estimated, is positive rather than normative, for the most part. It cannot be used to determine minimum costs of health service delivered to a given catchment population. Some quasi-normative applications are also possible, since actual costs in a facility might be compared to the costs predicted from the model and outliers identified. Pressure could be brought to bear on those facilities significantly above predicted values through adjustments to their capitation rates. For example, suppose a facility with a total budget of $2 million, has a catchment population of X ($= \Sigma_i X_i$, $i = 1 \ldots n$, where n is the total number of subgroups identified). Let $\$\hat{C}_i$ be the estimated average marginal cost of having a member of group i in a facility catchment population derived from our methodology. Suppose the methodology also estimates that $\$\hat{Y}^*$ are necessary to cover the costs of the facilities and staffing not directly associated with beneficiary care provision, where $Y = \Sigma_{j=1}^k Y_j$. Then k is the subset of the K total variables of this type "possessed" by, or applicable to, this facility. Thus Y will be different for various facilities or regions depending upon their specialized capabilities. Then $\$C = \Sigma_{i=1}^k \hat{c}_i x_i$ is the size of that portion of the budget the methodology would predict as "necessary" to care for the facilities beneficiary population. If ($2 million $- \$y)/\$\hat{C} > 1$, then there is the *possibility* that the facility is operating inefficiently. To the extent that this discrepancy was greater than 1 (e.g., suppose it is 2) and that the facility manager could not justify its magnitude, a portion of the difference ($2 million $- \$\hat{Y}$) could be deducted from the following year's budget, as is done in the recently restructured British NHS (West, 1973). The incentive would be for hospital administrators to determine the source of the suspected inefficiency and correct it (or innovate). In analytical terms, even though we may not be able to identify the actual long-run average cost curve for this catchment population and facility, we are "forcing" *them* to discover and move toward their overall cost minimizing positions. Periodic reestimation of the vectors $\hat{Y}$, $\hat{C}$, will tend to continually motivate this activity.

While we recognize that significant detail work and research remains before such a program could be implemented, we believe that the need and potential productivity for such a restructured PPGP/HMO sector has been clearly indicated.

ACKNOWLEDGMENTS

The research upon which this paper is based was supported by the Office of the Surgeon General of the U.S. Navy under a contract entitled "Analysis of Elements of the Military Health Care Delivery System." The analysis presented here was supported by the Office of Naval Research Foundation Research Program at the Postgraduate School and is gratefully acknowledged. The opinion and analyses presented are those of the author and not necessarily those of the Navy. Portions of this work were presented at the 1977 and 1978 meetings of the Eastern Economic Association and the 1978 meetings of the Western Economic Association. The comments of Michael Redisch and John Glasgow were extremely helpful.

REFERENCES

American Public Health Association, (1971), "Health Maintenance Organization: A Policy Paper," *American Journal of Public Health 61*,(12), 2529–2536.

Bailey, Richard M. (1968), "A Comparison of Internists in Solo and Fee-for-Service Group Practice in the San Francisco Bay Area," *Bulletin of N.Y. Academy of Medicine 44*(11).

Bauer, Katherine G., and Densen, Paul M. (1974), "Some Issues in the Incentive Reimbursement Approach to Cost Containment: An Overview," *Medical Care 31*(1), 61–100.

Berry, Ralph (1977), "Hospital Cost Containment: Some Thoughts About the Research Needs for Future Policy," in *Hospital Cost Containment: Selected Notes for Future Policy* M. Zubkoff and I. Raskin (eds.), New York: Milbank Memorial Fund.

Densen, Paul M., Jones, Ellen, Shapiro, Sam, and West, Howard (1971), "The Design for Evaluation of HIP's Incentive Reimbursement Experiment," *Uses of Epidemiology in Planning Health Services: Proceedings of the 6th International Scientific Meeting of the International Epidemiological Association, Belgrade, Yugoslavia*, Aug. 29–Sept. 3.

Donabedian, Avedis (1969), "An Evaluation of Prepaid Group Practice," *Inquiry 6*(3), 3–27.

Enthoven, Alain (1977), *Memorandum for Secretary Califano*, Sept. 22, 1977 (also in *The New England Journal of Medicine 298*(12,13)).

Dunlop, John T. (1965), "The Capacity of the United States to Provide and Finance Expanding Health Services," *New York Academy of Medicine Bulletin 41*(12), 1327.

Falk, I. S. (1973), "Financing for the Reorganization of Medical Care Services and Their Delivery," *The Economic Aspects of Health Care*. Prodist, pp. 159–189.

Freidson, Eliot (1964), "Physicians in Large Medical Groups: A Preliminary Report," *Journal of Chronic Disease 17*, 827–836.

Garfield, Sidney R., Collen, Morris, Feldman, Robert, Soghikian, Kriker, Richart, Robert, and Duncan, James H. (1976), "Evaluation of an Ambulatory Medical-Care Delivery System," *New England Journal of Medicine 294*(8), 426.

Gaus, Clifton (1976), *Health 17*(4).

Glaser, William A. (1970), *Paying the Doctor: Systems of Renumeration and Their Effect*. Baltimore: Johns Hopkins Press.

Golladay, F.L., Smith, Kenneth, Davenport, Esther, Hansen, Marc, and Over, A.M. (1976), "Policy Planning for the Mid-Level Health Worker: Economic Potentials and Barriers to Change," *Inquiry 13* Mar., 80–89.

Group Health Association of America (1976), "HMO Qualification Director Discusses the Federal Program," *Group Health and Welfare News 17*(5), 2.

Jones, Ellen W., Densen, Paul, Altman, Isidore, Shapiro, Sam, and West, Howard (1974), "HIP Incentives Reimbursement Experiment: Utilization and Costs of Medical Care, 1969 and 1970," *Social Security Bulletin* Dec., 3–34.

Luft, Harold S. (1975), "Designing Improved Health Maintenance Organizations: Policy Makers Needs for Data, Their Availability, and Methods to Obtain Them." Background paper submitted to Brookings Panel on Social Experimentation, Aug.

———. (1978), "How do Health-Maintenance Organizations Achieve Their Savings?" *New England Journal of Medicine 297*(24), 1336–1343.

McNamara, Mary E., and Todd, Clifford (1970), "A Survey of Group Practice in the United States, 1969," *American Journal of Public Health 60*(7), 1303–1313.

MCSA Consultant Group (1976), Final Report to Group Health of Puget Sound, MCSA, Seattle, Wash. Summer.

Military Health Care Study (1975), Final Report, OMB/HEW/DOD, Dec.

Montgomery, John E. (1974), "Economic Incentives for Health Care Providers and Consumers Under Various Reimbursement Systems, Working Paper No. 12, NSHCA, Bethesda, Md., Mar., pp. 39–40.

Newhouse, Joseph (1973), "The Economies of Group Practice," *Journal of Human Resources 8*(1).

Pauly, Mark V. (1970), "Efficiency, Incentives and Reimbursement for Health Care," *Inquiry 7*(1), 123.

Penchansky, Ray, and Berki, Sylvester E. (1976), "Evaluating HMO Development: Contributions from the Experience of the Community Health Network," Mimeo, Presented at APHA Miami Beach Meetings, Oct.

Pineault, Raynold (1976), "The Effect of Prepaid Group Practice on Physician's Utilization Behavior," *Medical Care 14*(2), 124.

"Professional Performances" *Medical Care Review 33*(3).

Reinhardt, U.E. (1973), "Proposed Changes in the Organization of Health-Care Delivery: An Overview and Critique," *Milbank Memorial Fund Quarterly 51*(2).

Roemer, Milton I., and Shonick, William (1973), "HMO Performance: The Recent Evidence," *Milbank Memorial Fund Quarterly 51*(3), 271–317.

Rosett, Richard A. (1974), "Proprietary Hospitals in the United States," in *The Economics of Health and Medical Care* (Mark Perlman, ed.). New York: Wiley, 57–65.

Scheffler, Richard (1975), "Further Considerations in the Economies of Group Practice in the Management Input," *Journal of Human Resources 10*(2), 258–263.

Shortell, Steven, and Brown, Montague, eds. (1976), *Organizational Research in Hospitals*. Chicago: Inquiry Books.

Sims, Joe (1978), *Public Interest Economics 3*(1).

Sloan, Frank A. (1974), "Effects of Incentives on Physician Performance," in *Health Manpower and Productivity,* (John Rafferty, ed.). Lexington, Mass.: Lexington Books, pp. 53–84.

Somers, Anne R., ed. (1971), *The Kaiser-Permanents Medical Care Program.* New York: Connecticut Printers, pp. 19–20.

Steinwachs, Donald M., Shapiro, Sam, Yaffe, Richard, Levine, David, and Siedel, Henry (1976), "The Role of New Health Practitioners in a Prepaid Group Practice," *Medical Care 14*(2), 99–101.

Strumpf, George B., (1976), "Health Maintenance Organizations, 1971–1976: Issues and Answers," Mimeo, Presented at APHA Miami Beach Meetings, Oct.

West, P.A. (1973), "Allocation and Equity in the Public Sector: The Hospital Revenue Allocation Formula," *Applied Economics 5*, 153–166.

Whipple, David (1975), "Doctors, Patients, and the Demand for Health Care," *Eastern Economic Journal 2*, July, 132–139.

Yankauer, Alfred (1970), "Physician Productivity in the Delivery of Ambulatory Care: Some Findings From a Survey of Pediatricians," *Medical Care 8*(1), 45.